Britain's glory: or, ship-building unveil'd. Being a general director, for building and compleating the said machines. By William Sutherland, ...

William Sutherland

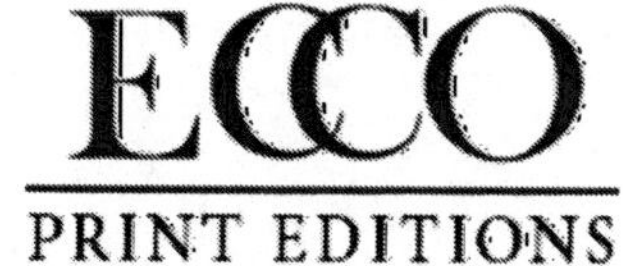

Britain's glory: or, ship-building unveil'd. Being a general director, for building and compleating the said machines. By William Sutherland, ...
Sutherland, William
ESTCID: T166915
Reproduction from National Library of Scotland
A second part was published separately later the same year, with the title: 'The prices of the labour in ship building adjusted: or, the mystery of ship-building unveiled'.
London : printed for John Clrak [sic], 1717.
xxvi,134p.,plates : port.,ill. ; 2°

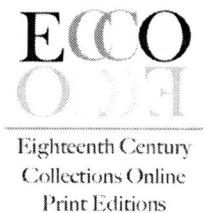

Gale ECCO Print Editions

Relive history with *Eighteenth Century Collections Online*, now available in print for the independent historian and collector. This series includes the most significant English-language and foreign-language works printed in Great Britain during the eighteenth century, and is organized in seven different subject areas including literature and language; medicine, science, and technology; and religion and philosophy. The collection also includes thousands of important works from the Americas.

The eighteenth century has been called "The Age of Enlightenment." It was a period of rapid advance in print culture and publishing, in world exploration, and in the rapid growth of science and technology – all of which had a profound impact on the political and cultural landscape. At the end of the century the American Revolution, French Revolution and Industrial Revolution, perhaps three of the most significant events in modern history, set in motion developments that eventually dominated world political, economic, and social life.

In a groundbreaking effort, Gale initiated a revolution of its own: digitization of epic proportions to preserve these invaluable works in the largest online archive of its kind. Contributions from major world libraries constitute over 175,000 original printed works. Scanned images of the actual pages, rather than transcriptions, recreate the works ***as they first appeared.***

Now for the first time, these high-quality digital scans of original works are available via print-on-demand, making them readily accessible to libraries, students, independent scholars, and readers of all ages.

For our initial release we have created seven robust collections to form one the world's most comprehensive catalogs of 18th century works.

Initial Gale ECCO Print Editions collections include:

History and Geography
Rich in titles on English life and social history, this collection spans the world as it was known to eighteenth-century historians and explorers. Titles include a wealth of travel accounts and diaries, histories of nations from throughout the world, and maps and charts of a world that was still being discovered. Students of the War of American Independence will find fascinating accounts from the British side of conflict.

Social Science

Delve into what it was like to live during the eighteenth century by reading the first-hand accounts of everyday people, including city dwellers and farmers, businessmen and bankers, artisans and merchants, artists and their patrons, politicians and their constituents. Original texts make the American, French, and Industrial revolutions vividly contemporary.

Medicine, Science and Technology

Medical theory and practice of the 1700s developed rapidly, as is evidenced by the extensive collection, which includes descriptions of diseases, their conditions, and treatments. Books on science and technology, agriculture, military technology, natural philosophy, even cookbooks, are all contained here.

Literature and Language

Western literary study flows out of eighteenth-century works by Alexander Pope, Daniel Defoe, Henry Fielding, Frances Burney, Denis Diderot, Johann Gottfried Herder, Johann Wolfgang von Goethe, and others. Experience the birth of the modern novel, or compare the development of language using dictionaries and grammar discourses.

Religion and Philosophy

The Age of Enlightenment profoundly enriched religious and philosophical understanding and continues to influence present-day thinking. Works collected here include masterpieces by David Hume, Immanuel Kant, and Jean-Jacques Rousseau, as well as religious sermons and moral debates on the issues of the day, such as the slave trade. The Age of Reason saw conflict between Protestantism and Catholicism transformed into one between faith and logic -- a debate that continues in the twenty-first century.

Law and Reference

This collection reveals the history of English common law and Empire law in a vastly changing world of British expansion. Dominating the legal field is the *Commentaries of the Law of England* by Sir William Blackstone, which first appeared in 1765. Reference works such as almanacs and catalogues continue to educate us by revealing the day-to-day workings of society.

Fine Arts

The eighteenth-century fascination with Greek and Roman antiquity followed the systematic excavation of the ruins at Pompeii and Herculaneum in southern Italy; and after 1750 a neoclassical style dominated all artistic fields. The titles here trace developments in mostly English-language works on painting, sculpture, architecture, music, theater, and other disciplines. Instructional works on musical instruments, catalogs of art objects, comic operas, and more are also included.

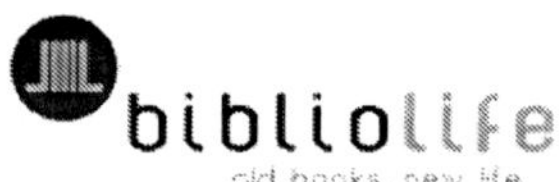
biblioLife
old books. new life.

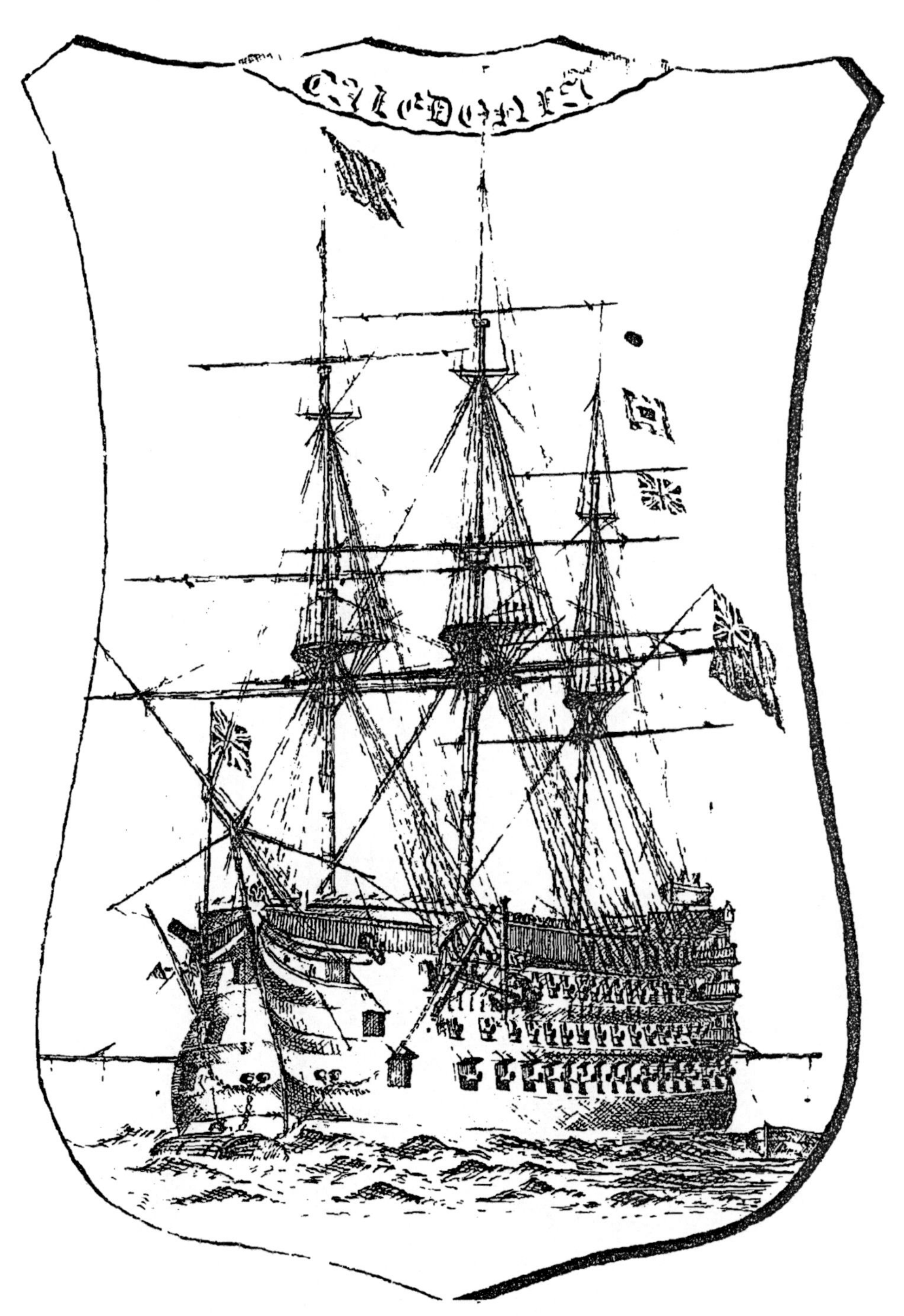
CALEDONIA

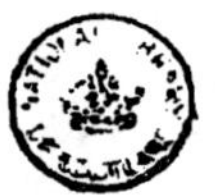

Scale of Capacity, for the Razee (

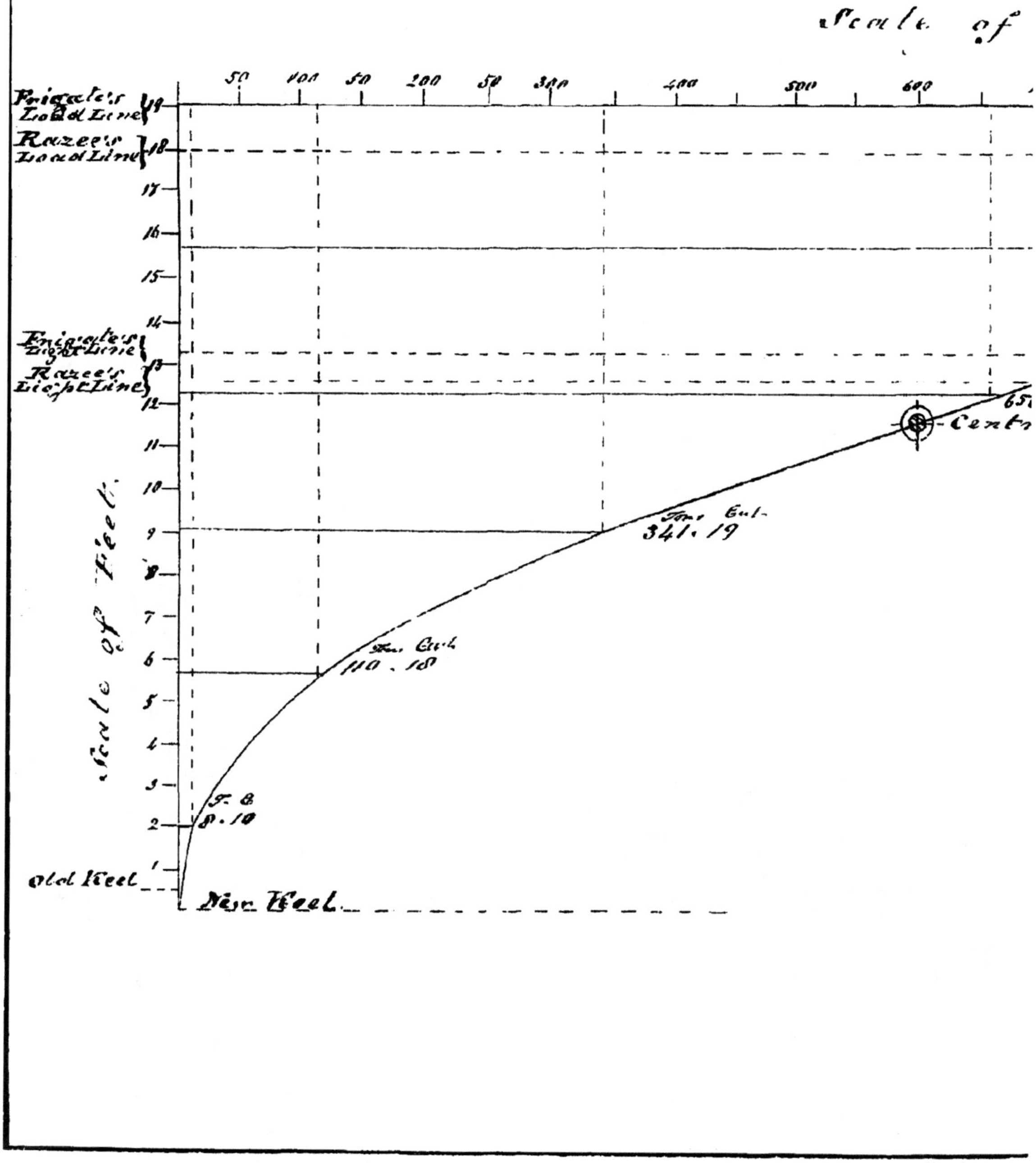

50 100 50 200 50 300 400 500 600

Frigate's Load Line 19
Razee's Load Line 18
17
16
15
14
Frigate's Light Line 13
Razee's Light Line
12
11
10
9
8
7
6
5
4
3
2
1
Old Keel
New Keel

Scale of Feet

T. C.
8.10

Tons Cub.
110.18

Tons Cub.
341.19

Centr

65

...orvette. Curacoa's Class of 26 Guns.

Tons.

Calculated Displacement &c per Draught	Tons . cwt
The Displacement of One Inch at the Light Line	9 . 18
Do Do Load Line	11 . 10
Do One foot at the Midship Section at the Light Line	6 . 10
Do Do Do Load Line	12 15
	Ft
Centre of Gravity of Displacement abaft the centre of Water Line	2 . 5
Do above the Lower side of Keel	11 . 8½
Do below the Load Water Line	6 0½
	Feet
Area in Feet of the Light Water Line	375[illegible]
Do Load Water Line	4734
Displacement in feet at Launching Line	24430
Do Load Line	44805
	Tons cwt
Displacement in Tons at the Light Line	698 . 0
Do Do Load Line	1280 . 0
The Corvette lighter than she was as a Frigate of 42 guns at the Light Line ft. in. 0 . 8	- 70 . 0
Do Load Line 1 . 2	- 161 . 3

The Weight of Every thing forming the Equipment of a 26 Gun Razee Corvette

		Tons cwt. qrs	Tons cwt. qrs
Hull	Iron Ballast & Tanks.		84 0 . 0
	Water.		106 . 0 . 0
	Provisions, Spirits, & Slops.		57 . 0 . 0
	Coals & Wood.		21 0 . 0
	Men & their Effects. No. 220–		20 . 0 0
	Cables { Hempen Bowers No. 3; Stream No. 1–		9 13 . 0
	Cables { Iron Do. " 3; " " 1–		26 . 2 . 0
	Anchors Do. " 4; " " 1; Kedge No. 1.		8 . 11 . 0
	Boats & their Gear		
	Boatswains & Carpenters Stores, Rope &c.		
	Gunners Stores with Breechings, Tackles &c.		
	Guns, Carronades, &c		68 8. 0
	Gun Powder &c.		9. 5 . 0
	Shot of every Sort		38. 15 . 0
Rigging	Bowsprit.	4 . 17. 3	
	Fore Mast	6. 2. 3	21 . 5 . .
	Main Mast	7. 16 . 1	
	Mizen Mast	2 . 8 . 2	
	Topmasts, Top Gallt. Masts, Yards, Caps &c.		18 . 12 . .
	Spare Topmasts, Booms, &c.		
	Standing Rigging		14 . 13 . .
	Running Do.		11 7 . 0
	Blocks		5 . 8 .
	Sails – No. of Yards on them –	7381	3. 17 . 0
	Spare set – Do.	5140	2 6 . 0

Total Weight recd. onboard.

Ships Hull.

Total Weight of Ship, when complete for Foreign Service.

, and her Total weight when complete, for Foreign Service.

Tons cwt qrs	Cost of Hull &c	£ s d	Remarks	Ft	in
			Length of Deck	145.	1½
290 0 0			" Keel for Tonnage	121.	9⅜
	Furniture &c, Sea Stores		Breadth for Do	38.	2
			" Extreme	38	6
			Depth in Hold	13.	3
74.6.0			Burthen in Tons	944	
3. 17. 0			Draught of Water, Light Forward (6 in above Keel)	10	11
31. 0 0			" Aft	14.	4
11. 10 0			Load Forward	17.	6½
			" Aft	18.	5½
116 8 0			Height of Ports, Fore	9.	4
			Midships	8.	5
			Aft	9.	10
39. 10. 0	Masts & Yards &c		No. of Men	220.	
			Guns 26		
7 10. 0			No. 26. 32 Pdrs	40 cwt.	
31. 8. 0	Rigging & Blocks				
6. 3 0					
592. 0. 0	Hull: Material				
695. 0. 0	Labour				
1280. 0. 0					

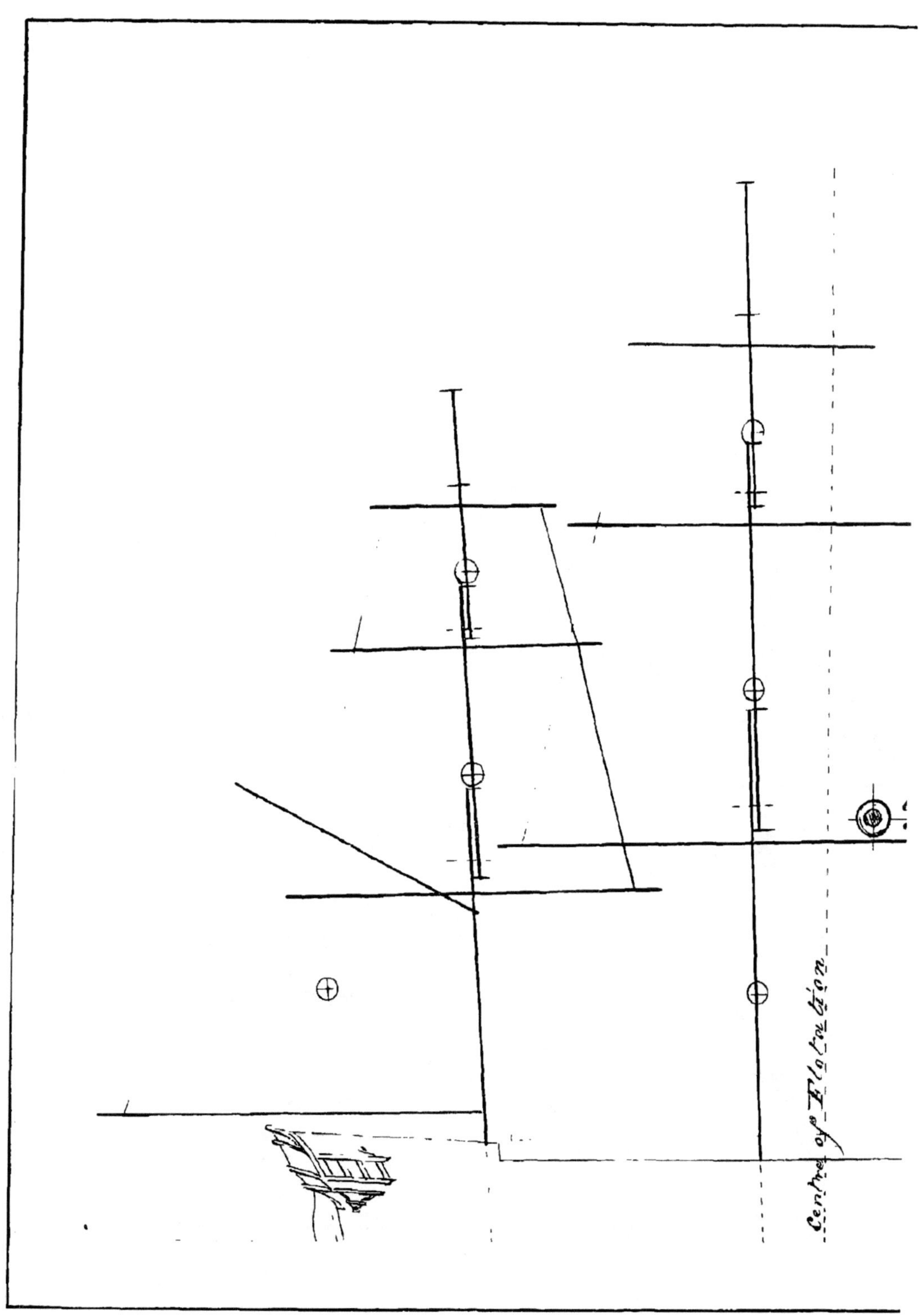
Centre of Flotation

The Razee Corvette of 26 Guns.

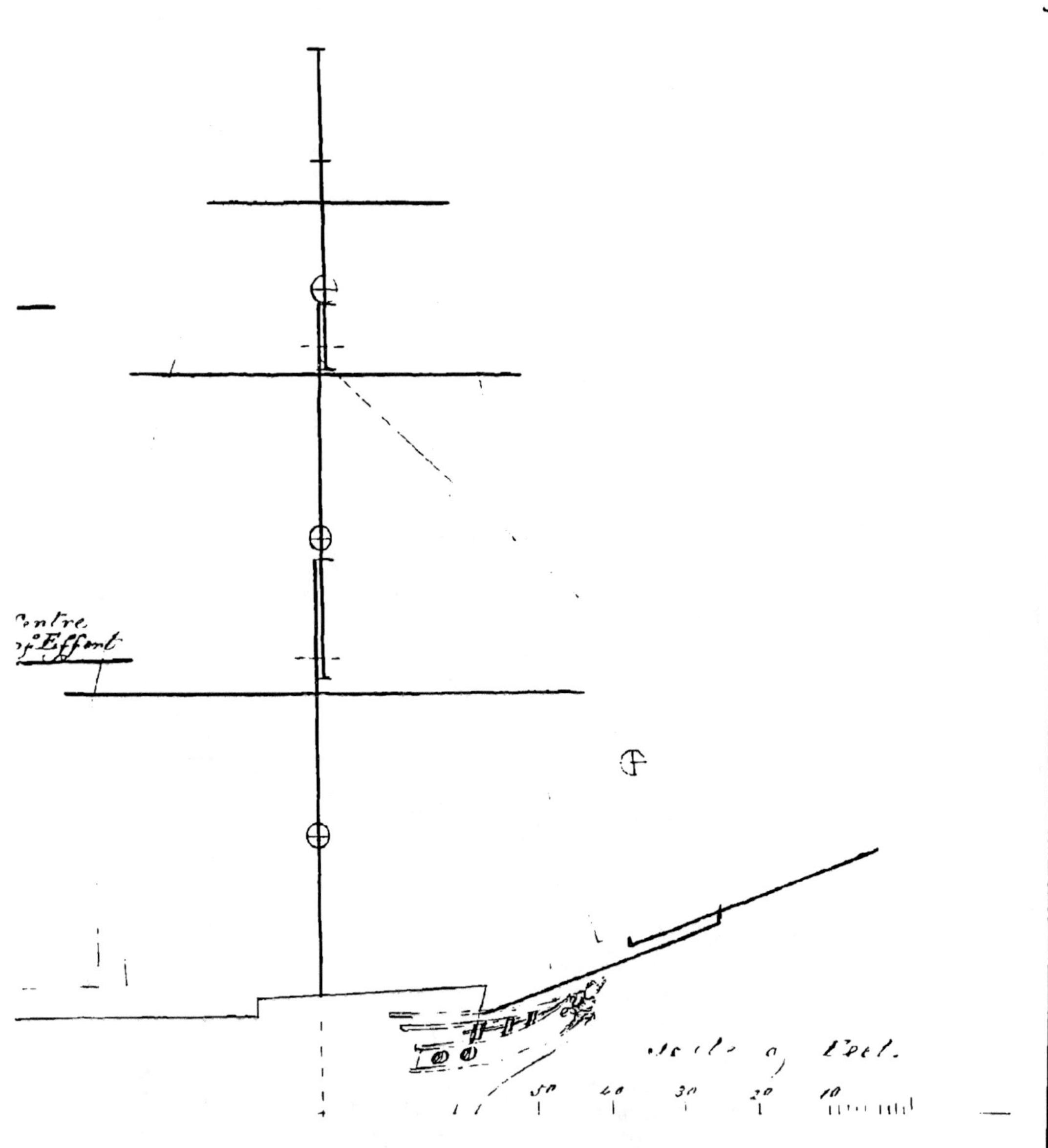

Dimensions & Area of the Principal Sails

Razee Corvette 26 Guns 644 Tons

Sails		Head		Foot		Depth		Area
		Ft	in	Ft	in	Ft	in	Feet
Jib		"		40.	0	64	0	121[illegible]
Fore	Course	63.	0	62.	0	35	6	2225
	Topsail	4[illegible].	0	65	0	41	0	214[illegible]
	Top Gall^t Sail	26.	0	44.	0	20	6	738
Main	Course	73	0	76	10	41	0	3075
	Topsail	46.	6	74	6	47.	0	2790
	Top Gall^t Sail	33	0	49.	0	23	6	972
Mizen	Topsail	34	0	49.	0	33.	0	1369
	Top Gall^t Sail	25.	0	36	0	18.	0	549
Driver		35	0	53	0	28 49	0 0	1694
Total Area of Sails								16873

Quantity of Timber [illegible] Number [illegible] [illegible] Ship

No. of Loads of Timber | [illegible]00 Loads

[illegible] One Man can work up in 12 Months is | [illegible]3¼ [illegible]

[illegible] to build a Razee 26 g[illegible] in [illegible] Months | 76 [illegible]

Size	Length	Circ.	Wool	Tar	Total	Cost £ s d
Riggings	[illegible]	[illegible]	[illegible]	[illegible]	[illegible]	
Fore	[illegible] 10	5 5/8	1 1 0	13 0	6 3 0	
Main	88 [illegible]	28	7 0 0 0	16 1 0	7 16 1 [illegible]	
Mizen	62 1	[illegible]/2	2 4 2 0	3 3 7	2 8 1 10	
[illegible]	32 4	6 2	4 6 3 0	11 [illegible] 1	4 7 3 1	
[illegible]	45 [illegible]	[illegible]	3 0 20	1 20	1 4 1 12	
[illegible] Do	23.4	7 ¼	3 [illegible] 24	.	3 [illegible] 24	
Staysail	70.4	6 4	1 3 2 26	2 3	10 1 26	
TS Do	[illegible]	11	2 [illegible] 6	26	6.1 1	
[illegible] Do	32 0	6 ¼	[illegible] 1 20	6	2. [illegible] 26	
Thick Cross[illegible]	"	"	"	"	2 1 0 5	
[illegible] mast	24 0	[illegible]	4 2 0	0 0	1 0 0	
[illegible] Do	27 0	1	4 2 1	"	4 2 4	
[illegible] Stay Yarn	80.10	1 [illegible]/8	2 7 2 10	2 3 14	2 10 1 24	
TS Do	[illegible]	[illegible]	[illegible] 21	3	4 2 20	
[illegible] Do	[illegible]	1 2	3 [illegible] 22	6	3 3 0	
[illegible]	"	.	"	"	4 1 0	
[illegible] mast	40 6	11 ¼	7 0 26	10	7 1 8	
[illegible] Do	20 3	6 ¼	2 0 0	.	2 0 0	
[illegible] Iron Yarn	56.0	12 ¼	[illegible]	[illegible]	[illegible] 12	
TS Do	40.0	8	4.1 4	26	4 .2	
[illegible] Do	28 0	5 ¼	1 0	4	1. [illegible] 4	
[illegible]	"		.	.	1 1 3 16	
[illegible] Boom	58.0	3 [illegible]/8	5.1 12	10	5 [illegible] 2	
[illegible]	40 10	4 3/4	7 1 4	2 0	1 3 4	
[illegible]	34.1	11 [illegible]/8	10 1 —	"	10 1 2	
[illegible] Yarn	[illegible] 8	4	[illegible] 1 6	20	12 1 26	
[illegible]					4 3 10	

[illegible] Average | 7 10 0 0

[illegible] Riggers [illegible] Rigging & Blocks of a 26 Gun [illegible] Ship [illegible] } 200 [illegible] [illegible]

GEOR

Dei Gratia, *MAGNÆ BRITANNI*
Rex, Fidei Defensor: *BRU*
Dux, SRI Arch-Thesaurarius
20. *Octobris*, 1714.

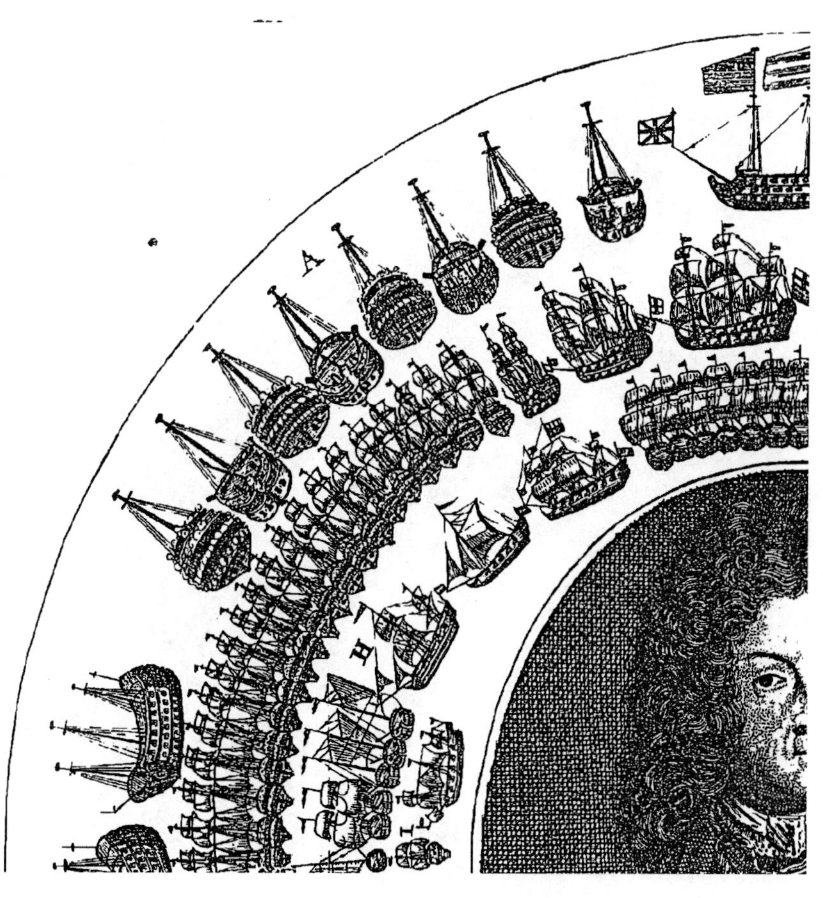

GIUS,

Æ, RANCIÆ & HIBERNIÆ

NSWICK & LUNENBURGH

s & Elector & Inauguratus,

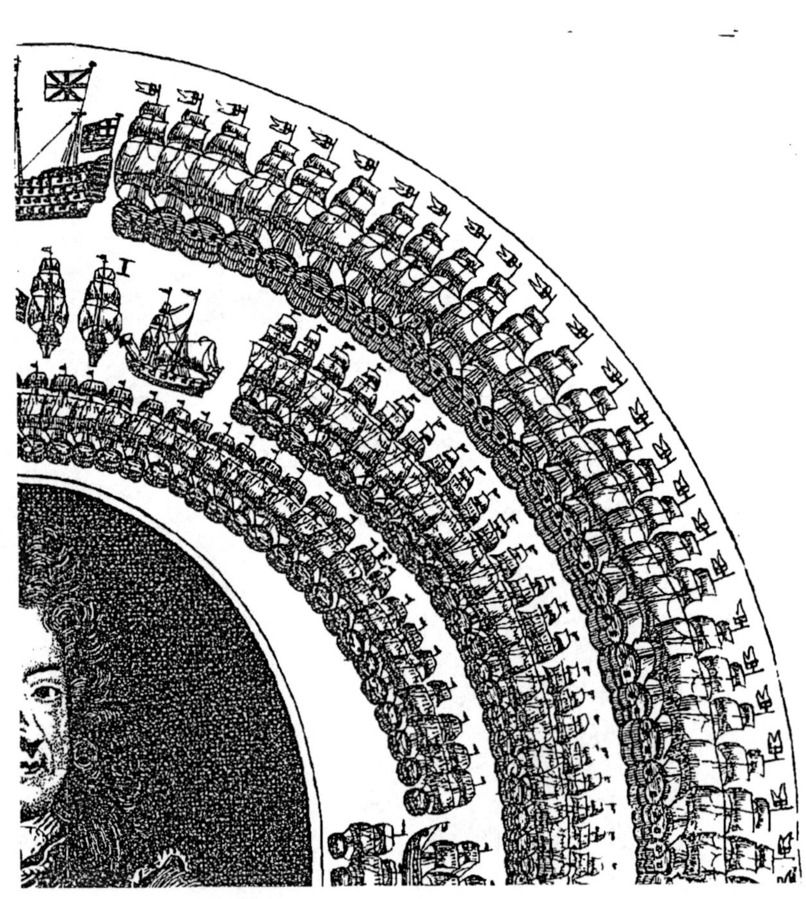

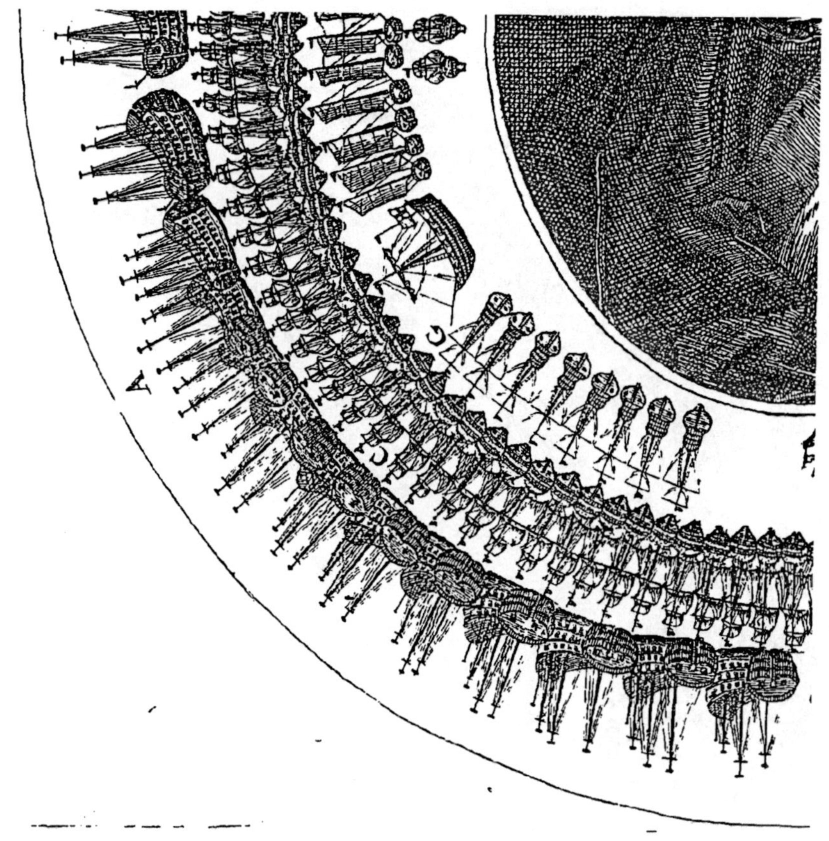

His MAJESTY

A. A. Is the Seven First Rates, and Fourteen Second Rates Unrigg'd, and Lying in a Harbour.

B. Is Five and Forty Third Rates Fore-shortned, with the Heads toward, Under-sail.

C. Is Three and Sixty Fourth Rates Fore-shortned, and with the Sterns toward.

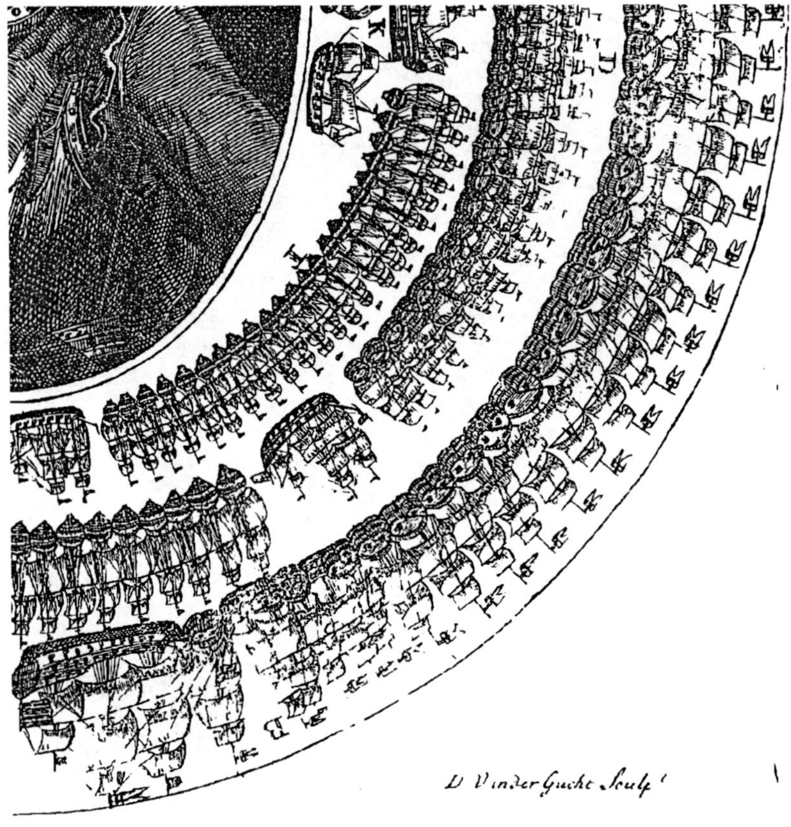

's Royal Navy.

D. Is Forty Fifth Rates, Under-ſail.

E. Is Thirty Fire Ships, Under-ſail.

F. Is Four and Twenty Sixth Rates.

G. Is Nine Bomb Veſſels.

H. Is Fifteen Yatchs, or Pleaſure Boats.

I. Is Ten Advice Boats.

Britain's Glory:

OR,

SHIP-BUILDING UNVEIL'D.

BEING

A General Director,

FOR

Building and Compleating

THE SAID

MACHINES.

By WILLIAM SUTHERLAND,

Author of *The Ship-Builder's Assistant*.

LONDON

Printed for JOHN CLRAK, at the *Royal Exchange*.

M.DCC.XVII.

A SA MAJESTÉ Tres Sacrée, GEORGE Roy DE LA *Grande Bretagne*, de la *France*, & de l'*Irlande*, &c.

SIRE,

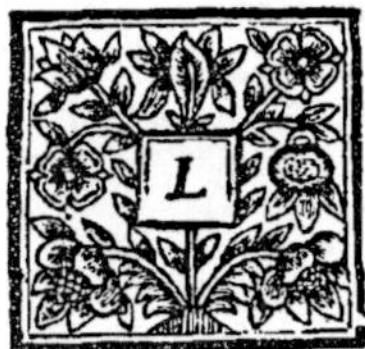

LA Flote Royale de Votre Majesté a été estimeé ces plusieurs Siecles passez, la plus Forte, & la plus Puissante de l' Univers; Vos Commandants, & Vos Officiers Braves & Courageux; Vos Mariniers fort hardi & entreprenants; Vos Royaumes (sur tout celuy de la Grande Bretagne *Meridionale) tres abondants en Bois de Charpente, d'une espece toute a faite differente d'aucun autre de l'* Europe, *le plus utile pour les Navires; & leurs Battiseurs, tant Artists, qu' Ouvriers, ont toutes les qualites requises pour des Talents si rares & excellents, que l'* Angléterre *peut vraiement pretendre a la Discipline Marine par desus tout autre Pais du Monde. Il ny a encore que peu d' années que la* France *etoit dependante des Ancetres Royaux de Votre Majeste pour sa liberté en d' Affaires Maritimes. Je n' entreprendray pas de dire comment elle s'y est appliqueé, mais par sa* Grande Puissance *sur mer depuis peu, il m'est facile de croire que cette liberté fatale luy a eté donnée par notre Nonchalance & Negligence de notre Titre Souverain de Maitre de la Mer étroite: De plus, etant bien assuré que la* France *pour plusieurs années a eu grande Assistance de l'* Angléterre *dans l' Art secret de l' Architecture des Vaisseaux, je ne diray pas absolument, que l'* Angléterre *luy a fourni de bon bois de* Charpente *propre a batir des Vaisseaux de Guerre; mais, comme je scay fort bien que les*

deux

deux Provinces voisines de Sussex *&* *de* Hampshire,*qui appartiennent a Votre Majesté sont tres abondantes en cette Commodité si rare & si choisie, elle peut fort bien (a ce qui me semble) etre transporteé en des Vaisseaux, dabors qu'elle est convertie & rendue propre pour l' usage. La relation suivante montrera clairement le peu de soin, ou plutot la grande Negligence de nos Directeurs icy, ce qui m'a obligé d'offrir ce petit Traité a un Prince si Excellent qu'est Votre Majesté, & j'ay même fait mon possible de prevenir un si grand mal, que celuy qui Arriveroit faut de chéne Anglois, les vrays nerfs de notre Force Maritime. Je presume (avec toute Humilité, toute Obeissance & Soumission) d' implorer la Faveur de Votre Majesté, pour obtenir quelque poste dans sa Flote Royale, selon le Caractere des Directeurs qui appartienent a Votre Majesté. Je suis d' une maniere la plus sensible de Fidelité, d' Obeissance & de Soumission assureé,*

SIRE,

De Votre Majesté,

Le plus Fidel & le plus Obeisant

Serviteur & Sujet,

Guiliaume Sutherland.

Grand

GRand *Monarch*, Arbitre de l'Element liquide,
Votre Flote Royale, qui donne aux Eaux la bride
D'un oeil favourable Regard, & la Soutiens,
Du monde la Merveille. Le monde même convient
Que la Puissance Marine avec l' Architecture
Sont sans dispute Votre droit, quoy qu'une obscure
Eclipse les fit aller un peu en decadence,
Jusqu'a du Conquerant *Nassau* la Vigilence
Remplit de la *Bretagne* le Trône Royal,
Et la Valeur d' *Orford* ce Brave Admiral,
Mortrerent a *Louis* derechef de reconnoitre
Que de la Mer étroite nous etions les Maitres,
Ou *Tourville* battu, fit quitter a la *France*
De revenir aux mains derechef toute *Esperance*.
Russel est Brave, est Juste, a la Couronne Fidelle,
Parmi les Admiraux pas un a tant de Zele
Mais, Maintenant que *GEORGE* possede de ses Ayeux
Les trois Royaumes, (ah ! quel bonheur pour eux,
Bonheur sans pareil pour tous ses bons Sujets,
Puisque le Ciel même y joint son Interest
En nous donant une Race si Nombreuse, si Belle
Que les Siecles passez n'en virent jamais telle,)
Pendant dis je que *GEORGE* possede son Trône en Paix,
A toute Rebellion adieu pour jamais :
Toutes les Cabales mechantes, toute Lacheté perira,
Et de la Flote *Angloise* la gloire fleurira.
Dieu d'en haut étale sur notre *Monarch* sa Grace
Sur le *Prince*, la *Princesse*, & toute l' *Illustre Race*.

COURTE
DESCRIPTION
De la Depenſe requiſe pour
L' Architecture & l' Equipement
DES
VAISSEAUX
DE LA
Flote Roiale
DE SA
MAJESTE,
Quand le Nombre en etoit 250.

AVEC
UN ESSAI,
Touchant le frais Neceſſaire a leur Radoubement, pour les mettre en etat de rendre Service.

Par *Guiliaume Sutherland*, Charpentier de Navire ;

Auteur de l' *Aide aux Architects*.

TABLE

TABLE

Des Matiers.

1. *REmarque sur la difference de la dureé de la Flote de sa Majesté, entre le tems passé, & celuy d'a present.*

2. *Description de la qualité & du nombre des Vaisseaux de sa Majesté : Et quel bois de Charpente est necessaire a l' Architecture de chac'un ; & le Total pour l' Architecture de toute la Flote.*

3. *Detail de la dureé des Vaisseaux de guerre au tems passé ; & de la, combien en doivent etre annuelment entre les mains du Charpentier ; Et quelle quantité de bois doit etre requise annuelment pour le radoubement de la Flote Roiale*

4 *Supputation du bois de Charpente que chaque Vaisseau contient quand fini, la juste pesanteur de chaque Vaisseau dans l'eau, la pesanteur du fer de chac'un : Quelle quantité du bois de Charpente se consume, ou est reduite en coupeaux : Et comment il doit etre appliqué.*

5. *La somme necessaire pour l' Architecture de chaque Vaisseau, avec le total pour celle de toute la Flote.*

6. *Detail des frais de chaque Navire : Aussi, tout le frais pour l'entier Equipement de la Flote Roiale en toute chose, hormis en canon, & son attirail ; En vivres aussi.*

7. *Interrogatoires pour prevenir la Depense en donnant a une telle Flote Royale son radoub necessaire Aussi pour preuve de son appointment.*

8. *Quelques Raisons pour faire la coupe de bois en la saison la plus propre, pour sa meilleure dureé, ou on fait voir que tout notre bois de chène est coupé hors de saison ; & commement on y 'en peut prevenir sans faire Dommage a qui que se soit.*

9. *Des Essais pour ajuster la Depense pour le Radoub de la Flote Royale, montrant les fautes Ordinaires de la Flote, & quel profit on peut tirer des materiaux par le troc : Et comment par un bon menage a Six pour Cent du premier prix, on peut seurement prolonguer la dureé des Vaisseaux a vingt huict ans, dont la Demolition se fait Maintenant en moitié de ce tems, avec les paralelles pour prouver la Depense qui se fait a cette heure aussi extravagante que deraisonnable.*

10. *Des Raisons pour faire un tel calcul, & tels essais, & les sommes differentes, entre ce qu'on a accordé pour batir, rebatir & radouber notre Flote Royale, & ce qui peut bien maintenir une telle Flote, avec un bon menage.*

THE INTRODUCTION.

HAVING obſerved a vaſt Difference in the Wear of Shipping, and that the generality of the Publick Ships are tore to pieces, and Rebuilt, in leſs than Fourteen Years; which in former Times uſed to continue Thirty Years, with but very ſlender Repairs. So that the Duration is more than Two to One I have therefore made it my Buſineſs to inquire what material Reaſons can be given for the ſame, and the ill Conſequence which may accrew from ſuch a Vulgar Practice. But firſt, for brevity ſake, I will ſhew two or three Characters which I ſhall make uſe of in ſuch a Deſcription.

= Stands for Diviſion, or Divide.
× Stands for Multiplied, or Multiply.
+ Stands for Addition, or Added.

I ſhall now proceed to ſhew the Quantity and Quality of His Majeſty's Ships, and the Quantity of Timber which will be requir'd to Build them.

The Firſt Rate, or largeſt Ship, is 1814 Tuns; which 1814 × by 1.6 is 2902; which number in Loads of Timber will Build ſuch a great Ship. The number of them being 7, × 2902 by 7, it is 20314 Loads of Timber; which Quantity will Build Seven ſuch Ships.

The Second Rate is 1438 Tuns; which 1438 × by 1·6 is 2300 Loads, which Quantity in Loads of Timber will Build ſuch a great Ship. The number of ſuch Ships is 14, which × into 2300, the ſum is 32200, which Quantity in Loads of Timber will Build Fourteen ſuch Ships

The Third Rate is 1064 Tuns, which 1064 × by 1:3 is 1383; which Quantity in Loads of Timber will Build ſuch a Ship The number of ſuch Ships is 45, which × into 1383, the ſum is 62235 · the Quantity in Loads of Timber which will be required to Build Forty five ſuch Ships.

The Fourth Rate is 677 Tuns; which 677 × by 1.3 is 880; which Quantity in Loads of Timber will Build ſuch a Ship. The number of ſuch Ships is 63; which × into 880 is 55440: the Quantity in Loads of Timber which will be required to Build Sixty-three ſuch Ships.

The Fifth Rate is 392 Tuns, which 392 × by 1.3 is 509; which Quantity in Loads of Timber will Build ſuch a Ship. The number of them Ships is 40; which × into 509 is 20360: the Quantity in Loads of Timber which will be required to Build Forty ſuch Ships.

The Sixth Rate is 246 Tuns; which 246 × by 1:0 is 246; which Quantity in Loads of Timber will Build ſuch a Ship. The number of ſuch Ships is 24; which × into 246 is 5904: the Quantity in Loads of Timber that will be required to Build Twenty-four ſuch Ships.

A Fireſhip is 270 Tuns, which 270 × by 1:3 is 351; which Quantity in Loads of Timber will Build ſuch a Ship. The number of them is 30; which × into 351 is 1053: the Quantity in Loads of Timber that will be required to Build Thirty ſuch Ships.

A Yacht is 150 Tuns; which 150 × by 1:0 is 150; which Quantity in Loads of Timber will Build ſuch a Yacht The number of Yachts was 15, which × into 150 is 2250 · the Quantity in Loads of Timber that will be required to Build Fifteen Yachts.

The Boomb-Veſſels are 260 Tuns; which 260 × by 1:2 is 312; which Quantity in Loads of Timber will Build ſuch a Boomb The number of them is 9; which × into 312 is 2808: the Quantity in Loads of Timber that will be required to Build Nine Boombs.

An Advice-Boat was 100 Tuns; which 100 × by 1·0 is 100, the Quantity in Loads of Timber which will be required to Build One ſuch Veſſel The number of them was 10; which × into 100 is 1000: the Quantity of Loads in Timber which will be required to Build Ten ſuch Veſſels

Then the whole Quantity of Timber which will be required to Build ſuch a Navy, will ſtand as follows:

		Loads	
Oak-Timber requiſite to Build	7 Firſt Rates will be	20314	Obſerving that there is contain'd in every Load of Timber 50 Foot, and in every Foot 1728 Inches.
	14 Second Rates will be	32200	
	35 Third Rates will be	62235	
	63 Fourth Rates will be	55440	
	40 Fifth Rates will be	20360	
	24 Sixth Rates will be	5904	
	30 Fireſhips will be	1053	
	15 Yachts will be	2250	
	9 Boomb Ketches is	2808	
	10 Advice-Boats is	1000	
	Total is	203564	

The Quantity of Timber required to Build the Royal Navy, when they conſiſted of 250 Ships, would be 203564 Loads of Timber; provided it be well Purvey'd, and brought as near the Uſe as it is in Private Yards for Ship-work: For if it is not, a double Quantity may be deficient for ſuch a great Deſign

And ſince I ſhall undertake to prove, that Ships may be made to continue (not wholly demoliſhed) Twenty-eight Years with ſome moderate Repairs, and that the ſaid Navy is compleated to hand, it will neceſſarily follow that 203564 Loads of Timber will ſupply the Uſe of Rebuilding the Royal Navy Twenty-eight Years, which is to have 9 Ships every Year in the Ship builders hands, and to expend the Quantity of 7608 Loads of Timber upon them: Which Quantity of Timber well Purvey'd, Inſpected, and Applied, will be ſufficient to Build, Rebuild, and Keep in neceſſary Repairs ſuch a Royal Navy; although they conſiſt of 250 Sail of Ships.

The number of Publick Yards, where His Majeſty's Ships are Manag'd, is ſix; four of which I count to be Capital, which are *Deptford*, *Woolwich*, *Chatham* and *Portſmouth*; *Plymouth* and *Sheerneſs* put together I deem equal with one of the others: ſo that I ſhall make 5 equal Diviſions of 7608 Loads of Timber; which will be 1521 Loads of Timber. A Sum I deem ſufficient to ſupply the Yearly Expence of Timber in the bigeſt of His Majeſty's Yards, for the Service of Building and Rebuilding his Majeſty's Ships.

In which Calculation it may be obſerved, that I allow of near half of all Timber to be waſte, as may be ſeen by my Trials mention'd in my *Ship-builders Aſſiſtant*, where the Weight of each ſeveral Rate is as follows:

	The Weight light at Launching (Tuns)	Weight of the Iron-work (Tuns)	(C)	Weight of the Wood (Tuns)	(C)	Quantity of Timber allow'd to each Rate (Tuns)	The Difference between the Tunage allow'd, and the Tunage of the Ship (Tuns)	(C)
A Firſt Rate is	2008	32	8	1975	8	3630	1654	12
A Second Rate is	1419	23	11	1395	9	2800	1405	11
A Third Rate is	900 7/10	15	0	885	3	1720	834	17
A Fourth Rate is	584 10/100	9	14	572	2	1100	525	18
A Fifth Rate is	329	5	10	323	10	638	315	12
A Sixth Rate is	170 11/100	2	17	167	14	305	137	6

It may be obſerved, that 40 Foot of Oak-Timber is 1 Tun in Weight, which is the principal Timber applied in Building *Engliſh* Ships By Waſte of Timber is not meant what is wholly loſt, or hewn to Chips; for then it may be obſerv'd

that

that half of all Timber, at the best Management, is served so · But by Waste is meant all such Timber, as in shaping and cutting up any Ship's Frame, cannot properly be used in that Ship, but ought to be preserved for another, which is vulgarly termed, *Building one Ship with another Ship's Chips*. such as Slabs and Ends of a large Ship's Timbers which may be too small for her Body, but probably may very well suit the Body of a Ship of a less Denomination. As in all likelihood a First Rate with a Fourth Rate may suit, a Second Rate with a Fifth, and a Third Rate with a Sixth, and so on And therefore it cannot be absolutely allowed that the $\frac{1}{6}$ part of all Ship Timber, applied in Building them, ought to be wasted, but may be useful in divers cases, and consequently my Calculations and Allowances made will be sufficient to supply the Publick Yards with Timber to Build, Rebuild, and Keep in necessary Repairs, His Majesty's Royal Navy (baring Sea Casualties and Extirpations) although the Number is, one with another, 250 Sail of Ships.

In the next place, I am to shew the whole Sum of Money which will Compleat the Building of such a Royal Navy, when it is Launched into the Water, in order to Rig and Equip.

A First Rate being 1814 Tuns, worth 17 *l.* 13 *s. per Tun* compleatly launched; which Sum amounts to 31110 *l* for one Ship — *l.* *s.*
The number of First Rates is 7, the Sum total to Build them will be -- 217770:00

A Second Rate is 1428 Tuns, worth 14 *l* 10 *s. per Tun* Building, and compleatly launch'd; which Sum is 20851 *l.* for one Ship.
The number of 2d Rates is 14, the Sum total to Build them will be -- 302339.10

A Third Rate is 1064 Tuns, worth 11 *l.* 18 *s. per Tun* compleatly launched; which Sum amounts to 12661 *l.* for one Ship.
The number of Third Rates is 45, the Sum total to Build them will be - 569745.00

A Fourth Rate is 677 Tuns, worth 9 *l* 4 *s. per Tun* compleatly launched; which Sum amounts to 6228 *l.* for one Ship
The number of 4th Rates is 63, the Sum total to Build them will be - 392364.00

A Fifth Rate is 392 Tuns, worth 7 *l.* 4 *s. per Tun* compleatly launched, which Sum amounts to 2822 *l* for one Ship.
The number of Fifth Rates is 40, the Sum total to Build them will be - 112880:00

A Sixth Rate is 246 Tuns, worth 6 *l* 4 *s. per Tun* compleatly launched; which Sum amounts to 1525 *l.* for one Ship.
The number of Sixth Rates is 24, the Sum total to Build them will be - 36600:00

A Fireship is 270 Tuns, worth 6 *l* 9 *s per Tun* compleatly launched, which Sum amounts to 1741 *l.* 10 *s.* for one Ship.
The number of Fireships is 30, the Sum total to Build them will be -- 52245:00

A Yacht is 150 Tuns, worth 5 *l.* 10 *s per Tun* compleatly launched, which Sum amounts to 825 *l.* for one Ship.
The number of Yachts was 15, the Sum total to Build them, with ordinary Accommodations, is —————— 12375:00

A Boomb Vessel is 260 Tuns, worth 6 *l.* 6 *s per Tun* compleatly launched; which Sum amounts to 1638 *l.* for one Ship.
The number of Boomb-Vessels is 9, the Sum total to Build them will be —————— 14742:00

An Advice-Boat is 100 Tuns, worth 5 *l.* 4 *s. per Tun* compleatly launched, which Sum amounts to 520 *l.* to Build one
The number of Advice-Boats is 10, the Sum total to Build them will be —————— 5200:00

Total—1716260:10

The Sum total for Building them all will stand as follows:

For

			l.	*s*
For Building	7	Firſt Rates	217770	00
	14	Second Rates	302339	10
	45	Third Rates	569745	00
	63	Fourth Rates	392364	00
	40	Fifth Rates	112880	00
	24	Sixth Rates	36600	00
	30	Fireſhips	52245	00
	15	Yachts	12375	00
	9	Boombs	14742	00
	10	Advice-boats	5200	00
		Total	1716260	10

The ſeveral and reſpective Sums added together are 1716260 *l* 10 *s* Which Sum well applied, would Build, and in every reſpect Compleat, the Hulls of His Majeſty's Royal Navy, as well as they are now perform'd: Nay, the Prices are much larger than what ſuch Ships may be built for in the Private Yards, with rather better Materials, and full as good Workmanſhip.

In the next place, I will ſet down the Charge of the Equiping, that the total Charge of ſuch a Number of Shiping may be adjuſted, when they are in every reſpect fitting to proceed to Sea, as to what belongs to the ſailing part; as the Charge of Maſts, Yards, Rigging and Blocks; for Boatſwain's and Carpenter's Stores: Which Materials will wholly Compleat the Machine for the Sea, excepting Guns, the Utenſils belonging thereto; alſo Victuals.

	l.	*s.*
The Charge of ſuch Equiping for a Firſt Rate will be—7290 *l.*		
Which Sum × by 7, the number of Firſt Rates, is	51030	00
The Charge of Equiping one Second Rate will be — 5608 *l.*		
Which Sum × by 14, the number of Second Rates, is	78512	00
The Charge of Equiping one Third Rate will be — 4080 *l.*		
Which Sum × by 45, the number of Third Rates, is	183600	00
The Charge of Equiping one Fourth Rate will be —2525 *l.*		
Which Sum × by 63, the number of Fourth Rates, is	159075	00
The Charge of Equiping one Fifth Rate will be —1381 *l.*		
Which Sum × by 40, the number of Fifth Rates, is	55240	00
The Charge of Equiping one Sixth Rate will be — 848 *l.*		
Which Sum × by 24, the number of Sixth Rates, is	20352	00
The Charge of Equiping one Fireſhip will be — 931 *l.*		
Which Sum × by 30, the number of Fireſhips, is	27930	00
The Charge of Equiping one Yacht will be — 518 *l.*		
Which Sum × by 15, the number of Yachts, is	7770	00
The Charge of Equiping one Boomb-Veſſel will be — 900 *l.*		
Which Sum × by 9, the number of Boomb-Veſſels, is	8100	00
The Charge of Equiping one Advice-Boat will be — 350 *l.*		
Which Sum × by 10, the number of Advice Boats, is	3500	00
The total Sum for Equiping the Royal Navy will be	595109	00
To which Sum add the Charge of Building the Hulls	1716260	10
The total Charge of the 250 Sail fit for Sea-ſervice will be	2311369	10

This Calculation ſhews plainly, that in Caſe ſuch a Royal Navy was to be new Built and Equip'd in every particular, the Charge would not amount to two Millions and half of Money.

And having demonſtrated what ſuch a Navy may be purchaſed for in every particular fitting for the ſailing part of the ſame, I ſhall proceed to illuſtrate in

as

as pathetical a manner as I can possible, how the Charge may be adjusted in Keeping them in necessary Repairs fitting for Sea-service, that so the direct Expence of our Royal Navy may be known.

Indeed I must confess this latter Part will not allow of a Definition so obvious as the former, since the variety of Accidents are so frequent in the Sea Management, that I will not pretend to give a positive Account of Casualties which are incident to the various Imployments of such a Navy; and therefore will only give Judgment how the Allowance may be stated for a common Wear, leaving the Accidents to be noted as they shall happen; notwithstanding I am really of Opinion, that the Allowance I shall make will comply with not only a small Casualty, but at sundry times a total Extirpation, to be put in with the Charge of the common Reparations

I shall first begin to draw a Parallel from the Repairs in Houses · Which altho' there is Land Taxes, Ground Rent, and pretty smart Repairs at divers times, a House whose Purchase is 100 *l* shall be Rented for 6 *l* a Year, that there cannot be at most allowed to the Landlord than 4 *l.* 10 *s per Annum* for such Repairs, and Interest of his Money And altho' this Comparison may seem very wide from our present Design, I do actually say, that there is a vast Advantage between bartering the Materials made use of in building Ships, (as Iron, Ropes, Canvas, nay, Wood too) over what there is in the Materials made use of in House-building, as Brick, Mortar, Tile and Slat; since the first mention'd Materials are composed with bodies of undissolvable Duration and Usefulness, to what the others are; as I have fully explain'd in several Places of the following Work: And therefore will pass on here with stating a Calculation for the Repairs, in allowing of 6 *l per Cent.* of the prime Charge in Building and Equiping the Royal Navy, for keeping it in such necessary Repairs, fitting in every respect for the Service of the Sea; observing that I will allow this 6 *l per Cent.* of the prime Cost of Building and Equiping the 250 Sail, without minding that it may always happen for 30 or 40 Sail of such a Number to be always in Harbour (by turns) and out of the Sea wear; which Allowance, I dare be positive, will do with good Management: Also shall allow that the Duration of all Shiping may be Twenty-eight Years (baring Casualties) which is a total Extirpation, or something almost as material. But to proceed,

The Interest of 2311369 *l.* 10 *s* at 6 *l per Cent.* is 138681 *l.* 3 *s.* which × by 28, is 3883072 *l.* 4 *s.* to which I shall add the first Charge of Building and Equiping the whole Navy, which is 2311369 *l.* 10 *s* that there may be an Allowance for wholly new Building them once in the Twenty-eight Years, the Sum will be 6194441 *l.* 14 *s.* which Sum being = by 28, the number of Years allowed for the duration of Ships well managed, the Sum will be 223372 *l.* 1 *s.* 5 *d* 2 *q* Which said Sum I will allow at present (without farther Consideration). A Sum sufficient, being carefully applied, to defray the Yearly Expence of Fitting, Refitting, and Keeping in necessary Repairs, His Majesty's Royal Navy one Year with another, during the number of Twenty-eight Years. But fearing several Objections against so material a Scheme as this will appear to be, well inspected, I shall endeavour to chalk it out a little plainer. And first, as to the Prices of Building which I have allowed in this Calculation, they are much larger than what such Ships may be every way as well perform'd in the Private Yards, and yet the Yard-keepers must stand to the necessary Repairs of their said Yards or otherwise pay Rent for the same, besides finding a Dwelling-house, and all other Necessaries for the Work; nay, they must provide Instruments, and perhaps bring up a large Family out of the Profit that is made by Building Ships, with less Prices than what I have here mention'd: Whereof in the Publick Service there is a Sum allowed for the ordinary Expence of the Navy, which includes several of such Stipendiaries herein mention'd.

If it be Objected, that Ships will not continue Twenty-eight Years without Rebuilding; but instead of that number, they must be tore to pieces and extirpated in Fourteen

I Answer, That they have formerly continued a much longer time than Twenty-eight Years; and if then, why not now? I am sure the Architects and Mechanicks in Ship building are much better than ever they were, and consequently if Time be given their Labour will be better perform'd; that such Machines will be better wrought and stronger connex'd, and undeniably will continue longer.

But then perhaps the Wear will be imputed to hasten their Decay, alledging that such moving Bodies are agitated more turbulently at Sea, than they are when lying in a Harbour, and at rest; and so by such long and assiduous Uses as are put upon them by constant acting at Sea, they cannot possibly endure so long, as when they are quietly laid up and moor'd in a Harbour. Which indeed at a single View, and without farther Consideration, will appear a great Topick, without any manner of Objection, and what might allow us in such a vulgar Practice of heaving a Ship away in half the time, as what with good Management they might reasonably last.

Indeed I cannot deny but that if Ships were as well look'd after in a Harbour as they are at Sea, there would be some difference in the Wear and Duration; since Ships and all their Equiping will be more affected (when in motion) by the Violence of the Sea and Wind, than when they are at rest, and no strain applied to them, also the Equiping in Harbour is useless, and the Expence that way saved. But then here is a great Advantage in the preservation at Sea more than there is in Harbour, since Ships are duely clean'd, scrub'd, air'd, wash'd with Salt-water, which is a sovereign Remedy for preserving Timber; also they have a number of Carpenters and Calkers on board, which are for ever inspecting the Defects, and amending every thing which they find out of its place, or amiss so that it cannot be a little tumbling in the Sea, that can alter the duration of a Ship so very much, provided she is well wrought and connex'd at the first Building And therefore,

I shall proceed to shew some other material Reasons for such a great Decay in Shiping, and the only Cause which hastens Rebuildings, other than what I have mention'd yet, which indeed by the Learned'st Architects is allow'd to be in the over-hasty Practice of Felling Timber at an improper season for the longest Duration, and that is when the Sap is up, and when the Bark will strip; which is for the Advantage of Tanning.

Vitruvius and other Learned Architects are for an Autumnal Fall, and throughout the whole Winter, as may be found by him Published, where he gives Reasons for the same. Others advise *December*. *Cato* says, when the Fruit is full ripe And several others commend the Opinion of such as advise for a Winter's Felling, that the Timber neither rifts, casts, nor twines, because the Cold of the Winter doth both dry and consolidate, when as in Spring, and when pregnant, so much of the Vertue gets into the Leaf and Branches: Happy therefore, they add, if some other Invention was for Tanning without so much Bark, (as the Honourable Mr. *Charles Howard* has most Ingeniously Offer'd) with several other Directions for preserving Timber by properly Felling of it; and yet something worthier of Note is still behind; whereas they tell you that a Method for making excellent Planks and Boards will be to unbark the Timber in a fit season for stripping, and let them stand naked a full Year before the Felling.

I say, If such an excellent Vertue is depending on so small a Difference in the Charge, and a little Trouble, it would be very proper to serve all Ship Timber so, since the Duration would be twice as long as that which is fell'd by our common Custom. Nay, something more may be offer'd on this Head, that Timber may much better be strip'd and stand naked seven Years, as to be cut down, strip'd, and lye naked on the Ground seven Years, as I have frequently observed. Therefore there can be no Objection made against felling Timber at a proper Season, that adds to its Duration; since it is matter of fact, and very demonstrable, that the Expence of Building Ships is made double (considering the Continuance) of what they would be, were Timber well and throughly season'd.

Neither

Neither is it impracticable to strip Timber standing, and the Expence of the same swell'd very little, perhaps not 6 *d* more in a Load of Timber, by that time it is brought to Use, I am pretty positive that the Publick Expence would be lessen'd near 100000 *l per Annum* by such a Practice and no Person damag'd one Penny, if the Bark were peel'd off two or three Years before the Felling, according as the *Tanner* may require the Bark, and the *Ship-builder* his Timber. I am positive for want of such a Practice, I have seen many a thousand Load of Timber laid, and perished on the Ground But I shall pass on to consider of another Objection, that perhaps may be made against this Scheme; which is, That Ships cannot be Kept in necessary Repairs for 6 *l. per Cent.* of the prime Cost, or as I have allowed, as aforesaid.

First, I shall give one Hint, a matter which will be easier proved, and that is, What Difference there is between the Price of the Publick and Private Ships at their first Building? For since such Difference is very wide, I shall borrow such an Advantage to prove this Calculation for Repairing them and Keeping them in Use; since a Defect may as well lye in the Fitting, as in the first Erecting and Building them.

I shall not be so tedious as to go through what ought to be necessarily applied in keeping every particular Ship (throughout His Majesty's Navy) in Repair, but shall take notice of one Ship in the medium, or a Ship of 677 Tuns carrying 50 Guns, which I am pretty positive will rather exceed the Charge requisite to repair the whole number, according to their different Magnitudes, than in the least manner lessen the medium Expence

The Charge I allow to compleat a Ship of 677 Tuns, in every respect fitting for the Sea-service, is 8753 *l.* and the Use Money of such a Sum at 6 *l per Cent.* is 525 *l* a Year; which for 7 Years is 3675 *l.* for 14 Years it is 7350 *l.* for 21 Years it is 11025 *l* and for 28 Years it is 14700 *l* I presume, that if such a Ship is well performed at the first Building (as I could demonstrate the manner very easily) she would require little to be done to her for the first seven Years, except to dress and preserve the weather Work, as Sides and upper Deck, also to pay her Bottom with Rosin or Pitch, according to the common Custom; also to paint the Work in the weather every Year, if it requires; to fit and preserve the Rigging, Masts and Yards, as occasion requires; otherwise the Wants will be very inconsiderable.

	l.
For Calking, or Searching, the upper Work and Decks, Dressing and Graving all over every Year	90
For refreshing the Paint in the weather, and small Jobbs within side every Year	15
For Docking three times in the Year, the *Shipwright*'s Work included	60
For preserving the Masts, Yards and Rigging, which is often done with the Crew, however I will allow	20
For repairing the Sails and a few Blocks	10
The Sum total for keeping such a Ship in Repair one Year	195
	7
The Sum total for keeping her in Repair seven Years	1365

But fearing it may be Objected, that such Ships, if on the Cruising station, will require Cleaning and Tallowing once in two Months, I shall therefore allow to tallow proper once in four Months, and Washing may suffice at the intervals of four Months; and this will be only for the Cruising Ships, which will not reach the 1/10 part of the whole Navy, considering the superficies of the largest Ships, which are only Cleaned once in every Year: However I will allow of three times Tallowing, which may help to make up some lame Article, if there should be one.

Then once Tallowing and Docking, to do it will be 30 *l.* and three times will be 90 *l.* for one Year. then 90 × by 7 is 630. So that the whole Charge will

	l
will be	1995
Which ſubtracted from the Sum amounting for the Intereſt	3675
The overplus remaining out of ſuch an Allowance is	1680
Which + to the Sum allow'd for the ſecond ſeven Years, it makes	5355

and ſome Money in bank

And now I proceed to conſider of ſome neceſſary Reparations for the ſecond ſeven Years; in which I muſt proceed to an Amendment for preſerving my Ship to the longeſt Duration: I will therefore allow of a competency of *Shipwright*'s Work, as in new hanging a Rudder, and ſhifting the Iron-work of the main and fore Channel, and placing three or four pair of Standards; ſhifting part of an upper Deck and lower Deck, for which I will allow the whole Charge of ſhifting the upper Deck, that is for the Planking part; obſerving that when Ships grow old, and patch'd, and cobbled, they are not fitting for Cruiſing, ſince Swiftneſs will be retarded by weight, and binding or doubling them, that I will rather propoſe a Method to ſtrengthen the Ship without ſuch an addition of Timber; which ſhall be to take off the lower and upper Deck Knees, and new fay and faſten them, which may be done at a very reaſonable Rate, conſidering that old Iron may be new wrought for five Shillings a Hundred, which in two ſuch Decks will be near four Tuns; which Method ſhall ſuffice for the ſecond ſeven Years. As to the Hull, and for the Equiping, I will allow a quarter of the firſt Charge of making it new for Repairing the ſame; and conſidering all ſuch Materials come eaſy by way of Barter, I believe it will very well ſuffice, ſince it will not be very ſhort of one third of the firſt Allowance.

	l	s.
The firſt ſeven Years Allowance I will ſet down here, without mentioning the Particulars, as Docking, Tallowing, Painting, and other Contingencies, as afore-mentioned	1995	00
To which I add the ſhifting ſix Tuns of new Iron, or new wrought, by Barter	50	00
For ſhifting an upper Deck, for Stuff and Workmanſhip	220	00
For other *Shipwright*'s Work in the courſe of ſeven Years	300	00
For ¼ of the Equiping	631	00
The total Sum for the neceſſary Repairs of the Ship the ſecond ſeven Years is	3196	05
Which ſubtracted from the Sum allotted for that Expence	5355	00
Remains	2158	15
Which being + to the Sum allowed for ſeven Years by our =, the Product is	3675	00
The Sum to be carried forward for the Expence of the third ſeven Years is	5833	15

And now I muſt begin to cobble up ſuch a Ship for the *Weſt-Indies*, or ſome other Foreign Voyage, and therefore I will apply a Sheathing, but may leave out the Charge of Tallowing and often Docking; which Sheathing well laid on, may laſt half ſeven Years; ſo that I muſt allow of the Charge of two Sheathings; I ſhall alſo allow of ten pair of Standards; to ſtrip the Ship above water, and put in new top Timbers, and new Gratings, and a doubling between the Wales; to new bolt the Riders, and fay them, and to ſhift any defective Plank as may be requiſite; alſo to allow of one third of the Equiping to be new by way of Barter.

Then

	l	s.
Then for Dressing and Graving wholly four times in seven Years, besides patching at divers times ———	360	co
For refreshing the Paint such a number of times ———	60	co
For Dock four times in the seven Years ———	80	co
For seven booter tops with Tallow ———	35	co
For repairing with top Timbers, Standers, and all other Jobbs, which will be found requisite in the time, I will allow of half the Charge of new Building the said Ship at first, which consider'd right it will be near ¼ of the said new Building, considering Barter -	3114	co
For two Sheathings, allowing each at 7 *d.* a Foot, according to the Custom ———	291	13
For ⅓ of the Equipping ———	841	14
But fearing an Objection here, I will allow Tallow and also to Careen four times in the Year, besides the Docking: Every Careen I will charge at 12 *l.* 10 *s* which with the Charge of the Tallow will be ———	980	co
The total Charge for the third seven Years to keep such a Ship in necessary Repairs, and to bring her to the Duration of Twenty-one Years is ———	5762	07
The Sum total allowed for it is ———	5833	15
Remains to be + to the fourth seven Years Expence is ———	71	c8
Sum allowed is ———	3675	co
The Sum remaining to keep the Ship in necessary Repairs the fourth seven Years, and bring her to the Duration of Twenty-eight Years is ———	3746	c8

And here perhaps will be an Admiration, before it is explain'd, how 3746 *l* 8 *s.* shall keep a Ship in necessary Repairs seven Years, when she is Twenty one Years old, and that she should require the Sum of 5762 *l.* 7 *s* to keep her in necessary Repairs when she was but Fourteen Years old!

I Answer, That there is an Old Ship with all the Equipping to be Barter'd, and then as I have fully explain'd under the several Heads of the following Work, that there will be nine Tuns of Iron-work, which if rightly applied, will be worth to the Owner, that can convert it again to smaller Uses, I'll say but 20 *l per Tun*; then there will be 25 Tuns of Cordage, which at 20 *l per Tun* is 500 *l.*, and 2270 Yards of Canvas, at 9 *d. per Yard* to the Owner, will be 85 *l* 2 *s.* 6 *d.*; then the Masts, Yards, Anchors, and the Hull of the Ship, where may be abundance of good Knees, Beams, Floor Timbers, Plank for divers Uses, which will not be worth less than 261 *l.* 10 *s*, since the Value of the serviceable Plank, and Deals, will be worth 2 *d per Foot* running Measure, which will be near one with another 40 *s per Tun*, the Timber I shall allow at 15 *s per Tun*, so that I may allow in the Medium 20 *s per Tun*, which if 77 Tuns is allowed for Waste, the remains will be 600 Tuns, or Pounds Sterling: However I will abate 10 *s per Tun* for pulling the Ship to pieces, which is 338 *l.* 10 *s*; which subtracted from 600 *l.* there remains 261 *l.* 10 *s* The Value of the Hull, abating the pulling her to pieces

Then the Value of the Hull will stand as follows

	l.	s	d
Value of the Hull is———	261	10	0
Masts and Yards ———	50	co	0
Anchors ———	120	00	c
Other Iron work ———	180	oc	0
Cordage ———	500	00	0
Canvas ———	85	02	6
	1196	12	6

Which several and respective Sums + together, then the Allowance for keeping the Ship in necessary Repairs the fourth 7 Years and bring her to the Duration of 28 Years, is 3746 *l.* 8 *s* + to 1196 *l* 12 *s* 6 *d.* makes 4943 *l* 00 *s* 6 *d.* for the fourth seven Years Expence.

 And

And now I am to consider of some frugal Management, to preserve the Old Ship at the Age of Twenty-one Years, and bring her to the Age of Twenty-eight Years with 4943 *l.* 00 *s.* 6 *d* And first I will give my Opinion of the most proper Station for her Ease, which I believe to be a Home Convoy, or in some serene Country, where her principal Use out of a Harbour will be in the Summer, or in a Line of Battle, and always pretty handy for to be Docked; not that I will be in the least manner observed to run Hazards, but had rather swell my Allowance as to the Charge of fitting her to the longest Duration of Twenty-eight Years, and therefore shall proceed in the following manner

I will allow of stripping off the Sheathing, and all the Plank, from the Keel to the upper Wale, and make all the out-board Plank new, since that upward has been once served so; which new Planking for Stuff and Workmanship, I will allow 20 *d. per Foot*, 10000 Foot being sufficient, will stand in 833 *l* 6 *s.* 8 *d.*; and for the Foot-hooks, which I presume may require to be shifted, I will allow such another Sum for that, and for shifting some of the Foot-waleing, which together will be 1666 *l* 13 *s.* 4 *d.* I will also drive out all my Iron-work, and new fit that; which 9 Tuns of Iron-work at 10 *l. per Tun* for new working it, is 90 *l*; and for other necessary *Shipwright*'s Work, I will allow 243 *l.* 6 *s.* 8 *d.* I shall also allow of ⅓ of the Equipping to be new; and of once Docking, and Dressing, and Painting every Year: And then the Expence of keeping such a Ship in necessary Repairs between the Age of Twenty-one and Twenty-eight Years, will be as follows:

	l.	*s.*	*d.*
For new Planking and Timbering under Water, the Charge will be	1666	13	4
For the Iron-work, the Charge is	90	00	0
For other *Shipwright*'s Work, the Charge will be	243	06	8
For ⅓ of the Equipping to be new	841	14	0
For new Dressing and Graving 7 times	630	00	0
For new Painting 7 times	105	00	0
For 7 times Docking	140	00	0
Sum total for the necessary Repairs for the last 7 Years is	3716	14	0
The Sum for the said seventh Year according to = is, with the old Ship included,	4943	00	6
The Sum remaining at the Expiration of 28 Years will be	1226	06	6

And now it appears by my Calculation, that after such a Ship of 677 Tuns has been in Use Twenty-eight Years, and kept in sufficient Reparations, there will be remaining 1226 *l.* 6 *s* 6 *d.* out of 6 *l. per Cent* of the first Charge in Building and Equipping her, and the total Sum added to it, when it is = by 28, the number of Years allowed for such a Ship's Duration, (baring large Casualties) which is above ⅛ part of the whole first Charge of Building and Equipping her. The ⅛ part of the first total Charge in Building and Equipping the Royal Navy, consisting of 250 Sail, is 288921 *l.* 2 *s* 4 *d* 2 *q.* which is more than One Years Expence for the whole number: And I am pretty positive, that such a Ship of 677 Tuns is more in Wear than Ships of any other Rate, especially in War, and all the Navy at Sea However having a due Consideration to the Vicissitudes of Publick Affairs, I will rather double such a Sum, and make 223372 *l* 1 *s.* 5 *d.* 2 *q.* 446744 *l.* 2 *s* 11 *d* for the Yearly Expence of such a Huge, Useful, and Supporting Navy; and proceed to shew my Reasons for making such Remarks on the Expence.

In the Year 1712, as I was walking by the *Royal Exchange*, at a *Bookseller*'s Shop I happen'd to see a Printed Paper hang out. The Title was thus,

An

An Anſwer of a Letter to a Friend, concerning the Publick Debts, particularly that of the Navy.

I ſhall not make large Repetitions on the ſame, but rather refer the over-curious to the Prints, only ſhall mention ſome Expreſſions and Remarks on the ſame Where, ſays he; "It is very well known that the Supply granted for the "Navy, is different from what is granted for the Land Service ſince the man-"ner of the latter is ſo abſolute, that it is ſubject to no Alterations or Enlarge-"ments; but the Annual Proviſion for the Navy is made by granting a general "Sum, not adjuſted or limited by any particular Eſtimate, but by Computa-"tion, that Four Pounds a Month for every Man will anſwer all the Expence "upon the ſeveral Heads, except the Ordinary of the Navy · But with ſuch a "Proviſo, that an exact or equal Sum ſhall not ſucceſſively anſwer Year after "Year; for if it ſhould, it would plainly appear that it lay in the Power of "the Manager

"But in order to ſtate a Method of Computing the Annual Charge, it will "be neceſſary to fix upon one certain Sum; and what has been moſt frequently "granted, is Two Millions Two Hundred Thouſand Pounds, for maintaining "Forty Thouſand Men imployed in the Sea Service · Which Proviſion is made "after the aforeſaid Rate, and the Proportion as follows:

l.	*s*	*d.*			*l.*	*s.*	*d*
1	07	0	A Man *per Month*	for Wear and Tear	707 000	0	0
1	10	0		for Wages	780,0~0	0	0
0	19	0		for Victuals	494,000	0	0
0	04	0		for Ordnance	1c4,000	0	0
				And for the Ordinary Expence	120,000	0	0
				The total Expence Yearly	2,200,000	0	0

By which Print it appears, that there was allowed in the late War for the Expence of Wear and Tear in His Majeſty's Royal Navy, the Sum of 700,000 *l.* a Year, one Year with another, beſides 120,000 *l* for the ordinary Expence of the ſame; which two Sums put together are 820,000 *l per Annum*

After I had conſidered theſe Prints, and obſerved that no Body had publickly confronted them, I took it for granted the Reports were true, and without making it my Buſineſs to inquire how far ſhort ſuch Sums fell in defraying the Annual Charge; and of Conſequence the Arrears ſunk into *South Sea* Stock to be very conſiderable; and having alſo been a Practical Man in ſuch Affairs for near Five and Thirty Years, was willing to pleaſe my Curioſity in inquiring how ſuch a Charge ſhould amount, and whether (in Caſe ever ſuch Trials ſhould happen again) the Charge might not be much abated, not only in Building and Equipping the Royal Navy, but alſo in Keeping it in neceſſary Repairs, every way fitting for Uſe

The difference between 223372 *l* 1 *s* 5 *d.* 2 *q.* (a Sum allotted to keep His Majeſty's Royal Navy in neceſſary Repairs One Year; which I am really apt to believe would, with very good Management, be every way fitting for any Branch of Sea Diſcipline) and 700000 *l.* is 476627 *l.* 18 *s* 6 *d* 2 *q* A large Sum to be waſted. And if I double my firſt Annual Charge, and make 223372 *l.* 1 *s* 5 *d* 2 *q.* 446744 *l.* 2 *s* 11 *d*; and ſubtract the double Sum from 700000 *l.* the remains will be 253255 *l* 17 *s* 1 *d.* A large Sum yet to be waſted So that upon the whole it cannot be otherwiſe allowed, than that inſtead of making 6 *l per Cent.* comply with the Annual Charge, 16 *l per Cent.* has not done, and inſtead of making the Royal Navy laſt *Twenty-eight Years*, there has been an Allowance to make a total Extirpation above twice in that time And having obſerved, nay proved, a prodigious Waſte of the Materials, eſpecially Timber, in ſome of His Majeſty's Yards, do believe the Management in His Majeſty's Navy has not been ſo nice as it ought to have been: But where the Fault lyes, I ſhall refer to be Examined, and remain in all Dutiful Obedience to Superiority, and in a Loving Reſpect to Equals and Inferiours.

To

To the Right Honourable

EDWARD, Earl of *ORFORD*, Baron *Barflur*, &c.

My Lord,

MAY it please your Lordship, The Reasons for my Dedicating the following *ESSAY* to your Lordship, is not only from Account of the Populace (but my own Observation) that your Lordship has been one of the Best and most Effectual Generals the *English* Royal Navy ever had, I having had the Honour of being very near your Lordship's Conduct in the *La Hoage* Engagement, and at Burning the *French* Fleet in that Bay: Which Unparallell'd Action I take to be very small, in comparison of your Lordship's Indefatigable Care in new Modeling the Royal Navy, and almost making it Invincible, both in the Strength and Activity of the Shipping, as well as in the due Order of Command.

My Lord, *France* was counted a petit Competitor in former Days, when our Old *English* Heroes spread their Laurels, and Triumphed over them and *Holland*, and assumed the Sovereignty of the Narrow Seas, maugre the Invention of those Two Maritime Powers: But this Glory was long eclipsed; and *England*, poor neglected *Britain*, must truckle to the Mighty *Lewis*! He singly did contend with *England* and *Holland* for the Sovereign Title at Sea: Not to mention *Bantry-bay* and *Beachy-head* Fights, when the *Frenchmen* rid in Triumph, first over the *English*, and next over the *English* and *Dutch* Fleets; nay, often have we been Beat with an inferiour Force of a single Ship, until your Lordship took up the Cudgels, and let *Lewis* know, that *England* had remaining a General that knew how to Conquer, and not only to Conquer, but absolutely Dispirit that Mighty Monarch, and bring him back to his old Opinion, that the *English* Navy was Invincible.

My Lord, This was not done desperately, or inhumanely, as in the *Holland*'s War, when half the Battle was gain'd by Fireships, and in destroying one number to confound another But our *La Hoage* Action was by Management in Battle and Device, preserving Thirteen tall *French* Ships to be fired in the Bay of

 La Hoage,

La Hoage, befides others at *Cherburg*, and that too without the Lofs of one Ship, or indeed fcarce of one Man.

My Lord, When the Mighty *William* deliver'd us from Popery, our Fleet was in a very mean Condition, out of One Hundred Sail fcarce Twenty of them were fitting for the Sea, let the Nation be in ever fo much Hazard ; and now thank God there may be One Hundred Twenty Nine Ships immediately Equip'd fit for Service, and none lefs than Fifty Gun Ships, which are full as good Ships as thofe that were put into the number of Seventy Gun Ships ; fo wonderfully are we fortified and barr'd by a Maritime Force, which Heaven preferve and blefs both them and your Lordfhip, as a Worthy Patriot and Preferver of your Country, maugre the Contrivance of fuch as would eclipfe you, and leffen the Luftre of fo Valiant, fo Wife, and fo Faithful a General.

My Lord, I could very much enlarge in celebrating your Lordfhip's Graces ; but believing my mean Capacity will not be fuitable to fo Worthy a Peer as your Lordfhip, and therefore fhall only pray for your Lordfhip's Health, and that you may continue a Bleffing to the Royal Navy. I am in all Dutiful Obedience,

Right Honourable,

Your Lordfhip's

Moft Obedient,

Ever Faithful,

Humble Servant,

William Sutherland.

THE

THE PREFACE.

IT'S *Reported, that when* Heraclitus's *Scholars found him in a Tradesman's Shop, into which they were ashamed to enter, He told them,* That the Gods were as conversant in such Places as in others. *Intimating, that a Divine Power and Wisdom might be discern'd in such common Arts, altho' so much despised: And tho' the Manual Exercise and Practice of them are esteemed ignoble, yet the Study of their general Causes and Principles cannot be prejudicial to any other (tho' the most sacred) Profession.*

This Observation plainly shews the Value which that great Man put upon the meanest Artificer, and how that the greatest Proficient in the most sublime Art may make some Improvements by the Conversation of a vulgar Mechanick.

Ramus *having observed the Reason that* Germany *has been so eminent for Mechanical Inventions, was because there has been Publick Lectures instituted amongst them of such kinds; and those not only in the Learned Languages, but also in the Vulgar Tongue, for the Capacity of every unletter'd ingenious Artificer.*

In a Treatise set forth by John Wilkins, *M. A. and Chaplain to the Elector* Palatine *is intimated the various Tempers and Opinions of the Ancients in divulging their Improvements in several Arts and Sciences. As more particularly, the Divine* Plato *is observed severely to dehort all his Followers from prostituting Mathematical Principles unto common Apprehension and Practice. Like the envious Emperour* Tiberius, *who, it's reported, caus'd an Artificer to be murdered for making Glass malleable, fearing thereby the Price of Metals might be debased.*

Aristotle *justly oppos'd* Plato *altho' his Scholar, being one of the first Authors that writ any Methodical Discourse concerning Mechanical Powers, chusing rather a certain and general Benefit, before the Hazard that might accrue from the vain and groundless Disrespect of some ignorant Persons. Since him there has been divers others; as,* Hero Alexandrinus, Hero Mechanicus, Pappus, Alexandrinus, Proclus Mathematicus, Vitruvius, Guidus, Ubaldus, Henricus Monantholius, Galileus, *&c. He instances likewise, that all the various Studies about which the Sons of Men do busy themselves may be comprised under three Kinds.*

Viz. { *Divine,* / *Natural, and* / *Artificial.* }

Which Arts alone may truly be stiled Liberal, since they set a Man at Liberty from his Lusts and Passions.

He goes on, and draws several Parallels between the Engines of the Ancients, and those made use of at this present Time, more particularly Archimedes's Ballista *for shooting or slinging Stones, and the* Catapulta *for shooting Darts or Arrows by* Dionysius, *drawing Comparisons betwixt them and our Gun-powder Instruments now in use.*

The Description he relates of a Sailing Chariot is very pleasing and admirable, with the Author's Notion of movable Sails, or such as will traverse as a Weather-cock, and so proceeds to explain the wonderful Contrivance of a submarine Ark, fitting for Navigation, or a Ship that Mersennus *doth very largely and pleasantly descant upon, wherein Men may safely swim under Water. With abundance of other very pleasant and plain Demonstrations in Mathematical Magick, as he stiles it.*

And now I proceed to shew some Necessities and Benefits that has induced us to Improve that most Useful and Necessary Art of Building and Equiping Ships.

And

And first to Instance, that wonderful Frame which is read of in Sacred History, that so miraculously preserved a certain number of Persons from a total Deluge: It was an Ark, or Ship, and Built with Gopher *Wood.*

The Proportion of that Ark was 300 *Cubits long,* 50 *broad, and* 30 *high; a Cubit being* 21 *Inches and* $\frac{888}{1000}$ *Parts. Which Dimensions far exceeded the biggest of our* English *Ships every way, since the biggest* English *Ship doth not exceed* 170 *Foot long on the longest Deck, and* 50 *Foot broad from the outside of one Plank to the outside of the other, and* 42 *Foot deep from the upper part of the Keel to the upper part of the Plansheer in the Midships.*

The Ark's Proportion was thus: Length to Breadth as 6 *to* 1, *and Length to Depth as* 10 *to* 1.

Now the largest of our English *Ships, Length to Breadth is as* 17 *to* 5, *and Length to Depth near as* 17 *to* 4.

Gopher *Wood, being a white Cedar, and is now commonly used amongst the* Turks, *it being very useful in Ship-Building. Let the Bodies of Ships be as various in their shape as they possibly can be, that it will be very hard to define whether* Noah's *Ark was altogether streight or circular.*

It had second and third Stories, or Decks, and finish'd in a Cubit upwards, having a Door in the side, somewhat like the Holland *Hoys, an Idea thereof I shall describe in the following Figure.*

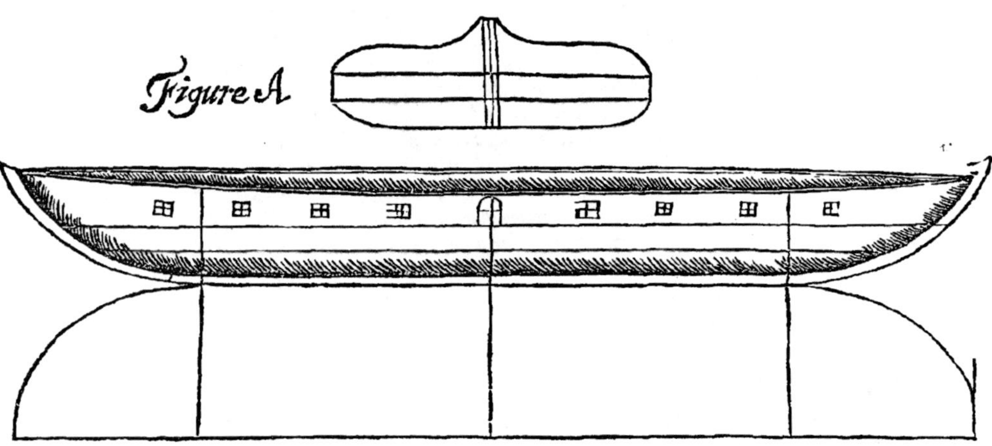

Fig. A *being drawn in proportion to that Ark which is believed to be the very Source of Ship-Building, naturally descending unto* Noah *for the Preservation of those Creatures he was commanded to take with him.*

After that Traffick and Commerce grew very desirable, as in the Case between King Solomon *and* Hieram, *the variety of Uses grew also more fashionable and general, tho' neither the Shape or Dimensions of Ships is any where absolutely defin'd, but by Simile in St* Paul's *anchoring at the Stern. It's very probable that Vessel was very acute forward, as the* Turks *and* Spanish *Galleys are at this day believed to be a Pattern for our River of* Thames *Wherries.*

And if the Angle of Incidence is the facilitating the Motion, without farther Consideration such Shapes will undeniably be the best, especially in such Climates where the Seas are so very serene, and the Vessels seldom used, except in the Summer season.

Precedent has no where absolutely proved the different shapes in Shipping, neither has the best of Authors made a decision of the same by clear Demonstration: But was it so, sharp Ships would not be proper for our Climates, where the Ocean is so violently agitated.

The Swing of any thing is stopp'd sooner by so much the farther you lay hold of it from the center of the Swing. Which Faculty may be applicable toward hindering Ships delving.

The

The Cono cuneus *has been highly recommended by some to be very proper in shaping Ships Bodies, and yet it's not made a general Method, neither doth it stand good with the Opinion of divers famous Writers; nor can it be naturally applied in the same.*

But such Digressions I allow rather as pro & con *for Table-talk, than a general Benefit, and proceed with a small Instance, that the solid of least Resistance, which has been so highly recommended, may be with vast Advantages applied in Building any Ship*

And since Projections in general, tho' grounded on ever so good a Basis, are nullified by those that should forward them, that same genuine Solid may continue unapplied, as long as it has been a discovering.

It is not for want of a Genius in Shipwrights *that the Practice is not exerted, although it's very rare to see an able* Shipwright *throughly skill'd in Learning; not but that there is very good Scholars in the Trade of Ship-Building, which will allow themselves to be Masters of the Practick Part, and throughly qualified to direct the Workman in Building or Rebuilding Ships. But the Qualifications requisite to make any Man such a Master are really so many, as well in the Theory as in the Practick Part, that it's almost impossible such Qualifications should be concenter'd*

But provided it was so, that Theory and Practice could be so easily interwoven, as imagined, the Experimental Part would be the most Noblest, without which no Man can properly call himself a Shipwright. *Neither is that all, since it's general for all Controversies to be determin'd by those in Vogue for the greatest Proficients in any Science; so that if they are Deficient for want of Learning, or Intricate through want of Practice, the Decision they make will be accordingly, which spoils Improvements, bars Societies, destroys our Studies, and, by consequence, confuses a Science.*

England'*s Shipping, and Sea Discipline, may be term'd their* Unum Necessarium *the only Center on which all their Riches and Safety are concentred; and to compleat it ought to be by the greatest Improvements, and not defend Errour because of a fanciful Temper.*

To observe the Largeness of our Navy, the Traffick of our Merchants, the vast Number of Sea-faring Men, as well as Mechanicks, are imployed, on that very Concern, and yet to exert on the same, is almost criminal, although divers famous Authors has hinted such Faculties as would improve our Art, were they but put in Practice

What Variety of Uses, as well as Shapes, may be observed in such Machines, and how admirably the Experimental Part has unvail'd it self; the Magnitude and Number, as well as the Difficult Voyages they have been lately exposed to, would have astonish'd our Predecessors in the very last Century

And having by Precedent shewn the variety of Temper in our former Ship-Builders, as well in Shapes as Proportioning the Parts, with some Remarks on the Miscarriages that has happened for lack of Standards in performing the same, also some private Opinions and principal Directions which has been publish'd (for Ship-Builders Assistance) by several famous Authors, and conclude my Preface in shewing the Advantages which may be made by the following Treatise.

From the Year 1617 *to* 1656, *Ships of three Decks were from* 38 *to* 40 *Foot broad; the* St. Michael *by Sir* John Tippets *but* 41 *Foot* 8 *Inches, the* London *by* Jonas Shish *but* 44 *Foot, and carried* 100 *Guns; since that several Ships of* 48 *Foot broad has been obliged to be Girdled*

The Monk *by Sir* John Tippets, Rupert *by Sir* Anthony Deane, Mary *by* Mr Pett, Dreadnought *by Sir* Henry Johnson, *all Third Rates, and but* 36 *Foot* 6 *Inches broad, the* Cambridge *by Mr.* Shish *but* 38 *Foot, and* Royal Oak *but* 40, *and both carrying* 70 *Guns each, as well as any of the size, and since them two Deck Ships of* 42 *Foot broad has miscarry'd, which is really a Paradox to most Men.*

And not to rake in the Ashes of some preceeding Builders that has verified the old Proverb in making the Addice the Reconciling Mould, there be several at this day that will engage to Build a Ship with little Assistance of such an Instrument.

The Royal Catherine *was Contrived by the* Royal Society, *and yet was Girdled, the double Keel'd* Experiment *was also made by the same* Society.

And since Miscarriages are frequently dismal, how curious ought our Inquiries to be either by infallible Demonstration, or general Precedents, and not to run the Hazard of such dismal Losses as has frequently happen'd in both Ship and Men

The Opinion of a great Proficient in Liberal Sciences is, that a Ship ought to be considered three principal ways.

First, says he, to try her Body below the deepest draught of Water, whether the Shape be truly Circular, according to the course of the Water, (and not by Horizontal Parallels) which will enable you to give true Judgment whether she shall sail swift, or otherwise

Secondly, to observe the Frame or Shape of the Ribs, as may be seen in my Ship-Builders Assistant, *in that Scheme at Page 82, which will inform you whether she will bear the Sail you design, term'd by* Shipwrights *to be stiff or tender sided.*

Thirdly, to consider the connexing of such a Machine, by drawing such a Scheme as may be seen in my Ship-Builders Assistant, *at Page 42. Which three Observations being throughly consider'd, will form the Hull of any Ship compleat.*

The Opinion of another Excellent Man is, that the Resistance is according to that Cross Section made by the Midship, or largest part of the Ship, only considering the Angle of Incidence; and that every Ship principally resists the Medium at the largest part of her, also that the mass of Water that resists a Ship, is not resisted by her until it's passed by her biggest Part, and that if two Ships were formed ever so various, one ever so Acute, and the other as Obtuse as possible she could be made, if their Cubic Inches under the surface of the Water, and the Power that drove them was equal, the Trim also with indifferency considered, their Velocity would be also equal.

The Honourable Mr Boyle's Hydrostaticks *is recommended by Dr.* Harris, *in his* Lexicon, *to be of the highest Importance to find the Gravity of Shipping.*

Leybourn *in his* Cursus Mathematicus, *mentions how the Parts of any Ship may be found, from the* Cube *and* Golden Rule of Proportion.

From such Observations, and some others that I mention'd in another place, I shall describe the Figures of Six Ships, and adapt their Shapes agreeable to the Proportion

First, I shall make a general Application of that admirable Solid of Least Resistance in Shaping them, and in doing it I shall briefly mention how a Center of Gravity may be obtain'd

Secondly, To make General Proportions for Equipping them, as to the Masts, Yards, Rigging, Cables, Anchors, Sails, Guns, and Men.

Thirdly, To calculate Tables for Scantling every individual Part of any Ship from 1700 Tuns to 100; also the Masts, and every Part belonging to them; so that any Man may be able to learn the Skill of making or providing such Materials with the greatest Exactness.

Fourthly, is fully considered the Advantage or Disadvantage that will accrue in Capstands, and how such Engines may be made Useful and more Beneficial than they have been made

Fifthly, The Law part, or making of Contracts, is described in a better Method than it ever was done, with different Cases to prevent such litigious Disputes as generally happen between Merchants, Owners, *and* Ship-Builders.

Sixthly, I have described the nature of converting Timber, and Rules how to adjust the different Value between Straight and Compass Timber.

Seventhly, I have described some particular Proportions for Rigging Vessels of a less Denomination than Three Mast Ships.

And Lastly, have Explained the Terms used in this Treatise.

SHIP-

SHIP-BUILDING IMPROVED.

A Is the Figure of a Ship measuring 1600 Tuns. Length on the lower Deck from the inside of the outward Plank at the Stem and Stern (measur'd on a direct Line in the middle) 170 Foot Breadth from the outside of the Plank between the Wales (at the extream breadth) 49 Foot. Depth in Hold, from the upper part of the Limber board, to the upper part of the lower Deck Beam (measur'd in the middle of the Ship by a Perpendicular Line) 19 Foot.

The usual Method to find the Tunnage I shall not mention here, only minding, that when the Depth in Hold, and half the Breadth was equal, the Depth was taken for a member to cast the Tunnage. But since the half Breadth has so far exceeded the Depth, that advantage is given to the *Vender* (to make the half Breadth a part) for that extraordinary Property of giving Ships a medium Breadth, notwithstanding two Ships may be equally long on the lower Deck, or equally broad, or equally deep in Hold, in the Mid-ships, and yet by their being Taper'd, one shall carry some score Tons more than the other: And therefore (although it's said that the Rule made use of to cast the Tunnage, is a medium Rule) it will be very hard for one Man to lose his Property, to help make up another Man's: And therefore, in another Place, I have considered how any Ship's Burthen may be exactly found

The next thing requisite is to lay down the Figure; and that as near as the Conveniency of such Shipping will allow, is laid down in the following Scheme. D E C is the rising Line, or Lipping of the Floor Timbers, and D B C the height of the breadth Line, L E K being Similar to D E C, which is the Narrowing or Tapering of the breadth. K I L is Similar to D B C, which is the Narrowing or Tapering of the Floor.

Now in consideration of Accommodating great Officers in their Apartments, I shall, instead of making a Pink, or round Stern Ship, make a square Stern'd Ship. So that L being prolong'd to M, that part at L H may imitate the cutting of a top part of a Conoid, and leave a Frustum of such a Figure behind, for the after part of any Ship upwards can be allow'd to be no other.

Then H E-K is now the narrowing of the breadth, or half breadth Line, and instead of the Floor Line narrowing aft, it will breadthen in all square stern'd Ships, according to N H. And after such a fashion may any Ship's body be turn'd out by one Rotation, according to the Demonstration of the Solid of least Resistance; only instead of making use of a straight Axis, it must be a crooked one, as D B C corresponding to the rising Line.

However, the transverse Lines will be Parallel one to another, and in a direct Current the Water will pass in such a body, where the whole weight of Water will equally affect the Ship, according to the distance from the extream part of the Ship's body.

And this part here mention'd, may be term'd the middle part of a Ship, since rightly considering her, she consists of three principal ones, which middle part naturally form'd is a hanging Conoid, the only part that helps or hinders the Motion of her, it being also the part that holds the Lading, and also bears the Ship,and her Utensils, and Lading: So that it really ought to be principally considered, since by the well or ill disposition thereof, depends the advantage or dis-

diſadvantage, which will undeniably accrew to the Uſe of either Ship, Bark or Boat.

The upper part of any Ship is only for accommodating and managing the Uſes requiſite to her Sailing and Loading, and to make Lodgings for Men.

The lower part, altho' ſeemingly of little Service, notwithſtanding without which part, both the other would be uſeleſs, ſince by this part ſhe is ſteady'd in the Sea, ſhe is laid in a Dock, or on the Ground ſafe. For if you conſider what cauſes that conſtant and uniform Motion in a Fiſh, it would be found to be nothing but her Fins; and therefore this lower part of a Ship doth partake of that Faculty.

And theſe are the Principal Conſiderations which ought to be made towards ſhaping the Log or Solid, which makes a Ship's Body, which will not be only the moſt profitable, but the true and genuine ſhape, which will naturally lead us to the Uſes, and Equipping the Machine.

When firſt it was obſerv'd, or rather conſider'd, that ſuch floating Bodies would be more expeditious, and much cheaper than any Animal could be hir'd, they were rowed with Oars, which is no other than lifting and ſhoving a weight fore-right; but by tryal and project, Sailing at length grew very faſhionable, and the uſes very intelligible. As to the Center of the Maſt's place, the magnitude of the ſame, as alſo the Yards, the faſhion of the Sails to the reſpective Maſts, the quantity of Rigging proper to ſecure the Maſts, and number of Ropes convenient to traverſe the Sails, and ſet them to the Wind, and alſo to furl them. And this has been wholly obtain'd by Practice, without the help of any Theory to improve them.

In ſmall Bodies where they uſe but one Maſt commonly call'd *Hoys*, the place of that Maſt has been generally found by dividing the extream length of the Veſſel at, or near the place of the Gun-deck, into three parts, and at the Period of one of thoſe parts from afore, that Maſt is plac'd; which place is as generally the place of the Midſhip Flat or Timber: And although a variety of temper will always be, this part in ſuch Veſſels is almoſt made Univerſal.

But in large Ships, where it's found directly oppoſite to Reaſon to have their Maſts in one Piece, it's divided into ſeveral, and ſeemingly plac'd otherwiſe, tho' in effect they all Concenter in the very place.

But before I proceed to ſhew how; I ſhall ſet down my Opinion concerning the placing of the Mid ſhip timber in three Maſt Ships. I divide the Ship on the lower Gun-deck into two halves, and ſet forward from that Diviſion half the extream breadth of the Ship from Out to Out of the Plank, ſo that there will be the whole breadth of the Ship conſidered as a Solid, with what is contain'd in it, to Ballance againſt the Power, or Sail, which in drawing the Ship forward alſo depreſſes her; ſo that when a Ship is drove with the greateſt impetuoſity, ſhe ſhall be equally poiz'd, which is what ought principally to be conſidered of a Center of Gravity.

Not that I aver this Opinion to be the abſolute Center of Gravity in the Ship, for the Point is really very weighty, and divers principal Conſiderations ought to be, before this can be made a general Maxim: As the weight of the Air, or the greateſt preſſure that can be on the Sail, according to what a Ship will bear, and how far ſhe will be depreſs'd forward, or end ways, in proportion of what the Ship will bear ſide-ways, or as it's term'd, to hold up her Side.

Now as to placing the Maſts, they ought to proceed from the ſingle Maſted Veſſel, altho' they be in ſeveral parts: However I ſhall not any ways mind the Bowſprit nor Mizen Maſt, ſince if I take them right, they are little otherwiſe than ſuper numeraries; and chiefly as Ballances one againſt another, to traverſe the Ship either this way or that way.

Then as to the Main maſt and Fore-maſt, and every part thereunto belonging, with every Sail uſed to thoſe Maſts, they ought altogether to be in proportion to a one Maſted Veſſel's Maſt and Sails, as the Bodies of the Ship and Veſſel is one to another, and ſo divided and ſub divided into parts, according to a direct proportion of what the Ship's body is one to another, at the two places where each reſpective Main maſt and Fore maſt ſtands. Alſo

Also the said Main-mast and Fore-mast, in such large Ships, ought to be plac'd one from another, after such a manner, that when the Sail is Bunted out and fill'd with Wind, it shall have the same effect on such a large Body, as if both those Masts, with every Respective part belonging thereto, were united in one, and plac'd in the very Center (according to a direct Proportion of the Ship) as it would be in a Hoy, or such a small fashion'd Vessel.

But before I proceed to shew the Proportion of the Equipping and Managing, I shall describe the Figure of the largest Ship, and set down her Proportions, as Length, Breadth, Depths, Draughts of Water, number of Men, and Guns, according to Custom: Also an Index to lead you to each respective part.

Figure A. *First to the Dimensions and Proportions of the Parts*

	Feet	Inc
Length of the Keel 2. *a.* from the Touch of the Stem to the back of the main Post	139	1
Height from the top of the Keel, to the top of the Plansheer Midship	41	0
Rake of the main Post to the top of the Plansheer	12	5
Breadth at the Fashion-pieces, at the Wing-transum, from inside of the Plank	30	10
Breadth extream afore, at ⅓ of the Load Mark Line, Divided between the inside of the Rabbits, } 26, 27.	45	3
Draught of Water loaded { afore	21	8
Draught of Water loaded { abaft	23	3
Rake of the Stem from the touch to the outside aloft, *a. w*	29	9
Figure B Breadth of the Floor, *a. b.*	12	0
This Ship may be esteem'd to be worth *per* Tun building 17 *l.* 13 *s.*		
What Guns, as to number according to the Establishment, 100		
What Men accordingly, 717.		
Stern to project and lay Parallel from the main Post aloft Round of the Rail included.	2	10

An Index to the several Parts in the Figure A.

a. 2. Length of the Keel from the back of the main Post to touch of the Stem

f 1. Ditto from the back of the false Post, to the extream fore part of the Keel or Tread

10 11 From the aft-side of the Rabbit of the Post, to the fore-side of the Rabbit of the Stem, for the length on the Lower Gundeck measured there.

Fig. B 12, 13. Breadth of the Ship's Timber from Out to Out, in the Midships, term'd Moulded

14, 15 Extream breadth from Out to Out of Plank, or Thickstuff, allowed in Measure.

4 *e* From the Limber-board to the upper Edge of the Gundeck beam, in the Midships, term'd the Depth in Hold, and formerly allowed in Measure.

3 1. Half breadth of Floor in the Mid-ships.

L I K Narrowing of Floor Line.

L ⊖ K. Narrowing of the Breadth Line.

D C ⊖. Rising Line, being Similar thereto.

B C D. Rising of the Breadth Line.

H E Narrowing of the Breadth aft with a broad Stern.

H L. Breadth of the Transum within the Plank.

N H Narrowing of the Floor Line with a broad Stern, breadthens as the

Line, N H And in such a Position the Narrowing of the breadth Line may be prolong'd to M

w a $\frac{1}{3}$ of the Breadth set back from *w* to *a* for the Rake of the Stem allowed in measuring the Tunnage of any Ship

C. 16. 15. Sheering-line, or the Hanging-line, of the upper breadth, from whence the sweep of the Top-timber commences

Lower Gun Deck 41, middle ditto 51, upper ditto 61, Quarter Deck 81, Forecastle Deck 100, Poop Deck 91: all which Decks ought to lye Parallel one from another, and the greatest Perpendicular height between any two of them need not exceed seven Feet, at the side.

R. The Lyon, or other Figure

Q. Knee of the Head or Cut Water.

S. Upper Rail of the Head.

T. The Steaving, or Angle, the Bowsprit makes with the Stem.

5. The Partners, or step of the Bowsprit.

P. The Stem in three Pieces.

O. 1. Depth of the Keel abaft, proposed to raise the Sheer, and to have less Dead Wood, and better fastning

3 The Foremost part of the Stern-post.

16 7. The corner Side Timber of the upright of the Stern.

Figure B. x x x x. The Midship Bend of Timbers.

A. z. The Fore Castle, where is Lodgings for the Carpenter, Boatswain, and their Mates.

B z. A Cook-room, for dressing Victuals for the Commanders, and other Officers

C z The Furnaces for boiling the Seamens Provisions

D z Apartments for Boatswain's and Carpenters Stores.

F. z. Ditto for the Powder, and for the Gunners Stores.

F z A filling Room to empt the Powder out of the Barrels into the Cartridges, alſo Chests and Troughs, and a Lanthorn fix'd to hold a Candle.

H z The place of the Jeer, Capstand and treble Jeer on the upper Deck.

I z. The Slop Room, to hold Seamens Slop-cloths.

K. z. L z. Captains and the Flag-Officers Store Rooms, with the Pursers and the Surgeons Cabbin.

M z. The Bread Room.

After Powder Room. K. z. L. z. Fish Room and Captains Store Room.

N. z. Gunners, and Gunners Mate's Cabbin, in the Gun Room.

O z The Ward Room and Volunteers Cabbins.

P. z. The great Cabbin.

Q z A Lobby, with some Pantries.

R. z The lower Coach.

S z. The upper Coach.

T z The Round House.

u. w. z. Belcony's, or Walks in the Stern.

I shall

A Scale of feet and Inches

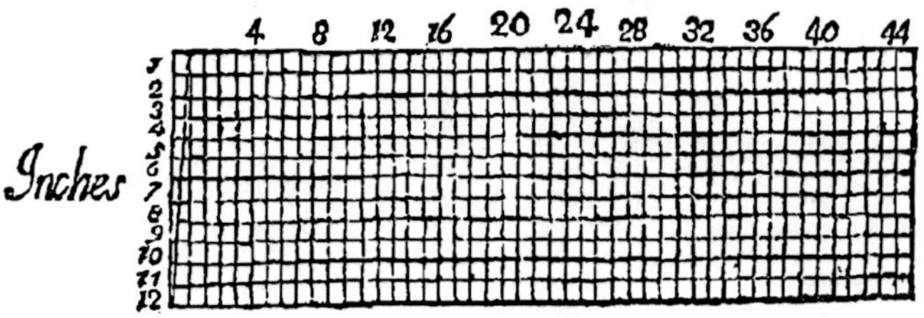

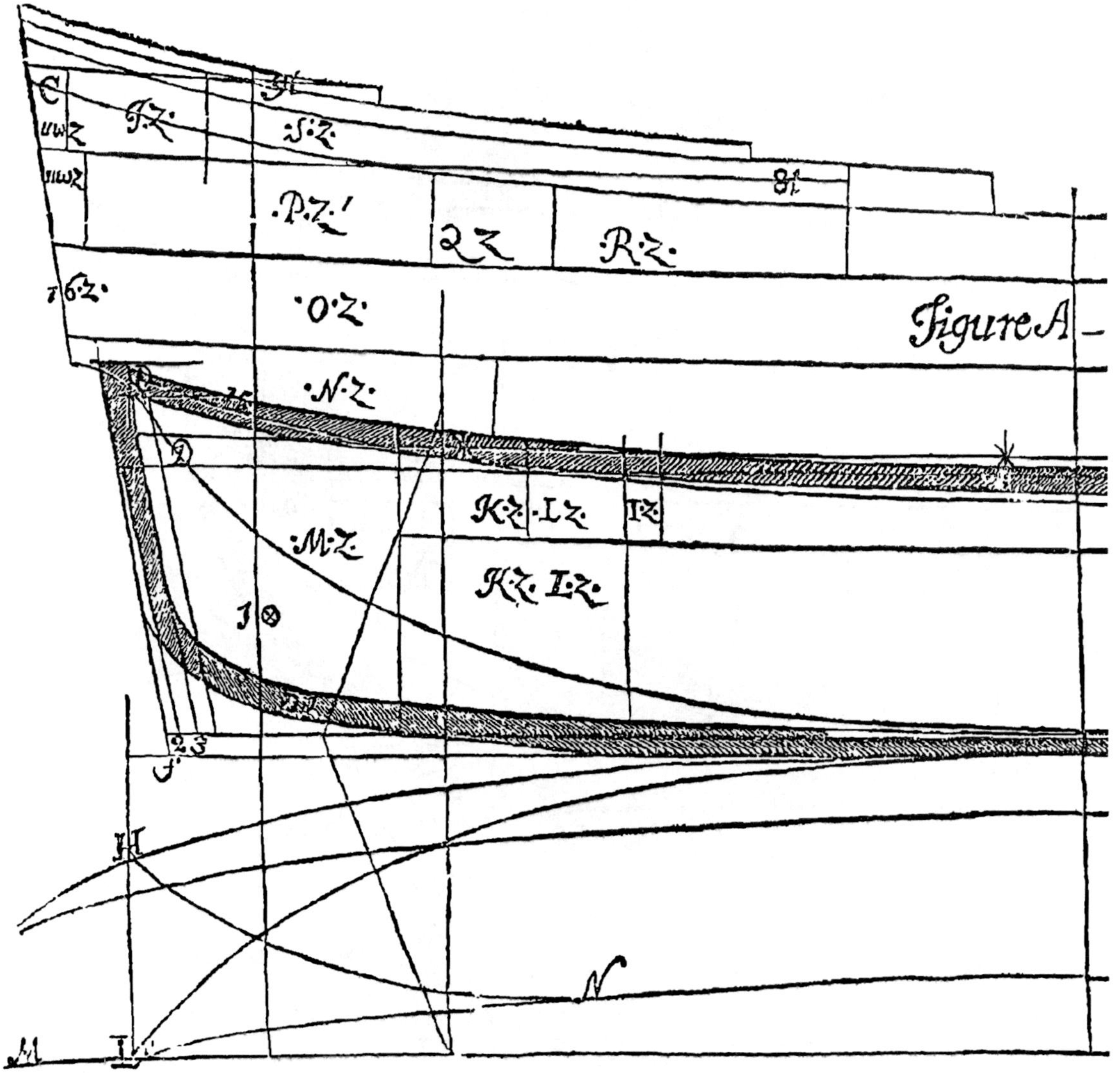

Figure A

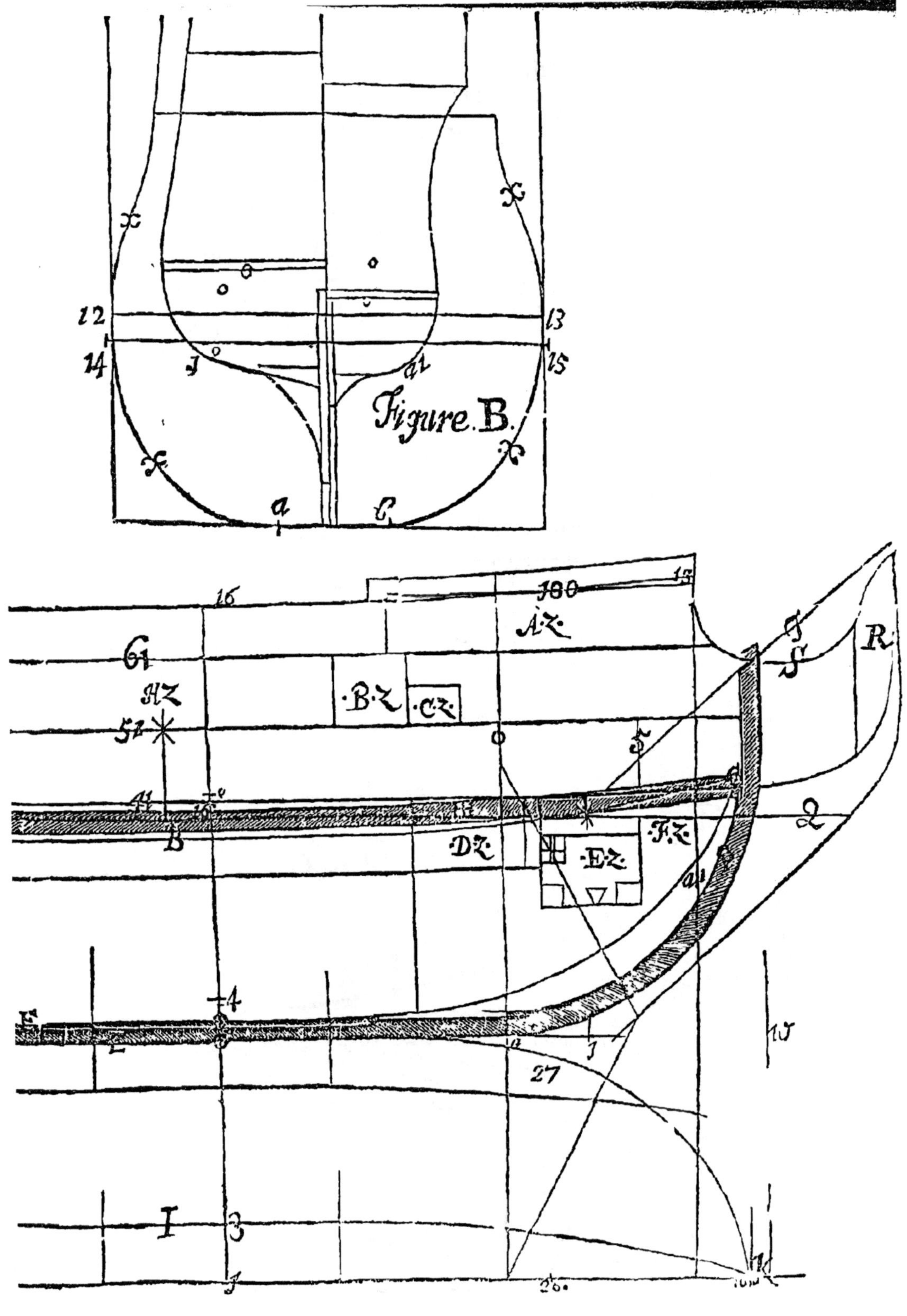

Figure.B.
12
13
14
15
a
b
16
180
17
A.Z.
G
B.Z.
C.Z.
H.Z
51
R
S
D.Z.
E.Z.
F.Z.
Q
E
4
27
I
3
26

I ſhall not here inſert the Scantling of each part, but ſhall put the Scantling of the Six Sizes together, and having ſhewn the Dimenſions, and Shape, and Contrivance of the largeſt ſiz'd Ship, I ſhall endeavour to ſhew a univerſal Rule to find the proportion of the Equipping and Managing: And alſo the proportion of any other Ship, and their Equipping, from the parts of ſuch a Ship, ſuitable and agreeable one to the other in every reſpect

Firſt, I ſhall draw a Parallel between a Ship of 1677 Tuns, carrying three Maſts, and a Hoy of 27 Tuns, carrying one Maſt.

Cube Root of 1677 is 11 $\frac{9}{10}$, Main maſt and Fore maſt together, 43 Inches Diameter.

Length in Yards 69.

Cube Root of 27 is 3· Diameter of the Maſt 11 Inches $\frac{3}{4}$, length 54 Feet. And from that Rule the Main-maſt and Fore-maſt together, of ſuch a great Ship, muſt be 44 Inches and $\frac{1}{2}$ Diameter, and 71 Yards and $\frac{1}{2}$ long.

Now according to Cuſtom { the Main-maſt is 39 Inches and $\frac{1}{2}$ Diameter.
the Fore-maſt is 34 Inches.

Length of the ſtanding Maſts, Top-maſts, Topgallant-maſts, abating Heads, is 63 Yards, for the Main-maſt and the Fore-maſt is 55 Yards.

Diameter 39 Inches, Circumference 122 $\frac{4}{10}$, Area 1197 $\frac{3}{10}$ Main-maſt.
Diameter 34 Circumference 106 $\frac{9}{10}$, Area 904-5 Fore-maſt.
Main-maſt and Fore-maſt put together, Diameter 44 Inches $\frac{1}{2}$, Circumference 140, Area 1575.

Content in Cubic Feet in the Main-maſt, Top-maſt, Top-gallant-maſt, according to Cuſtom, 527 Feet, and in the Fore maſt, *&c* 345 4, which total is 872.4

In both, according to a new Obſervation, 783 Feet, the difference is 89 Feet $\frac{4}{10}$, Heads and Heels, only one meaſur'd, that is, to meaſure from Head to Heel of each Maſt, as a Fruſtum of a Cone.

Then the diſtance of the Centers of theſe Maſts are found as follows. From the Center of the Main-maſt for 3 Maſts to the Center for 1. Maſt, is 35 Feet, and from the Center of the Fore-maſt to the ſaid Center is 40 Feet

Breadth of the Ship Extream at the Main-maſt is 49 Feet.
Ditto at the Fore-maſt, accordingly ———— 43 Feet.

That the ſaid diſtances is as 7. to 8. as well as the Breadth of the Ship and Diameter of each Maſt; ſo that the diſtance of the three Maſts Center, and the breadth of the Ship Extream, where they do center, and Diameter of each reſpective Maſts are Reciprocal, and bear the ſame proportion.

That according to the Proportion of our accuſtomary Tunnage, it's found, that the Main-maſt will be but,

Main-maſt Diameter 23 Inches $\frac{68}{100}$, Length 38 Yards.
Fore-maſt Diameter 20 $\frac{18}{100}$, Length 35-5 Yards.

However I ſhall conſider it farther, of the weight of Water, which is reſiſted by ſuch a great Ship of 50 foot broad, and 21 foot deep in the Water, which if ſhe was ſhaped in every reſpect as a Cylinder, or Parallelopipedon, then the weight of Water reſiſted would be equal to half that Solid, whoſe Area is equal to the depth and breadth of ſuch a Ship in the Water, ſo that × 50 by 21, and by 32, the ſquare Root of thoſe two Numbers, the Product is 33600, the half of which

which is 16800 feet, which would be the weight of Water resisted by the Ship, provided she was fashion'd by any of the preceeding shapes: But since the Ship's body doth converge into Angles, which in such a body is equal every way, which Angulations is most certainly the facilitating of the Resistance of the Ship: Besides we have it by Information, that the absolute resistance is to the relative resistance, as the Radius is to the Angle of Incidence. But waving such nice demonstrations at present, with observing, that the weight of Water is not resisted absolutely 'till it's past the broadest or biggest part of the Ship, and in some Ships chiefly resisted there.

However let 16800 feet of Water, or 509 Tuns 3 feet be allowed to be the weight of Water, resisted by such a Ship, which is shaped according to the Incurvations in the preceeding Figure, and that a small Boat of 6 foot broad, and 1 foot deep in the Water, resists (by such a Calculation) 15 foot: The Mast or Leaver in the small Boat, is, from Experience, allowed to be 4 Inches Diameter, and 19 Foot long From which it appears, that the weight to be removed in the large Ship is, 16800 feet, and in the Boat, 7 foot and half, which is as 2506 is to 1; and the Leaver ought to be of equal strength, and as artificially applied, to lift the large weight as to lift the small weight: Then square 4 the Diameter of the small Leaver it's 16, which × 2506, and it's 40156, the square Root of which is 200, the Diameter of a Leaver suitable to lift the great weight, provided they were both to be of equal length 19 foot, but since the great Leaver will be 10 times as long, it ought to be 10 times as big, which will then be 633 Inches.

Then the Dimensions of the Masts will stand thus. { Main-mast 343 Inches / Fore mast 300 Inches } Diameter.

And the Dimensions will agree to the resistance or weight to be removed.

The lengths will also be standing Masts, Topmasts, Topgallant Masts, as they stand Rigg'd.

Main-mast — 190 feet, or 63 Yards 1 foot.
Fore-mast — 178 feet, or 58 Yards.

But if the Power or Sail of those two Bodies were considered, they would be found to be one to another, as 90 to 1; as I shall instance something of that Nature hereafter

According to the present Establishment, the Main mast and Fore-mast put together, is to the 4 Inch Mast, as 167 to 1; and therefore without some other Consideration to prove this Property, the Dimensions of such great Ships Masts to small ones, are false either way: And therefore, I shall rather reduce the Power to the Resistance, than the Resistance to the Power, which must be done by some other Additiments besides the bare strength of the Mast, which is done with Stays and Shrouds to double the Mast, and add to it's strength; of which I shall consider as follows.

The Shrouds allowed for such a great Ship's Main-mast is 18 of 10 Inches and half Circumference, and a Stay of 19 Inches and half Circumference, which Shrouds and Stay added to the Mast, will make him 42 Inches, three Inches bigger than what he was before such Addition.

Now if these Shrouds and Stays were placed directly perpendicular by the side of the Mast, they would add to the strength thereof 1 Inch and half of a side; but on the other hand, if they were placed directly Horizontal from the Head of the Mast, they would double the Mast, and add to it's strength the whole length of the Shrouds, or 740 Inches But they standing at a certain Angle, according to conveniency, and the tumbling home of the Ship side, which in this I shall allow to be 18, from a Perpendicular made by the side of the Mast; so that the Mast is doubled and strengthened by the Stay and Shrouds in such a Position, as 18 is to 90, or $\frac{18}{90}$ parts of 740 Inches, which is 148 Inches for

I the

the Main-maſt each way, which, with the Diameter of the Maſt according to the preſent Eſtabliſhment, is 335 Inches, within 8 Inches of our Calculation.

And from ſuch Conſiderations may be drawn a general method to find the Dimenſions of Leavers, ſuitable in ſtrength to ſupport a Power to drive its reſpective Solid on its Paſſage of which I ſhall ſet down as follows

Take the depth from the upper Edge of the Keel to the Gun-deck line at the Side, and the breadth of the Ship from Outſide to Outſide at the broadeſt place, and the girt of the Body from the Gun-deck line to the middle line at the Keel, and add them together, Divide the Sum by 3, gives the Diameter in Inches and Parts, and for the length, take the extream length from the forepart of the Lyon, or Figure of the Head, to the aftſide of the upright Stern Timber, meaſur'd on the upper Gun-deck, which ſhall give the length in feet from the Step of the Standing-maſt to the Top-gallant-maſt Head, as they ſtand rigg'd: Which Rule may be made general for all ſorts of Ships

The Opinion of a great Philoſopher is, that a Ship may be underſtood to be all from the Keel to the Vane, and from the Extremity of the Bowſprit to the Poop-lanthorns, and therefore it may be allow'd, that there may be as much Canvas converted to any Ship's Sails as is equal to a Superficies, whoſe length ſhall be equal to the whole length of the Ship, from the foreſide of the Head to the Stern, as was before ſaid · And depth ſhall be equal to the depth of the Ship from the Keel to the Top gallant-maſt head.

Firſt, to find the length of the Main-maſt, from which all the other Maſts and Yards ought to be found.

		Feet	*Inch.*
Tuns 1677	Depth from the Upper-edge of the Keel to the Gun deck line at the ſide	21	6
	Breadth from Out to Outſide at the Extream breadth	49	
	Girt of the Body or Ring, at the Outſide, from the lower Deck to the Keel	40	0
	Length of the Main-maſt in Feet and Inches	110	6

Then for the Diameter of the Main-maſt

Tunnage of ſix ſeveral ſizes of Ships			*Inches*	Diameter of the Main-maſt in Inches and parts.
	1677	Square-root is	41	
	1488		38 $\frac{6}{10}$	
	969		31 $\frac{1}{10}$	
	625		25	
	364		19 $\frac{2}{10}$	
	225		15	

Then for the length of the Main-maſt, Top-maſt, Top-gallant-maſt's, as they ſtand rigg'd.

Length of the Upper-deck. *Feet*	Length of thoſe Maſts accordingly meaſur'd, as they are now made by Cuſtom,
190	189
183	180
164	168
142	144
117	111
104	105

That the length of the Upper-deck nearly correſponds to the length of the Main-maſt, from the Heel to the Top gallant-maſt's head, as they ſtand Rigg'd.

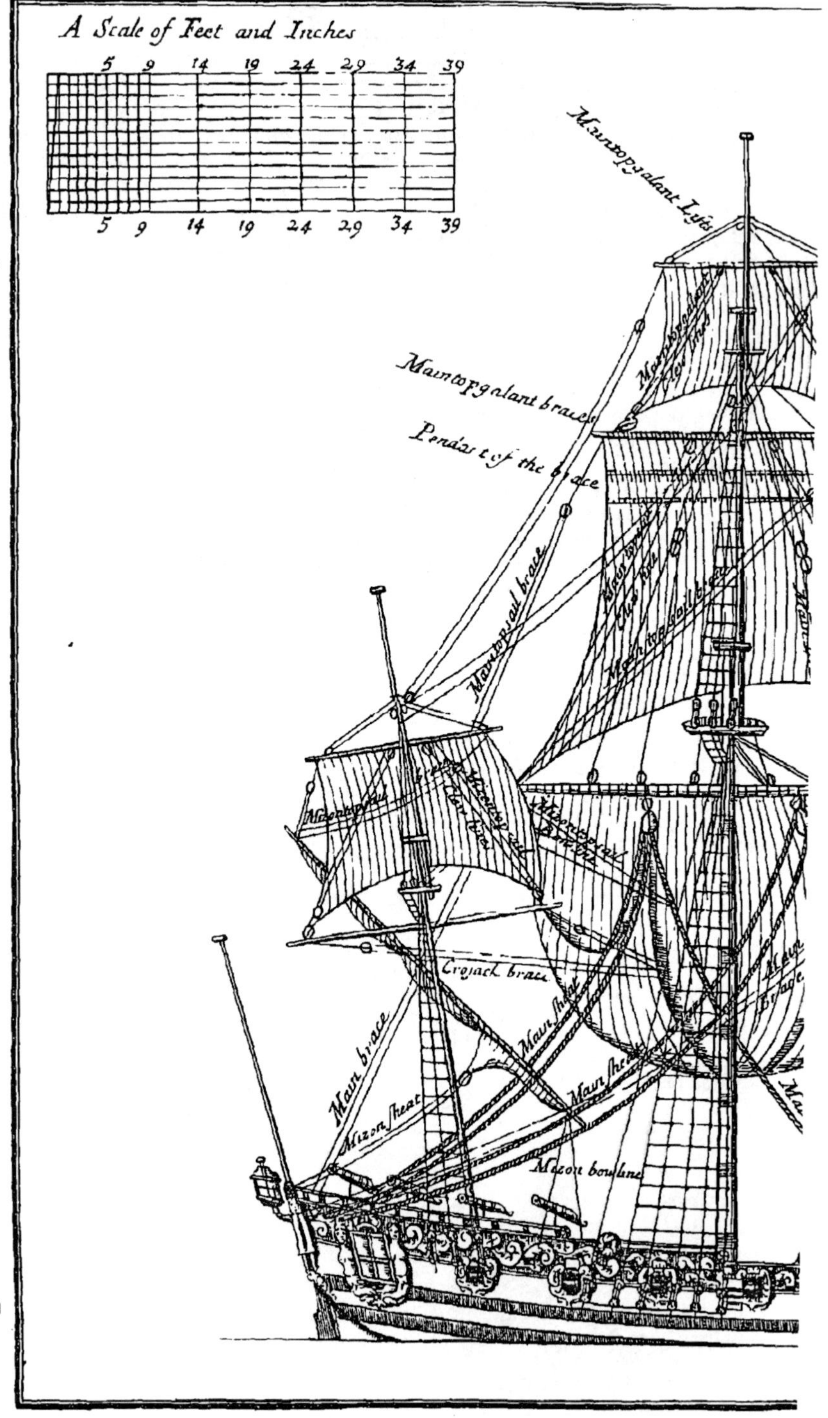

A Scale of Feet and Inches
5 9 14 19 24 29 34 39
5 9 14 19 24 29 34 39
Maintopgalant Lifts
Maintopgalant brace
Pendant of the brace
Maintopsail brace
Crojack brace
Main brace
Mizon sheat
Main sheat
Main sheat
Mizon bowline

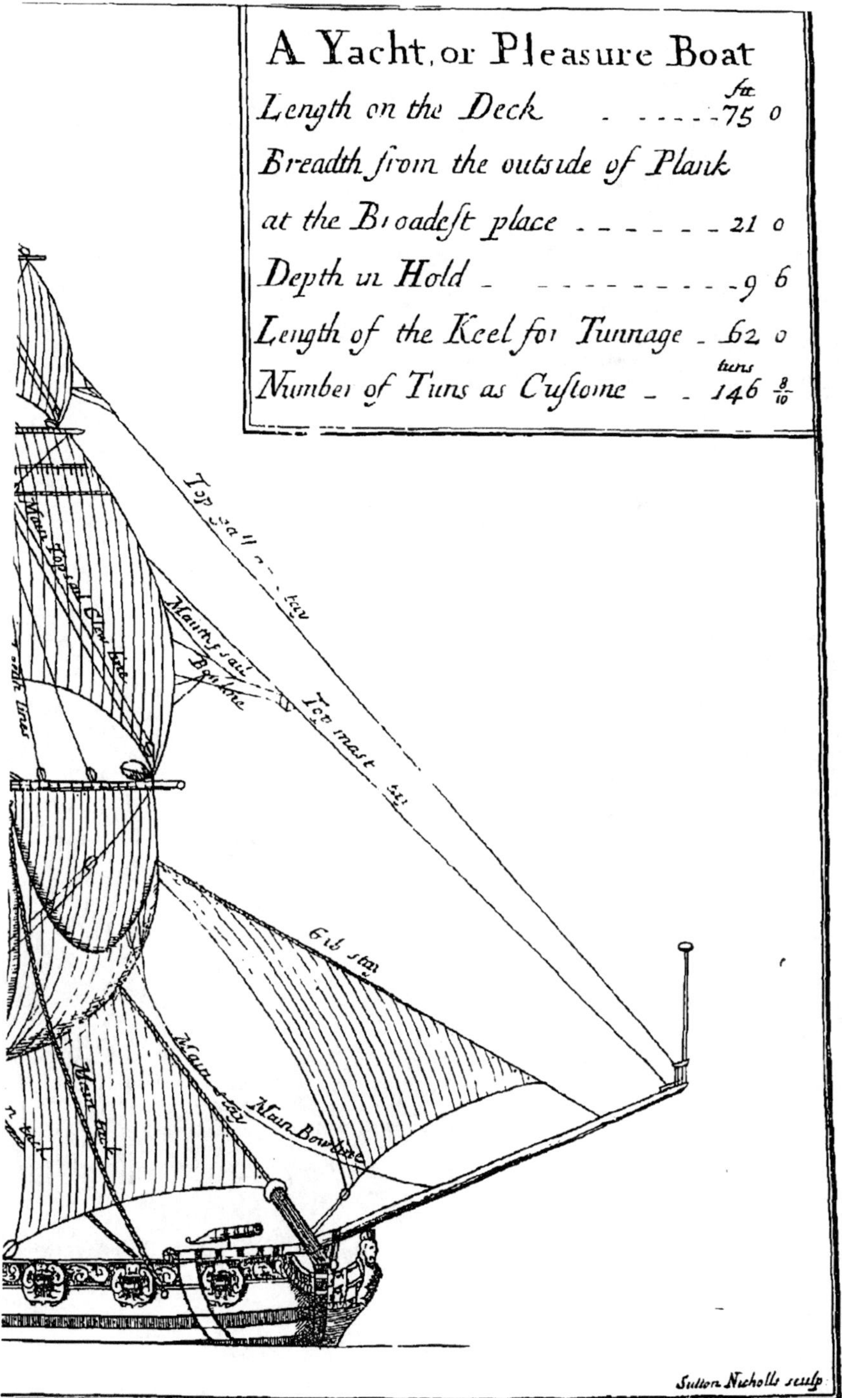
A Yacht, or Pleasure Boat
Length on the Deck - - - - - - ft. 75 0
Breadth from the outside of Plank
at the Broadest place - - - - - - - 21 0
Depth in Hold - - - - - - - - - - - 9 6
Length of the Keel for Tunnage - 62 0
Number of Tuns as Custome - - tuns 146 8/10
Top sail - - stay
Top mast stay
Main top sail Clew line
Maintopsail Bowline
Gib stay
Main stay
Main Bowline
Main Back
Sutton Nicholls sculp

And now I proceed to the Rigging that secures the Masts, which is call'd Stays and Shrouds, which ought to be plac'd in a circular Position, that the assistance may equally effect the Masts: For such Strings may be properly called doubling the Masts, and adding to their strength, which otherwise would not be sufficient to carry a Power suitable to the Resistance of such huge large Bodied Ships, which may help to make good my Parallel, drawn between a large Ship's Mast and a Boat's.

There's one Mr *Miller* of *North Yarmouth*, Mariner and Master, in the Art of raising the Model, as he stiles himself, says, *That a Mast of* 34 *Inches, has a Stay of* 17 *Inches and half, and Shrouds of* 8 *and half: As also a Mast of* 30 *Inches, a Stay of* 15 *Inches, and Shrouds of* 7 *and half, that is, the Circumference of the Rigging and Diameter of the Mast*

From which I shall draw the following Proportions.

Ship's Tunnage	Number of Shrouds	Length of each (*Yards*)	The whole Length of both Sides Multiplied by	is	Whole length (*Yards*)
1677	9	26	18		468
1488	9	24	18		433
969	8	22	16		396
625	7	19	14		351
364	7	16	14		288
225	6	14	12		252

Since the general Rule is to allow the Stay to be as long as the Mast and the Shroud, each to be ½ of the Mast, 468 Yards is the whole length of the Shrouds for the biggest Ship, and so on

Length of the Main-mast (*Yards*)	Diameter of the said Masts (*Inches*)	Circumference of the Shrouds (*Inches*)	Ditto of the Stay (*Inches*)
39	39	97	194
36 ½	36 ½	90	179
33 ½	30 ½	75	150
29	26	68	137
24	21 ½	53	105
21	16	40	79

Number of Fathoms in all the Shrouds
234
216 ½
198
175 ½
144
126

It being generally allowed that there is spun in length, in every Cable 106 Fathoms, and so very near of any other Rope

Then if 106 Fathoms weighs	C	q	l	Then one Fathom will weigh (l)
	20	1	12	21 ½
	17	3	7	19
	12	1	14	13
	10	0	0	10 ½
	6	0	20	6 ½
	3	3	0	4

If (l wt.)	Weight of 106 Fathom, one Fathom shall weigh (l)	Then (Fathom)	weighs (l)	Which is the Weight of all the Shrouds to the Main-mast
2280	21 ½	234	5031	
1995	19	216 ½	4113 5	
1386	13	198	2508	
1120	10 ½	175	1840	
692	6 ½	144	933	
420	4	126	504	

	Divided by 2240, or 1 Tun is	Tuns and the		or (l)	Which Fraction added to the Sum is (Tu)	C	qrs	l	The whole Weight of all the Shrouds
5031	2		[illegible]	537 ½	2	5	1	9 ½	
4113	1		[illegible]	1881 ½	2	18	2	24 ½	
2508	1		[illegible]	269	1	2	2	13	
1840	0		[illegible]	1881 ½	0	18	2	24 ½	
933	0		[illegible]	941	0	9	1	13	
504	0		[illegible]	495	0	4	3	11	

Circum-

Circumference of the Stay to the Main-mast (*Inches*)	Length in Fathoms is	The weight of 106 Fathom is	
194	19	8550	Pounds wt
179	18 $\frac{1}{2}$	7280	
150	13 $\frac{3}{4}$	5115	
137	14 $\frac{1}{2}$	4260	
105	12	2502	
79	10 $\frac{1}{2}$	1410	

Then if 106 Fathom weighs as aforemention'd, what shall 1 Fathom weigh? (*l*)		Then what shall the Number of Fathoms weigh? (*Fathoms*)		
80 [illegible]	The weight of one Fathom	19 $\frac{1}{2}$	will weigh	1569
68 $\frac{1}{2}$		18 $\frac{1}{4}$		1265
48		16 $\frac{3}{4}$		738
40		14 $\frac{1}{2}$		850
23 $\frac{3}{4}$		12		285
13 $\frac{1}{4}$		10 $\frac{1}{2}$		140

Pound weight of the Main-stay

Note, That all these Six Divisions refer to the Six several Tunnages as abovesaid, and so along successively.

Square of	is		Divided by 2240 is C	qrs	l	added to Tu	C	qrs	l
194	376 $\frac{36}{100}$	1569	15	2	13	2	5	1	9 $\frac{1}{2}$
179	320 $\frac{41}{100}$	1265	12	2	0	1	18	2	24 $\frac{1}{2}$
150	225	758	7	2	4	1	2	2	13
137	187 $\frac{69}{100}$	580	5	2	26	0	18	2	24
105	110 $\frac{25}{100}$	285	2	2	17	0	9	1	13
79	62 $\frac{41}{100}$	140	1	1	13	0	4	3	11

Both Sums is	*Tuns*	*C*	*qrs*	*l*
	3	0	3	22 $\frac{1}{2}$
	2	10	0	24
	1	9	0	17
	1	4	1	22
	0	12	0	10
	0	6	0	24

The whole Weight of all the Shrouds and Stay to the Main-mast

I now proceed to shew the Dimensions and Weight of the Main-mast

Diameter of the Mast (*Inches*)	Circumference	Area (*Inches*)	Or (*Feet*)
39	122 $\frac{1}{2}$	1189	8 [illegible]
36 $\frac{1}{2}$	113	1063	7 [illegible]
30 $\frac{1}{2}$	96	732	5 [illegible]
26 $\frac{1}{2}$	83 $\frac{1}{2}$	555	3 [illegible]
21	67 $\frac{1}{2}$	362	2 [illegible]
16	50 $\frac{26}{100}$	200	1 [illegible]

Multiply by the length in feet	is	Content of the Main-mast in feet × by 40 the Content of a Square-foot of Fir (*Pounds*)	*Tuns*	
117	9717	38868	17 [illegible]	Weight in tuns and parts
108 $\frac{1}{4}$	785	31400	14	
100 $\frac{1}{2}$	510	20400	9 [illegible]	
87	340	13600	6	
72	180	7200	3 [illegible]	
63	87 $\frac{1}{2}$	3500	1 [illegible]	

To compute the measure of the Main-mast as a long Parallelopipedon or Frustum of a Pyramid from end to end (*Inches*)	Area as so, or (*Feet*)	× by the length in feet is (*Feet*)	× by 40 is (*Pounds*)
1520	10 [illegible]	1233	49320
1335	9 [illegible]	990	39600
935	6 [illegible]	653	26120
703	4 [illegible]	426	17040
463	3 [illegible]	230	9200
256	1 [illegible]	110	4440

In

In Tuns is (*Tuns*)			In a Square or Frustum of a Pyramid
22	Weight of the Main-mast in a Square, or Frustum of a Pyramid	Cube Root of the Weight in a Round Position or Frustum of a Cone	
176		2 $\frac{58}{100}$	2 $\frac{8}{10}$
116		2 $\frac{45}{100}$	2 $\frac{0}{10}$
76		2 $\frac{09}{100}$	2 $\frac{27}{100}$
41		1 $\frac{82}{100}$	1 $\frac{95}{100}$
18		1 $\frac{41}{100}$	1 $\frac{8}{10}$
		1 $\frac{16}{100}$	1 $\frac{22}{100}$

Observing that the Circle to the Conscrib'd Square is as 11 to 14, the Area

And since a Mast that's cheek'd with Oak is heavier than if it was all Fir, (or as we term it) a Mast that heads it self, that instead of computing the Mast as the Frustum of a Cone, it ought to be computed as the Frustum of a Pyramid, or rather as a Parallelopipedon, according to the Area made by squaring the Diameter at the Partners, or biggest place, and that multiplied into the length. But for a Mast that heads it self, compute it as a perfect Cylinder, which will very nearly do, considering the Cap, Top, Cross and Tressle-trees, and Iron-work.

And from such Observations it will appear, that in all Shipping that has Masts cheek'd with Oak, the Rigging to each respective Mast will bear a Proportion as follows.

The weight of all the standing Rigging, as Stays and Shrouds, will be in direct Proportion to the weight of the Mast, as their respective Cube Roots are to its respective Cube · So that after you have computed the weight of your Mast, the Cube Root thereof will give the weight of the standing Rigging.

From which may arise a general method to size the weight of the Rigging from the magnitude of the Mast; that as Masts are, or ought to be, in direct Proportion to the magnitude of the Ship's Body or Burthen thereof, and every Mast suitable and agreeable to each other, according to the Bulk of the Ship's Body, where each Mast centers, so the Rigging according to such Proportion, ought to be sized to the Bulk of the Masts, Yards and Superficies of the Sail that drives the Body or Ship.

Next I shall consider the Area of the Sails or Power that drives the Log or Solid of the Ship's Body And since the Velocities are as the Square-roots of the Power, which either drives or draws the Body, that Quadruple Sail is requisite to double Swiftness, so that Ships ought to have (for that extraordinary faculty of Swiftness, and mighty advantage which may accrue from Nimbleness in Ships or Vessels, Bodies of either sort) as much Sail as they possibly can bear, with conveniency and security to the other parts and uses requisite, which in running Ships may be considered accordingly.

Tunnage		*Yards*	*Yards*		*Yards*	
1677	The length of the Ship on the upperDeck from the inside of the Stern-side Timber, to the Fore-side of the Figure of the Head	63	— 63	Length of all the Main-masts as they stand Rigg'd multiplied one into another is the Area of the Sail	3969	Area
1488		61	— 60		3660	
969		55	— 56		3080	
625		$47\frac{1}{2}$	— 48		2270	
364		39	— 37		1441	
225		35	— 35		1225	

Area of the Sails is one to another, as 1 is to the Numbers following,		Their Resistances is one to another as 1 is to the Numbers following,		Without considering nicely, the Angle of Incidence
	3 $\frac{22}{100}$		7 5	
	2 $\frac{98}{100}$		6 6	
	2 $\frac{15}{100}$		4 3	
	1 $\frac{85}{100}$		2 $\frac{74}{100}$	
	1 $\frac{18}{100}$		1 6	
	1		1	

The Proportion or Disproportion between the Power and the Resistance is as		to			So that instead of allowing the Number of Yards of Canvas to be as follows, to make every Ships Velocity equal,
3	[illegible]	to	7	5	3969
2	[illegible]		6	6	3660
2	[illegible]		4	3	3080
1	[illegible]		2	[illegible]	2270
1	[illegible]		1	6	1441
1			1		1225

The Number of Yards ought to be
9157
8100
5300
3360
1950
1225

From which it plainly appears, that the large Ships Sails are not in Proportion to their Resistance, without exactly considering the various Angles of Incidence and Reflection in their several Bodies, for then the Disproportion will be still larger, since great Ships are more obtuse, according to their Dimensions, than small Ships are.

Area of the Sail allowed according to the Length and Breadth as aforesaid, Yards	Required to make the Velocity equal Yards	Difference or want Yards
3969	9157	5188
3600	8100	4440
3080	5300	2220
2270	3360	1090
1441	1950	509
1225	1225	

So that to make the Velocity of all these several Sizes equal to the Resistance of each respective Ship, (provided that the Angulation and Gravitating was Similar, according to the Bulk of each Ships Body) there ought to be an Additional Quantity of Canvas, or some other matter, in Equilibro to the Resistance, which ought to be made out in either Length, Breadth, or Thickness, but Thickness would be most agreeable to the use.

The Main Sail will be [illegible] of the whole Area of Canvas required for all the Sails, Fore Sail [illegible] of the Main Sail, Maintop Sail [illegible] of the Main Sail, Foretop Sail [illegible] of the Fore Sail, Top gallant Sails [illegible] of the Top Sails, Mizon [illegible] of the Main Sail, Mizon top Sail to the Main top gallant Sail, as 11 to 9, Sprit-sail [illegible] the Fore-sail, Sprit-sail Top-sail [illegible] the Sprit-sail, Studing-sails together [illegible] of their respective Sails, flying Gib as big as the Sprit-sail top-sail, Foretop-sail stay sail [illegible] of the Foretop-gallant-sail, Main-stay-sail [illegible] of the Main-sail, Maintop-sail-stay sail [illegible] of the Maintop-gallant-sail, Mizon-stay-sail [illegible] of the Main-stay-sail, Mizon-top-sail-stay-sail [illegible] of the Mizon-stay-sail. And now I proceed to demonstrate the shape.

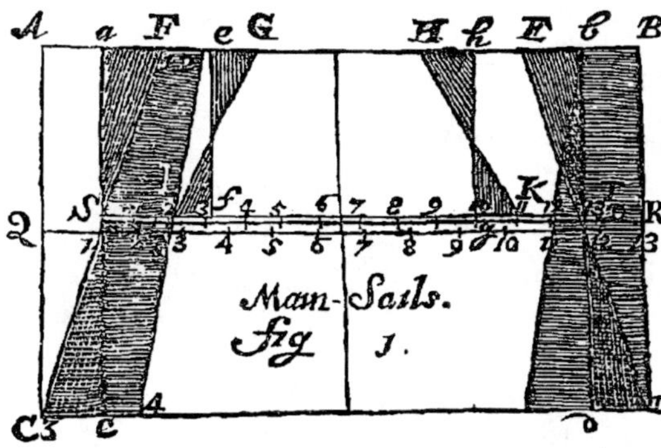

Figure 1. A B C. D. is the Area of the Main-sail, D C F E is the Maintop-sail, which Figure is the Face of a Frustum of a square Pyramid, a.b.c d. is the superficial Area of the Maintop-sail, in square Cloths, considered as a Parallelogram, as the Main sail is such, but the Top sails are cut taper, and the Angle E b o is equal to the Angle D d o. G. H I.K. is the Maintop-gallant-sail, and e f. g h the Maintop-gallant sail in square Cloth. 1 2 3. 4. the Main top sail Studing sail, which is also the face of a Frustum of a square Pyramid, and is divided by the Line S T being the middle of the Maintop sail, and dividing that Line into 13 equal parts, two of them parts is the bigness of the Studing-sail, the Main-studing-sail is divided after the same manner on the Line Q. R. which is the breadth of the Main-sail, e h. f g. is the square Cloth that will make the Top-gallant-sail, but the Sail in its perfect shape is a Frustum of a Pyramid, and after such a manner may the Fore-sails be demonstrated and cut, with having a due respect to the Length of each Yard, and the Hoist of the Sail

Figure 2

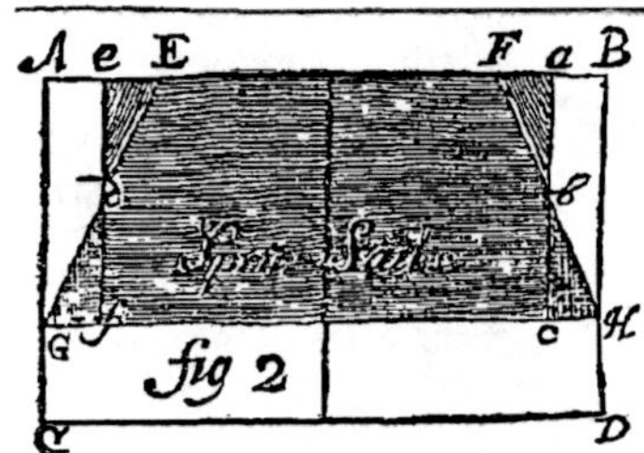

Figure 2 The next is the Figure of the Sprit-ſail, A. B C D being the ſuperficies of the Sprit-ſail, and E. F G. H. the ſuperficies of the Sprit-ſail-top ſail, which is cut as the Topgallant ſails

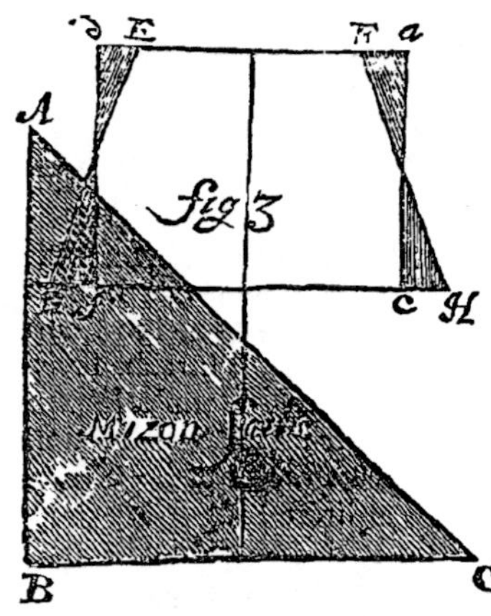

Figure 3 Next I deſcribe the Figure of the Mizon, and Mizontop-ſail. The Mizon is a direct Rectangled Triangle: The Hypotenuſe is deſcribed by the Mizon Yard A. C. That this Sail is half a Parallelogram, which is equal to the Baſe, B. C. and A. B the Perpendicular, multiplied one into the other.

And by ſuch a Conſideration is every Stay-ſail cut, and the Proportion that the Baſe and Perpendicular will bear to each other, may be found by the Proportion of the length of the Stay, and the diſtance that one Stay is off from the other: Alſo to obſerve the conveniency of ſetting the Sail, and haleing the Sheet aft, which in my Opinion cannot be better obtain'd, than by drawing Figures of the Ship you deſign to Rig, as is done in my *Ship-Builders Aſſiſtant*

The Mizon top-ſails are cut after the ſame manner as the other Top-ſails are cut, with having reſpect to the length and difference of the Yards, alſo the length of the Hoiſt of the Sail.

Main-ſails Hoiſt to the ſquare of the Yard is as 4 to 7.
Fore-ſails is as 8 to 13.
Maintopſails Hoiſt to the length of the Topſail-yard is as 18 is to 17
Foretopſail is ditto
Maintopgallant-ſails Hoiſt to the ſaid yard is as 26 to 25.
Foretopgallant-yard is ditto
Mizontopſail-yards length is to the Hoiſt as 6 to 7
Spritſail-yards length to the Hoiſt is as 5 to 3.
Topſail-yard of ditto length to Hoiſt is as 11 is to 9.
For the Main and Fore yard Arms, take out the [illegible] of the length of the Yard for the length of both Arms.
For the Mizon-yard ditto.
For the Topſail-yards, Main and Fore, take the [illegible] of the Yards length for both Yard Arms, obſerving that for as many Reefs above one, as there is to be in the Topſail, add ſo many times [illegible] of the length of your Yard extraordinary for that conveniency Spritſail yard Arms [illegible] of the Yard, Topgallant-yard-Arms, Mizontopſail, Spritſail-topſail and Croſs-jack the ſame.

As to the running Rigging which is uſed to traverſe the Sails, that ought to be conſider'd as Tackles and Pulleys, and proportion'd from the Maſts and variety of Uſes, ſo that in the next Place ſhall be conſider'd the Guns or Weight of Metal

From

From Obfervation its found, that a Ship of near 1000 Tuns, carries 70 Guns containing in Weight 104 Tuns, being 26 of 25 *C.* in the Medium, and 26 of 46 *C* and 14 of about 15 *C.* and 4 of 7 *C.*

A Ship of near 600 Tuns carrying 50 Guns, containing 64 *Tuns* $\frac{1}{2}$ *C.*

Tuns		*Tuns*	*Number*		*Tuns*	*Tuns*		
1677	Divide by 95 is	177 $\frac{4}{10}$	100	Then if 969 gives 104 *Tuns* what fhall	1677	170 $\frac{4}{10}$	100	N° of Guns
1488		157	90		1488	150	90	
969		102	70		969	104	70	
625		65 $\frac{7}{10}$	50	And if 625 give 64 *Tuns*, what fhall	625	64	50	
364		38 $\frac{3}{10}$	34		364	37 [illegible]	34	
225		23 $\frac{7}{10}$	24		225	23	24	

It has been lately allowed as a general Rule, that the biggeft of our Ships fhall carry 100 Guns, and called a Firft Rate, the next being a Second Rate of 90 Guns, however the Difproportion of thefe two Rates is far larger than they ought to be, fince one has near as much Accommodation as the other in every refpect: The next is call'd a Third Rate of 70 Guns, the next a 50 Gun Fourth Rate, next a 34 Gun Fifth Rate, next a 24 Gun Sixth Rate. There be feveral other Men of War, which are different in degrees, and may be term'd Intermedium Bodies; as Third Rates of 80 Guns, having three Decks, and Fourth Rates of 60 Guns, and Fifth Rates of 40 Guns, and therefore in fuch Cafes, all the Utenfils, and Equipping, ought to be fiz'd from a direct Proportion drawn from the Magnitude of each Ship's Body.

The fix that are here mentioned may properly be look'd on as an ancient Standard in the Navy, being in the general (excepting a Fifth Rate) as properly fixed as any Ships can well be, for the Ufes incident to them; but as to their Shapes, and other Additaments, which may be applied to them, to make them more fafe and ufeful, will take up far larger Confiderations, or will take up more Time than what at prefent can be allowed for doing the fame, only minding, that dividing any Ship's Tunnage by 9 $\frac{1}{10}$ will give the Weight of Metal of their Guns, fuitable to the magnitude of the Ship.

Next I fhall confider the Weight of the Anchors, that is, the Weight of them together, or in part; but firft fhall fet down the Dimenfions of the Anchors according to Cuftom, belonging to a Ship near 600 Tuns.

	C	*q.s*	*l*	
Sheet-Anchor	32	2	0	Weight of them altogether is 132 *C* 2 *q.s* 14 *l.*
Beft Bower	31	1	0	
Small Bower	25	3	0	
Spare-Anchor	31	3	14	
Stream ditto	8	0	0	
Kedg ditto	3	1	0	

Ship's Tunnage		*Tuns*		*C*				*C*	
1677	Divide by 94	17 $\frac{9}{10}$	or	358	Then Divide the Weight of all the Anchors by	41	it's	87	Which will be the Weight of the biggeft Anchor
1488		15 $\frac{8}{10}$		318		42		76	
969		10 $\frac{3}{10}$		206		41		50	
625		6 $\frac{6}{10}$		132		41		32	
364		3 $\frac{9}{10}$		78		41		18 $\frac{9}{10}$	
225		2 $\frac{4}{10}$		48		41		11 $\frac{7}{10}$	

However I fhall confider it farther, according to the fize of the Cable generally allowed to each Rate.

Hundreds

In Tuns is (Tuns)			
22	Weight of the Main-maſt in a Square, or Fruſtum of a Pyramid	Cube Root of the Weight in a Round Poſition or Fruſtum of a Cone	2 $\frac{58}{100}$
176			2 $\frac{45}{100}$
116			2 $\frac{9}{100}$
76			1 $\frac{81}{100}$
41			1 $\frac{47}{100}$
18			1 $\frac{16}{100}$

In a Square or Fruſtum of a Pyramid
2 $\frac{8}{10}$
2 [illegible]
2 $\frac{32}{100}$
1 $\frac{95}{100}$
1 [illegible]
1 $\frac{32}{100}$

Obſerving that the Circle to the Conſcrib'd Square is as 11 to 14, the Area

And ſince a Maſt that's cheek'd with Oak is heavier than if it was all Fir, (or as we term it) a Maſt that heads it ſelf, that inſtead of computing the Maſt as the Fruſtum of a Cone, it ought to be computed as the Fruſtum of a Pyramid, or rather as a Parallelopipedon, according to the Area made by ſquaring the Diameter at the Partners, or biggeſt place, and that multiplied into the length: But for a Maſt that heads it ſelf, compute it as a perfect Cylinder, which will very nearly do, conſidering the Cap, Top, Croſs and Treſle-trees, and Iron-work.

And from ſuch Obſervations it will appear, that in all Shipping that has Maſts cheek'd with Oak, the Rigging to each reſpective Maſt will bear a Proportion as follows.

The weight of all the ſtanding Rigging, as Stays and Shrouds, will be in direct Proportion to the weight of the Maſt, as their reſpective Cube Roots are to its reſpective Cube: So that after you have computed the weight of your Maſt, the Cube Root thereof will give the weight of the ſtanding Rigging.

From which may ariſe a general method to ſize the weight of the Rigging from the magnitude of the Maſt; that as Maſts are, or ought to be, in direct Proportion to the magnitude of the Ship's Body or Burthen thereof, and every Maſt ſuitable and agreeable to each other, according to the Bulk of the Ship's Body, where each Maſt centers; ſo the Rigging according to ſuch Proportion, ought to be ſized to the Bulk of the Maſts, Yards and Superficies of the Sail that drives the Body or Ship.

Next I ſhall conſider the Area of the Sails of Power that drives the Log or Solid of the Ship's Body: And ſince the Velocities are as the Square-roots of the Power, which either drives or draws the Body, that Quadruple Sail is requiſite to double Swiftneſs; ſo that Ships ought to have (for that extraordinary faculty of Swiftneſs, and mighty advantage which may accrue from Nimbleneſs in Ships or Veſſels, Bodies of either ſort) as much Sail as they poſſibly can bear, with conveniency and ſecurity to the other parts and uſes requiſite, which in running Ships may be conſidered accordingly.

Tunnage		Yards	Yards		Yards	
1677	The length of the Ship on the upperDeck from the inſide of the Stern-ſide Timber, to the Fore-ſide of the Figure of the Head	63	— 63	Length of all the Main-maſts as they ſtand Rigg'd multiplied one into another is the Area of the Sail	3969	Area
1488		61	— 60		3660	
969		55	— 56		3080	
625		47½	— 48		2270	
364		39	— 37		1441	
225		35	— 35		1225	

Area of the Sails is one to another, as 1 is to the Numbers following,		Their Reſiſtances is one to another as 1 is to the Numbers following,			Without conſidering nicely, the Angle of Incidence.
	3 $\frac{31}{100}$		7	5	
	2 $\frac{98}{100}$		6	6	
	2 $\frac{50}{100}$		4	3	
	1 $\frac{85}{100}$		2	$\frac{74}{100}$	
	1 $\frac{38}{100}$		1	6	
	1		1		

K	The

The Proportion or Disproportion between the Power and the Resistance is as		is to		So that instead of allowing the Number of Yards of Canvas to be as follows, to make every Ships Velocity equal,
	3 [illegible]		7 5	3969
	2 [illegible]		6 6	3660
	2 [illegible]		4 3	3080
	1 [illegible]		2 [illegible]	2270
	1 [illegible]		1 6	1441
	1		1	1225

The Number of Yards ought to be
9157
8100
5300
3360
1950
1225

From which it plainly appears, that the large Ships Sails are not in Proportion to their Resistance, without exactly considering the various Angles of Incidence and Reflection in their several Bodies for then the Disproportion will be still larger, since great shipping are more obtuse, according to their Dimensions, than small Ships are

Area of the Sail allowed according to the Length and Breadth as aforesaid,	Yards	Required to make the Velocity equal	Yards	Difference or want	Yards
	3969		9157		5188
	3660		8100		4440
	3080		5300		2220
	2270		3360		1090
	1441		1950		509
	1225		1225		

So that to make the Velocity of all these several Sizes equal to the Resistance of each respective Ship, (provided that the Angulation and Gravitating was Similar, according to the Bulk of each Ships Body) there ought to be an Additional Quantity of Canvas, or some other matter, in Equilibro to the Resistance, which ought to be made out in either Length, Breadth, or Thickness; but Thickness would be most agreeable to the use.

The Main Sail will be [illegible] of the whole Area of Canvas required for all the Sails, Fore Sail [illegible] of the Main Sail, Maintop Sail [illegible] of the Main Sail, Foretop Sail [illegible] of the Fore Sail, Top gallant Sails [illegible] of the Top Sails, Mizon [illegible] of the Main Sail, Mizon top Sail to the Main top gallant Sail, as 11 to 9, Sprit-sail [illegible] the Fore-sail, Sprit-sail Top-sail [illegible] the Sprit-sail, Studing-sails together [illegible] of their respective Sails; flying Gib as big as the Sprit-sail top-sail, Foretop-sail-stay sail [illegible] of the Foretop-gallant-sail, Main-stay-sail [illegible] of the Main-sail, Maintop-sail-stay-sail [illegible] of the Maintop-gallant-sail, Mizon-stay-sail [illegible] of the Main-stay-sail, Mizontop-sail-stay-sail [illegible] of the Mizon-stay-sail. And now I proceed to demonstrate the shape.

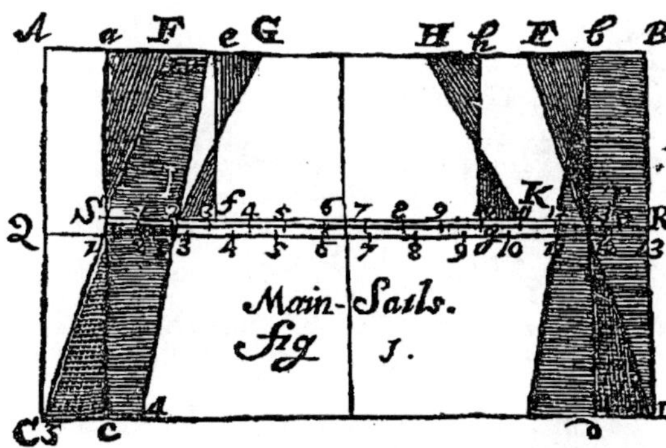

Figure 1 A. B. C. D. is the Area of the Main-sail, D C F E. is the Maintop-sail, which Figure is the Face of a Frustum of a square Pyramid, a.b.c.d. is the superficial Area of the Maintop-sail, in square Cloths, considered as a Parallelogram, as the Main sail is such, but the Top sails are cut taper, and the Angle E. b o is equal to the Angle D d o. G. H. I. K. is the Maintop-gallant-sail, and e. f. g h the Maintop-gallant-sail in square Cloth. 1 2 3. 4. the Main-top sail Studing-sail, which is also the face of a Frustum of a square Pyramid, and is divided by the Line S T. being the middle of the Maintop sail, and dividing that Line into 13 equal parts, two of them parts is the bigness of the Studing-sail; the Main-studing-sail is divided after the same manner on the Line Q. R. which is the breadth of the Main-sail; e h. f. g. is the square Cloth that will make the Top-gallant-sail, but the Sail in its perfect shape is a Frustum of a Pyramid; and after such a manner may the Fore-sails be demonstrated and cut, with having a due respect to the Length of each Yard, and the Hoist of the Sail.

Figure 2.

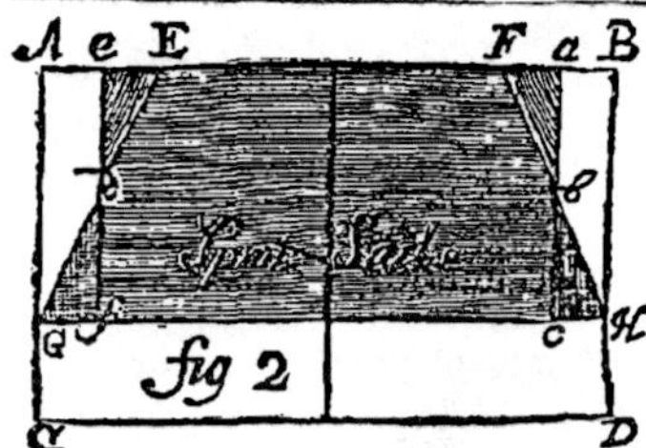

Figure 2 The next is the Figure of the Sprit-sail, A. B. C D. being the superficies of the Sprit-sail, and E. F G. H. the superficies of the Sprit-sail-top sail, which is cut as the Topgallant-sails

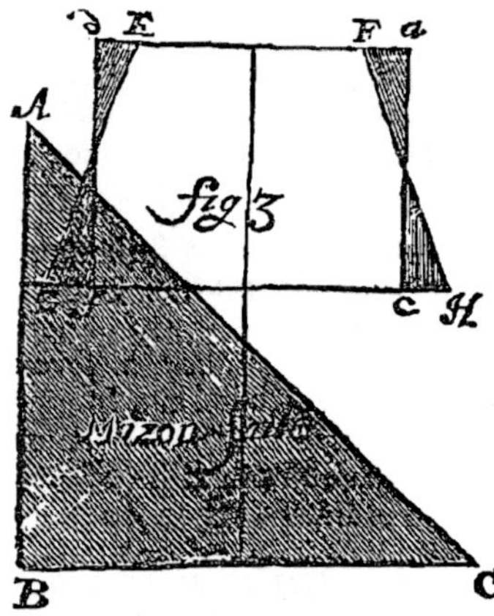

Figure 3. Next I describe the Figure of the Mizon, and Mizontop-sail The Mizon is a direct Rectangled Triangle: The Hypotenuse is described by the Mizon Yard A. C. That this Sail is half a Parallelogram, which is equal to the Base, B. C. and A. B the Perpendicular, multiplied one into the other.

And by such a Consideration is every Stay-sail cut; and the Proportion that the Base and Perpendicular will bear to each other, may be found by the Proportion of the length of the Stay, and the distance that one Stay is off from the other: Also to observe the conveniency of setting the Sail, and haleing the Sheet aft; which in my Opinion cannot be better obtain'd, than by drawing Figures of the Ship you design to Rig, as is done in my *Ship-Builders Assistant*.

The Mizon top-sails are cut after the same manner as the other Top-sails are cut, with having respect to the length and difference of the Yards, also the length of the Hoist of the Sail.

Main-sails Hoist to the square of the Yard is as 4 to 7.
Fore-sails is as 8 to 13.
Maintopsails Hoist to the length of the Topsail-yard is as 18 is to 17
Foretopsail is ditto
Maintopgallant-sails Hoist to the said yard is as 26 to 25.
Foretopgallant-yard is ditto.
Mizontopsail-yards length is to the Hoist as 6 to 7.
Spritsail-yards length to the Hoist is as 5 to 3.
Topsail-yard of ditto length to Hoist is as 11 is to 9
For the Main and Fore-yard Arms, take out the $\frac{1}{2}$ of the length of the Yard for the length of both Arms.
For the Mizon-yard ditto.
For the Topsail-yards, Main and Fore, take the $\frac{1}{2}$ of the Yards length for both Yard Arms, observing that for as many Reefs above one, as there is to be in the Topsail, add so many times $\frac{1}{2}$' of the length of your Yard extraordinary for that conveniency. Spritsail yard Arms $\frac{1}{2}$ of the Yard, Topgallant-yard-Arms, Mizontopsail, Spritsail-topsail and Cross-jack the same.

As to the running Rigging which is used to traverse the Sails, that ought to be consider'd as Tackles and Pulleys, and proportion'd from the Masts and variety of Uses, so that in the next Place shall be consider'd the Guns or Weight of Metal.

From

From Obſervation its found, that a Ship of near 1000 Tuns, carries 70 Guns containing in Weight 104 Tuns, being 26 of 25 *C* in the Medium, and 26 of 46 *C.* and 14 of about 15 *C.* and 4 of 7 *C.*

A Ship of near 600 Tuns carrying 50 Guns, containing 64 *Tuns* ÷ *C.*

Tuns	Divide by 95 is	*Tuns*	*Number*		*Tuns*	*Tuns*	N° of Guns
1677		177 6/10	100	Then if 969	1677	170 4/10	100
1488		157	90	gives 104 *Tuns*	1488	150	90
969		102	70	what ſhall	969	104	70
625		65 7/10	50	And if 625 give	625	64	50
364		38 3/10	34	64 *Tuns*, what	364	37 1/10	34
225		23 7/10	24	ſhall	225	23	24

It has been lately allowed as a general Rule, that the biggeſt of our Ships ſhall carry 100 Guns, and called a Firſt Rate, the next being a Second Rate of 90 Guns, however the Diſproportion of theſe two Rates is far larger than they ought to be, ſince one has near as much Accommodation as the other in every reſpect. The next is call'd a Third Rate of 70 Guns, the next a 50 Gun Fourth Rate, next a 34 Gun Fifth Rate, next a 24 Gun Sixth Rate There be ſeveral other Men of War, which are different in degrees, and may be term'd Intermedium Bodies; as Third Rates of 80 Guns, having three Decks, and Fourth Rates of 60 Guns, and Fifth Rates of 40 Guns; and therefore in ſuch Caſes, all the Utenſils, and Equipping, ought to be ſiz'd from a direct Proportion drawn from the Magnitude of each Ship's Body.

The ſix that are here mentioned may properly be look'd on as an ancient Standard in the Navy, being in the general (excepting a Fifth Rate) as properly ſized as any Ships can well be, for the Uſes incident to them; but as to their Shapes, and other Additaments, which may be applied to them, to make them more ſafe and uſeful, will take up far larger Conſiderations, or will take up more Time than what at preſent can be allowed for doing the ſame, only minding, that dividing any Ship's Tunnage by 9 5/10 will give the Weight of Metal of their Guns, ſuitable to the magnitude of the Ship.

Next I ſhall conſider the Weight of the Anchors, that is, the Weight of them together, or in part, but firſt ſhall ſet down the Dimenſions of the Anchors according to Cuſtom, belonging to a Ship near 600 Tuns

	C	*qrs*	*l*	
Sheet-Anchor —	32	2	0	Weight of them altogether is 132 *C* 2 *qrs* 14 *l*
Beſt Bower —	31	1	0	
Small Bower —	25	3	0	
Spare-Anchor —	31	3	14	
Stream ditto —	8	0	0	
Kedg ditto —	3	1	0	

Ship's Tunnage	Divide by 94	*Tuns*	or	*C*	Then Divide the Weight of all the Anchors by		it's	*C*	Which will be the Weight of the biggeſt Anchor
1677		17 9/10		358		41		87	
1488		15 8/10		318		42		76	
969		10 3/10		206		41		50	
625		6 6/10		132		41		32	
364		3 9/10		78		41		18 1/10	
225		2 4/10		48		41		11 7/10	

However I ſhall conſider it farther, according to the ſize of the Cable generally allowed to each Rate.

Hundreds

Hundreds: Anch.	Turn	Inch.
87	1677	32 [illegible]
76	1488	30 [illegible]
50	969	24 $\frac{9}{10}$
32	625	19 $\frac{8}{10}$
18 $\frac{2}{10}$	364	15 $\frac{1}{10}$
11 $\frac{7}{10}$	225	12

The Size of a Cable suitable for a Ship capable to carry a Main-mast of 16 Inches Diameter is 12 Inch Circumference, and an Anchor of 11 C weight

But since the Cables and Anchors ought to be sized from the Resistance of the Ship, and Wind loft, I shall go on accordingly.

The Square of 12 is 144 × by { 7 5 · 6 6 · 4 3 · 2 [illegible] · 1 6 } is { 1080 · 950 · 620 · 394 · 226 } Square Root of which is { Inches: 32 8 · 30 4 · 24 9 · 19 8 · 15 1 }

For since a 12 Inch Cable is sufficient for a Ship of 225 Tuns, square and × that by the Proportion of Resistance of one Ship to another, the Square Root of that Number shall be the size of the Cable, equal to the Resistance of a Body, provided the Cables are strong in Arithmetical Proportion, but since Timber is strong according to the Root of the Doubling, it may be also expected in Cables.

So that if a Cable be augmented in bigness as 4 to 1, it will be strong as 4 to 1. Four times 144 being 576, the Square Root thereof is 24.

Cables Augmented as 4 to 1, will be strong as 4 to 1 Then if 75 gives 24 what shall { 7 5 · 6 6 · 4 3 · 2 $\frac{74}{100}$ · 1 6 } is { 24 · 22 $\frac{3}{10}$ · 18 2 · 14 · 11 $\frac{1}{10}$ } Then if 12 gives 12 what shall { 7 5 · 6 6 · 4 3 · 2 $\frac{74}{100}$ · 1 6 } gives { 30 · 28 $\frac{2}{10}$ · 22 $\frac{1}{10}$ · 18 $\frac{1}{10}$ · 13 $\frac{9}{10}$ }

Add the Products of 24 and 30, and 22 $\frac{3}{10}$ and 28 $\frac{2}{10}$, and 18 $\frac{2}{10}$ and 22 $\frac{1}{10}$ together { 54 · 50 $\frac{5}{10}$ · 40 $\frac{9}{10}$ · 32 $\frac{1}{10}$ · 25 } Half that is { 27 · 25 $\frac{5}{100}$ · 20 $\frac{45}{100}$ · 16 $\frac{5}{100}$ · 12 $\frac{5}{10}$ }

But since the strength is according to the Root of the Doubling, and that a 1st Rate to a 6th is near as 8 to 1, but the Windloft is near as 12 to 1, it may be allowed, that such a great Ship requires a Cable 10 times as strong as the small Ship

If 7.5 gives 12, what shall { 7 5 · 6 6 · 4 3 · 2 $\frac{74}{100}$ · 1 6 · 0 } it gives { 12 · 10 $\frac{11}{20}$ · 6 9 · 4 4 · 2 $\frac{53}{100}$ · 0 } The Square Root of which is { 3 $\frac{46}{100}$ · 3 $\frac{24}{100}$ · 2 $\frac{65}{100}$ · 2 1 · 1 $\frac{66}{100}$ · 0 } Which × into 144 the Square of the Circumference of the small Ships Cable 12, its { 500 · 466 · 382 · 302 · 235 · 144 }

The Square Root of the last Product shall be the size of the Cable { Inches: 500—22 $\frac{7}{10}$ · 466—21 $\frac{6}{10}$ · 382—19 · 302—17 $\frac{4}{10}$ · 235—15 $\frac{9}{10}$ · 144—12 } The Circumference of the Cables to each Rate in Inches and Tenths

And from the Sizes of Cables may be drawn the Size of the Anchors.

{ 22 $\frac{7}{10}$ · 21 $\frac{6}{10}$ · 19 · 17 $\frac{4}{10}$ · 15 $\frac{9}{10}$ · 12 } Size of the Cable, Square Root thereof is { 4 $\frac{71}{100}$ · 4 $\frac{62}{100}$ · 4 5 · 4 $\frac{20}{100}$ · 3 9 · 3 $\frac{41}{100}$ } The first Size of the Cables is as was aforesaid { Inches: 32 8 · 30 4 · 24 9 · 19 8 · 15 1 · 12 0 } Square Root of which is { 5 $\frac{71}{100}$ · 5 $\frac{51}{100}$ · 5 0 · 4 $\frac{46}{100}$ · 3 $\frac{8}{100}$ · 3 $\frac{43}{100}$ }

Then

Then as the Root 4 ÷ is to the Root 5 ÷ so is all the other

C		C
87		71
76		64
50	to	45
32		30
18 9		18 8
1 7		11 7

That the Weight of the biggest Anchor is very nearly proportioned from the Tunnage of the Ship That for every Hundred Tun any Ship Measures may be allowed 5 C for the Weight of the biggest Anchor

And consequently a Cable of the several Sizes mentioned, must have Anchors of the several Sizes following

Inches		C		Tunnage
22 3	Size of Cables in Inches and parts	71	Weight of the Anchors from the several Sizes of the biggest Cable	1677
21 7		64		1488
20 1		45		969
17 7		30		625
15 4		18		364
12 0		11		225

In the last place may be considered, from the preceeding Observations, what Number of Men will mannage all the said Uses, in every respect.

It is very observable, that in the Merchant's Service, where they carry no more Cats than can catch Mice, that 14 Men will very well manage a Ship of 100 Tuns, and to perform the hardest Service in her, which is to heave up the Anchor, and as it's term'd, to bring the Ship to sail; but then their Equipping is not so Bulky, as the Equipping is generally on Board of Men of War.

From the Observation of the Merchant Ships say, if 14 Men will manage 100 Tuns, what will the Tunnage as follows?

Tuns		
225	—	32
364	—	51
625	—	88
969	—	137
1488	—	208
1677	—	238

Men that will be required to manage them

However its observ'd that the Fireships has 50 Men allowed, and all little enough to act and do the Uses requisite at sundry times.

Notwithstanding 40 very good Men would make a shift to do the Services required on Board of such a Ship, which is near 250 Tuns

So that if 250 requires 40, what shall

Tuns		Men
225	Require, and it will be	36
364		58
625		100
969		155
1488		239
1677		269

Now for the Guns which on Board a Sixth Rate is 24, and will require 60 Men to manage them well

Weight of Metal		Men
23 [illegible]	—	60
38 1/10	—	97
65 7/10	—	157
102	—	258
157	—	398
177	—	447

That the Number of Men which will be required to manage the Guns, Sails, Anchors, and all other Services (provided that they were all required to be managed together) in Ships of the several Magnitudes, as follows

Tuns		Men requisite
1677	—	716
1488	—	637
969	—	413
625	—	257
364	—	155
225	—	96

Next I shall proceed to lay down the particular Dimensions of Masts and Yards.

For the Area												
7 22	So is	39	to	121	Then half	39	its	19½	Then half	121	its	60½
7 22		36½		115		36½		18¼		115		57½
7 22		30½		96		30½		15¼		96		48
7 22		26½		82		26		13		82		41
7 22		21¼		67		21½		10¾		67		33½
7 22		16		50		16		8		50		[illegible]

Mul-

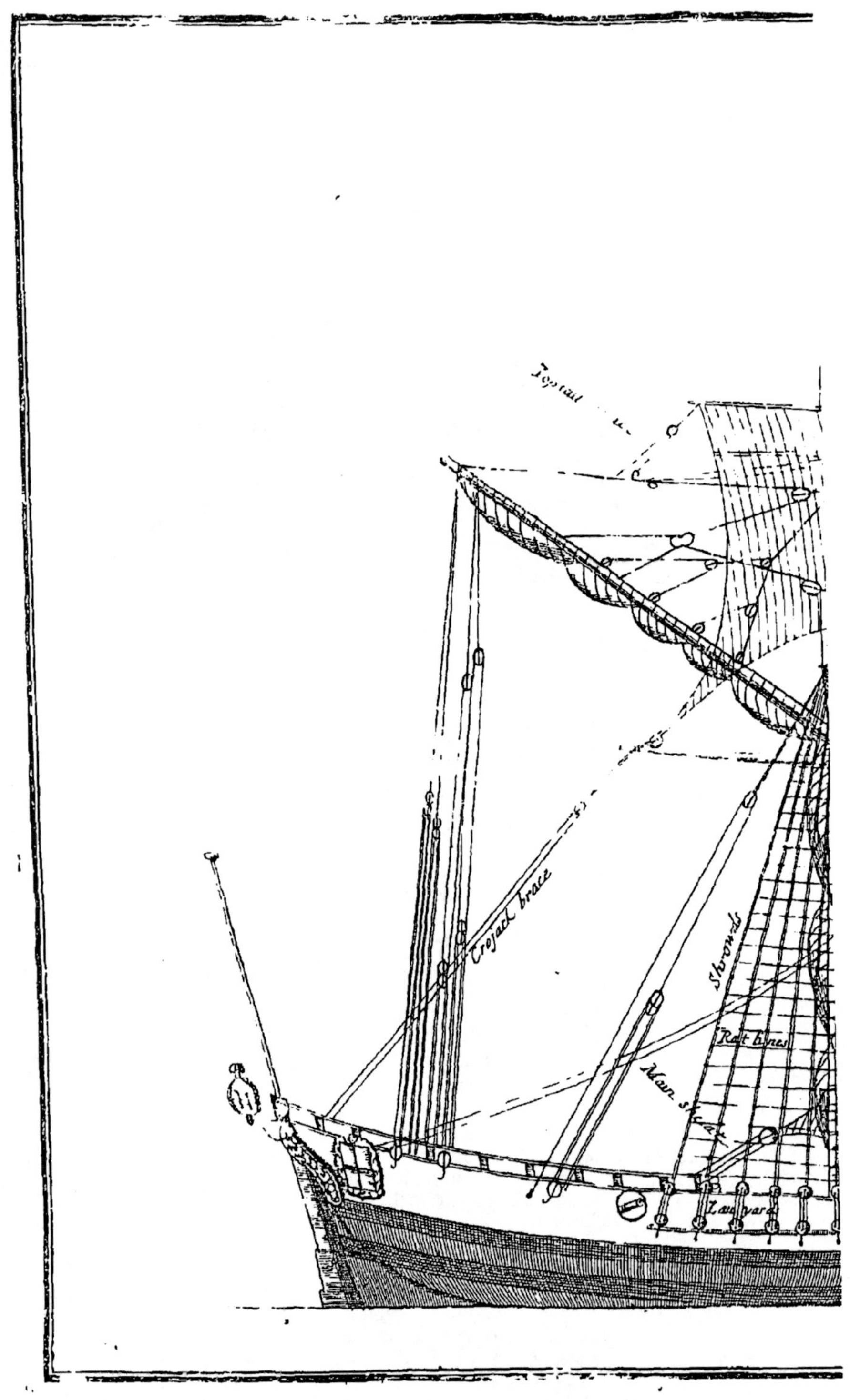
Crojack brace
Shrowds
Rat lines
Laniyards

A Hoy for Burden, *Drawn by the same Scale of the Yacht*

	ft	
Length on the Deck - - - - - - - - - - - -	79	0
Breadth from the outside of the Plank at the Broadest place - - - - - - - - - - - -	21	0
Depth in Hold - - - - - - - - - - - -	11	0
Length of the Keal for Tunnage - - - - -	65	0
	tuns	
Numb. of Tuns as Custome - - - - - - -	153	$\frac{9}{10}$

and may be made to Carry neer Twice as much

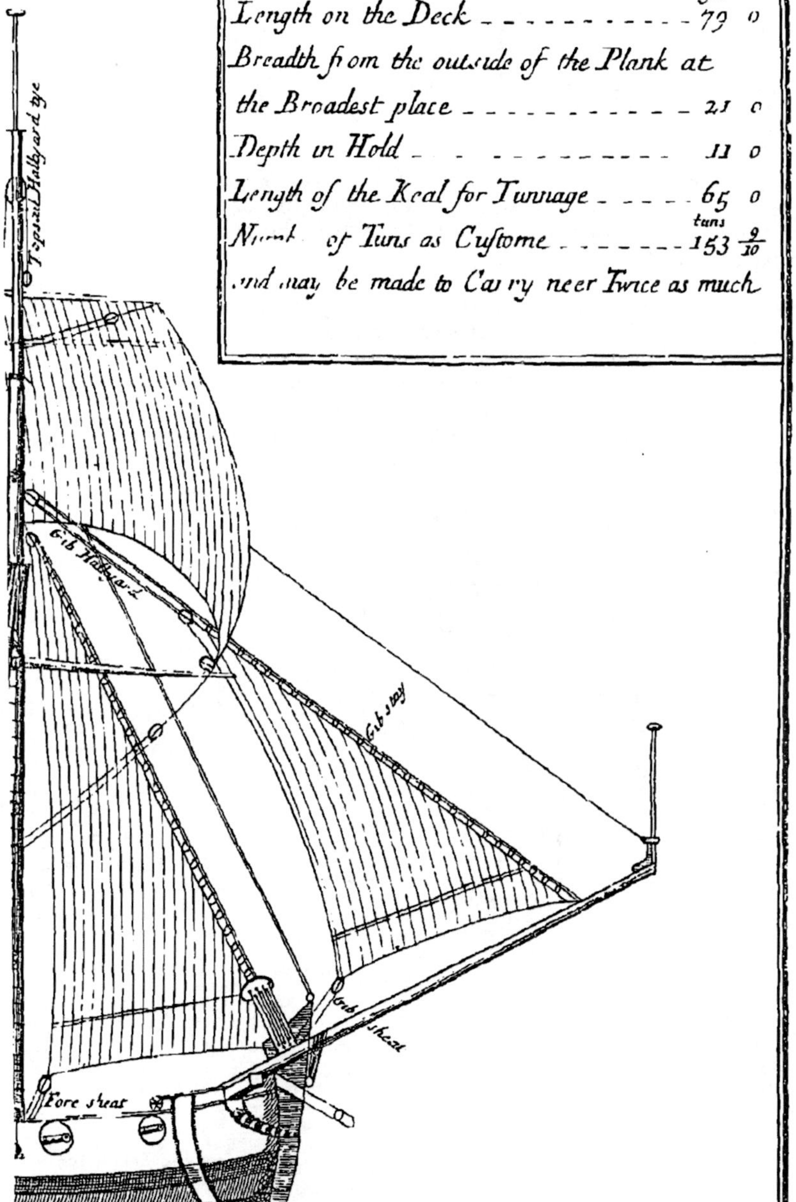

Topsail Halliard
Gib Halliard
Gib stay
Gib sheat
Fore sheat

Sutton Nicholls sculp

Multiply		by		its			Then divide		
	19½		60 5		1180	The Area of the Circle of the Diameter of each Mast		1180	by 200 and its
	18½		57½		1046			1046	
	15¼		48		735			735	
	13		41		530			530	
	10¼		38½		410			410	
	8		25		200				

			Yards		Inches
5 [illegible]	Which is the Proportion that all the other sized Ships Masts bears to the smallest sized	Length according to the Establishment	38½	Diameter according	39
5 [illegible]			36½		36½
3 [illegible]			33¼		30½
2 [illegible]			29		26¼
2			24		21½
			21		16

It's found by this, that the large sized, Ships Mast is 39 Inches big, and the small one 16 Now was the large one but 32 Inches, or the small 19 one ½, and of equal length, they would be in Quadruple Porportion in Magnitude, and strong ss 1 to 16.

But since they are in length near as 1 to 2, they are strong as 1 to 4, and in Content as 1 to 8, however the Diameters make the Area near as 1 to 6, so that one contains six times as much as the other, and if they were of equal length, would be strong according to the Square of the doubling, which is as 1 to 36, but being of double length, the Proportion is as 1 to 18 But the small Mast being 21 Yards long, and the other 38 ½, they are not exactly as 1 to 2, and therefore I shall lay down a Proportion suitable to their lengths.

			is to			it will be	
38½	The length of the large Ships Mast to the small one is as	1		1 [illegible]	Then if a Quadruple Proportion in doubling be strong with equal length as 1 to 4, what will	5 9	11 8
36½		1		1 [illegible]		5 2	10 4
33½		1		1 [illegible]		3 7	7 4
29		1		1 [illegible]		2 [illegible]	5 6
24		1		1 [illegible]		2 [illegible]	4 [illegible]
21		1					

	From 42 remains		then if 21 gives		what shall		give & it gives		which
38½		3 [illegible]		5 9		3 [illegible]		8 [illegible]	
36		5 [illegible]		5 2		5 [illegible]		1 [illegible]	
33		8 [illegible]		3 7		8 [illegible]		1 [illegible]	
29		13		2 [illegible]		13		1 [illegible]	
24		18		2 [illegible]		18		1 [illegible]	
21		21							

added to		is			
	5 9		6 [illegible]	Which is the Proportion of Strength according to the length of each Mast	Then for the Diameter of the Mast, and what ought to be allowed in a Yards length for the bigness
	5 2		6 [illegible]		
	3 7		5 2		
	2 [illegible]		4 [illegible]		
	2 [illegible]		3 [illegible]		

	The Square Root of which is				
38½		6 2	Then if 62 require 1 Inch in Diameter to every Yard long, what shall the other Square Roots	100	They require the several 100 parts of an Inch to a Yard in Length
36½		6 [illegible]		[illegible]	
33½		5 8		[illegible]	
29		5 4		[illegible]	
24		4 9		79	
21		4 6		74	

Then × the several 100 parts by		its		which divided by 100 its		
	38½		3875		38 [illegible]	Which is the Diameter of the Main-masts, in Inches and Parts at the Partners, or biggest place of him
	36½		3516		35 [illegible]	
	33½		3115		31 [illegible]	
	29		2523		25 [illegible]	
	24		1896		18 [illegible]	
	21		1551		15 [illegible]	

Area's

Area's of the Masts, or Square of the Diameter, is	They are one to another, as		as	
1521		First to Second		1 to 1 [illegible]
1332 2		First to Third		1 to 1 [illegible]
930		First to Fourth		1 to 2 [illegible]
588		First to Fifth		1 to [illegible]
462		First to Sixth		1 to 6
256				

Their lengths are one to another, as		as		Then the Areas will be to make them equally strong	
	First to Second		1 to 1 [illegible]		1521
	First to Third		1 to 1 [illegible]		1433
	First to Fourth		1 to 1 [illegible]		1320
	First to Fifth		1 to 1 [illegible]		1120
	First to Sixth		1 to 1 [illegible]		932
					835

The Diameters are, to make them equally strong		The length to make them equally strong is	
	39		38 [illegible]
	37 [illegible]		33 [illegible]
	36 [illegible]		23 [illegible]
	33 [illegible]		15 [illegible]
	30 [illegible]		12
	28 [illegible]		6 [illegible]

And now I shall set down the length of every Mast and Yard from a Proportion of the largest Size, and drawn from the Cube of the Tunnage.

Tuns		*Cube Root*	*Tuns*		*Cube Root*
1677	is	11 [illegible]	625	is	8 [illegible]
1488		11 [illegible]	364		7 [illegible]
969		9 [illegible]	225		6 [illegible]

	1st size Cube Root 11 [illegible]	*2d. size* Cube Roo. 11 [illegible]	*3d size* Cube Root 9 [illegible]	*4th. size* Cube Root 8 [illegible]	*5th size* Cube Root 7 [illegible]	*6th. size* Cube Root 6 [illegible]
	Yards and Parts	Yards and Parts	Yards and Parts	Yards and Parts	Yards and Parts	Yards and Parts
Main mast	38 3/4	37 1/4	32 [illegible]	28 [illegible]	23 [illegible]	20
Ditto Top-mast	22 3/4	21 [illegible]	18 [illegible]	16 [illegible]	14 [illegible]	12 [illegible]
Ditto Topgallant-mast	9 [illegible]	9 [illegible]	8 [illegible]	7 [illegible]	5 [illegible]	4 [illegible]
Fore-mast	33 [illegible]	32 6	28 [illegible]	24 [illegible]	20 [illegible]	17 [illegible]
Ditto Top-mast	20	19 [illegible]	16 [illegible]	14 [illegible]	12 [illegible]	10 [illegible]
Ditto Topgallant-mast	8 1/2	8 [illegible]	7 [illegible]	6 [illegible]	5 [illegible]	4 [illegible]
Mizon-mast	32 1/4	31 [illegible]	27	24 [illegible]	20 [illegible]	17 [illegible]
Ditto Top-mast	12 [illegible]	11 [illegible]	10 [illegible]	9 [illegible]	7 [illegible]	6 [illegible]
Bowsprit	27	26 [illegible]	22 [illegible]	20 [illegible]	16 [illegible]	14
Sprit Sail Topmast	7 [illegible]	6 [illegible]	5 [illegible]	5 [illegible]	4 [illegible]	4
Main yard	34	33 [illegible]	28 [illegible]	24 [illegible]	20 [illegible]	17 [illegible]
Ditto Top-sail yard	19	18 [illegible]	15 [illegible]	13 [illegible]	11 [illegible]	9 [illegible]
Ditto Topgallant yard	9	9 [illegible]	8 [illegible]	6	5 [illegible]	4 [illegible]
Fore-yard	30	29 [illegible]	25 [illegible]	21 [illegible]	15 [illegible]	15 [illegible]
Ditto Top sail-yard	16 [illegible]	16 [illegible]	14	12 [illegible]	[illegible]	8 [illegible]
Ditto Topgallant yard	8	8 [illegible]	8 [illegible]	7 [illegible]	6 [illegible]	5 [illegible]
Mizon-yard	30	29	25	21 [illegible]	18 [illegible]	15 [illegible]
Top-sail-yard	9 [illegible]	9 [illegible]	8	6 [illegible]	5 [illegible]	4 [illegible]
Crossjack yard	19 [illegible]	18 [illegible]	16	13 [illegible]	11 [illegible]	9
Spritsail-yard	21 1/4	20 [illegible]	17 [illegible]	15 [illegible]	12 [illegible]	10 [illegible]
Ditto Top sail yard	11	10 [illegible]	9 [illegible]	7 [illegible]	6 [illegible]	5 [illegible]

Then for the Diameter of each Mast, it may be found from the Cube Root of the length, that is, as the Cube Root of the Masts length are one to another, so is the allowance of the bigness to a Yard in length, divided into 100 parts to each other

And indeed it cannot well be adjusted better, than from a Proportion drawn from the length; since the Proportion of strength is according to a Proportion of the length, observing that the biggest Mast that's made, has no more than an Inch allowed for the Diameter to every Yard the Mast is long.

Then

Then to proceed and draw a Calculation from the Cube of the Length

Cube Root of the Length.		Then if 3 38/100 give 1 Inch, divided into one 100 parts, what shall the other Roots give?	Which × by the lengths, is	Divided by 100 is	Diameter according to the Establishment
Main-maſt	3 38/100	100	3875	38 3/4	39
Top-maſt	2 84/100	84/100	1900	19	20
Topgallant-maſt	2 15/100	61/100	620	6 2/10	8 1/4
Fore maſt	3 23/100	97/100	3260	32 1/10	34
Foretop-maſt	2 72/100	81/100	1620	16 2/10	17 [illegible]
Topgallant-maſt	2 4/100	41/100	520	5 2/10	7 1/4
Mizon-maſt	2 98/100	88/100	2320	23 2/10	22
Top-maſt	2 31/100	69/100	840	8 4/10	10 [illegible]
Bowſprit	3	89/100	2400	24	36 1/4
Sprit-ſail-top-maſt	1 92/100	57/100	424	4 5/[illegible]	7 1/2

So that it appears, that the Proportion of all Maſts which ſhall fall under 12 Yards long, may be calculated from a Root of a higher Power, for the Cube Root reduces them too low Alſo the Bowſprit, that can be counted little otherwiſe than as an Out-licker, to ſtay and ſecure the other Maſts. And ſince he is placed at ſome certain Angle, neither Perpendicular, nor Horizontal, without an aſſiſtance of Stays or Shrouds, as the other Maſts have, he will require a larger allowance of Bigneſs to his Length; and the Cuſtom has been to allow his Diameter between the Diameter of the Main-maſt and Fore-maſt · However, to ſquare the Length of the Bowſprit and double it, the ſquare Root of that Number will give the Diameter very near, from the largeſt Ship, as low as one of a 1000 Tuns; and for all Ships below that bigneſs, to the ſquare of the Length, add half the ſquare of the Length, and extract the ſquare Root will give the Diameter. And ſince the Sprit-ſail Top maſt has neither Stays nor Shrouds materially placed, let there be an Inch allowed in Diameter for every Yard the ſaid Maſt is long, which may be made general. Obſerve alſo that the Length of the Mizon-maſt, in this Cuſtom, is conſidered no lower than the lower Gun-deck.

Main-maſts, *Yards long*	Cube Root is	Then if 3 38/100 give one Inch, what ſhall the other Roots give	Multiply'd by the length is	Divided by 100 is, *Inches*	*Inches*, Cuſtom
38 3/4	3 38/100	100	3875	38 3/4	38 3/4
36 1/4	3 [illegible]/100	98/100	3540	35 4/10	36 [illegible]
33	3 [illegible]/100	95/100	3135	31 35/100	30
28	3 4/100	90/100	2520	25 2/10	24
23 6/7	2 88/100	85/100	2020	20 2/10	19
21	2 [illegible]/100	78/100	1680	16 8/10	16 1/4

Bowſprits, *length yds*	Squared is			The Square Root of which is,	Diameter in Inches & Parts	Diameter in Inches, &c as Cuſtom
27	729	Doubled is	1458	38 2		36 1/2
25	625		1251	35 3		34
21 1/4	425		850	29 3		30
17 1/2	360	1/2 doubled is	540	23 2		22
15 4/5	237		355	18 27/100		17 3/4
13	169		253	15 9/10		15

The Length of the biggeſt Ship's Main yard, ſhall be the Length of the Main-maſt, excepting Head, which to every Yard the Maſt is long, there ought to be taken out at leaſt 4 Inches, or 4 and half, and all other Ships Main-yards ſhall be in Proportion to the large Ships, as their lower Gun-decks are one to another; and for the Diameter of ſuch Yards, ſay, As the Cube Root of the Length on the Ships Gun-deck is to the Cube Roots of the Ships Breadth, and half the Breadth, ſo is the Length of the Yards in Yards, to the Diameter in Inches.

Length of the Main-yards	Yards	Diameter of the Yards drawn from the Cube Roots	Diameter of the Yards as Cuſtom
34 1/2	25 1/2	24	
32	24	22 1/2	
30	22 1/2	20	
26	19 1/2	16 1/2	
21 1/2	15 15/100	14	
18 1/4	13 1/2	12 1/2	

The Mizon-yard may be proportion'd from the whole Length of the Mizon mast, excepting Head, which Head in those Masts, ought to be 3 Inches at least, or 3 Inches and half in Length, for every Yard the Mast is long

The Crossjack yards Diameter will bear the same Proportion as the Mizon-yard, he being for no other Service than to Clew out the Mizon top-sail Sheets. And after such a manner may every particular Mast and Yard be proportion'd, and shap'd according to its particular Service, by first considering the Bulk and Magnitude of the Ship, and not only so, but the shape also.

And then to subdivide the whole allowance of the Masts, which will be found proper to drive the Body onward, and also what it will bear; which subdivision, is only to be divided between Main-mast and Fore-mast, and their parts, without considering the Bowsprit and Mizon-mast

Next to consider the Superficies of the Sails, or quantity of Canvas proper to be converted into Sails, and to subdivide that according to the Dimensions of the Masts and Yards. As also to consider the Tractive or Pulsive Force of Wind on the several Sails, from which may be exactly proportion'd every individual Mast and Yard, and fashion of the Sail, from the shape of the Log or Ships Body. Which to give a nice and particular Account of every part thereof, would fill a large Volume. And therefore I only mention this as a Breviate of what may follow

And shall lay down some particular Demonstrations, to shape a Mast or a Yard, which ought to be exactly Circular, according to their respective Lengths and Bigness.

Gunters's Line has been a general Method for setting of any Mast or Yard, which is no other than a Sweep, which is, from the Partners, Caps or Slings, to the Head or Yard Arm, to make them truly Circular, as the [illegible], the [illegible], the [illegible], the [illegible], the [illegible] part of the Biggest place of the Mast or Yard, for the intermedium places or quarters between the Extreams, as I shall shew in the old customary Methods.

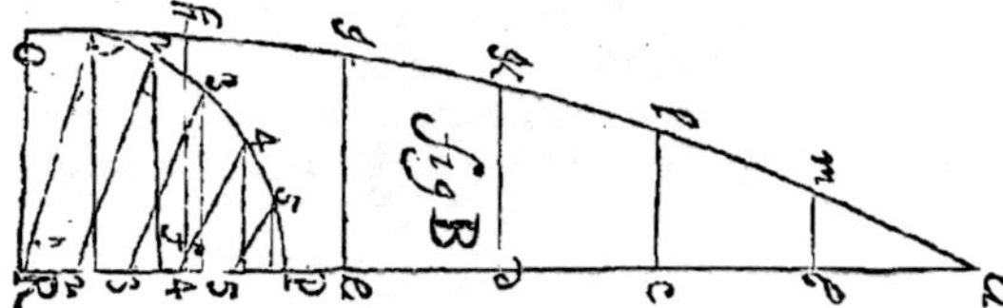

Figure B. Shews a Method to set off a Mast, Beam Mould, or any other Circular Sweep, proposing *o. R.* to be the Diameter of the Sweep, from the straight part or Spindle of the Mast or Yard. Then describing the Quadrant *R P o* into parts, as 1. 2. 3 4 5. and propose the length of the Mast, Yard, or Beam mould, to be from *R.* to *a.* divide that Line into an equal Number of equal Parts to the Quadrant; then set off 1.1 at *b f.* 2.2 at *I e.* 3 3 at *K. d* 4.4. at *l. c.* 5.5 at *m. b* which may mark out any of the abovesaid Particulars.

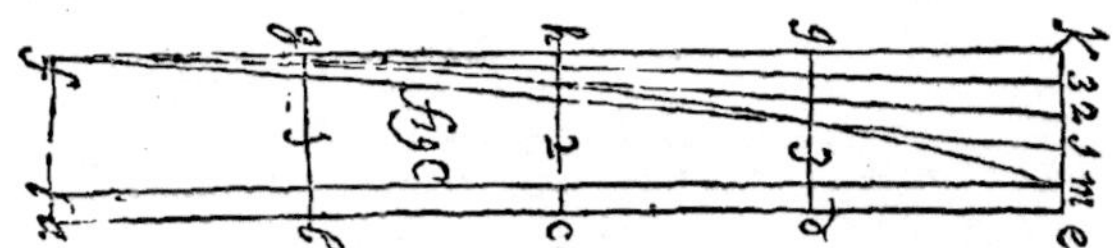

Figure C Shews another Method Supposing *f l.* to be the Diameter of the Sweep, and *l. a.* the Spindle or streight Part of any Mast or Yard, then the length of the Part let be from *a* to *e.* Mark out the Quarters 1. 2 3. on the Lines *g. b h. c. I. d* and *K. m* then strike streight Lines from 1 2. and 3. to *f.* and where those streight Lines intersect on the Lines *g. b. h. c. I. d.* will be the Height of the Sweep.

Figure A.

Figure A being another fashion: Supposing the Line *A B.* to be the Diameter of the Mast or Yard in the Partners, and 2. 1 the bigness at the Head, Heel, or Yard Arm, and the Lines 2 2 and 1.1 to be the Spindle of the particular Part, then describing the Semicircle *A. B. C* and dividing it at Pleasure into any Number of equal Parts from *B.* to *C.* or *A* to *C* divide the length into as many, then taking the distances from the Line *C* P. to 1 *a b c*, and set them off on the Lines *c.c b b a.a* will shape you out any Mast or Yard, according to the Magnitude thereof, either upwards or downwards, towards Head or Heel.

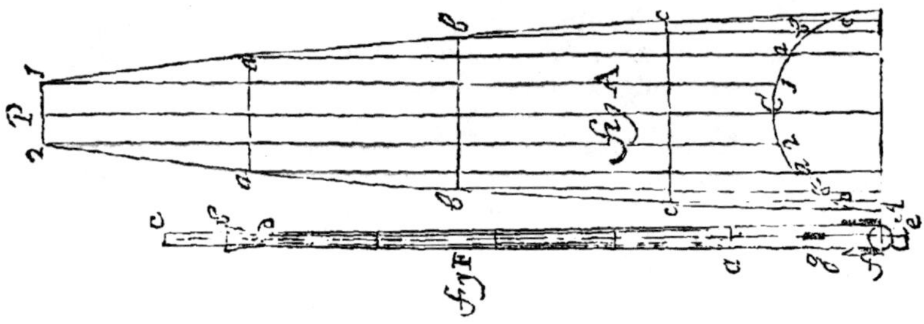

Figure F is the Top-mast, *f* is the Heel, and *e.* the Block, where the top Rope goes through to hoist or heave the Top-mast up, *g* is another part where a Shiver is fitted for the same purpose; *a* is the Cap or place of the Top mast, that fits in the Cap, *c b.* the Head or Scarph for the Top-gallant-mast; *b. d.* the Hounds, where it has been usual to have a shiver to hoist up the Top-sail, but now wholly left off, observing it to be much better to have a Block lash'd for such a use, that it may yield to the moving of the Ship, and also to the Purchase

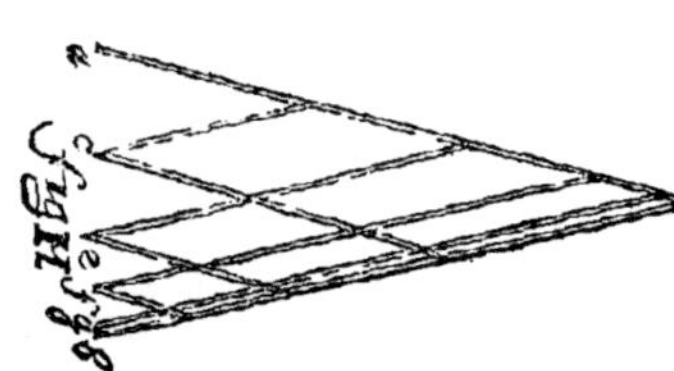

Figure H. may be made a universal Instrument to set off any Sweep, by only having it to be Riveted at every Intersection, almost in the nature of Compasses, so that opening of it to make *a b* the greatest Diameter of the Sweep; then *a g.* shall be next, or *c. d a. f e f a. c g b.* and *a. c* in Figure *H.* 1 *k.* in Figure G And this would be made a very concise Instrument, and in divers Cases be made Portable.

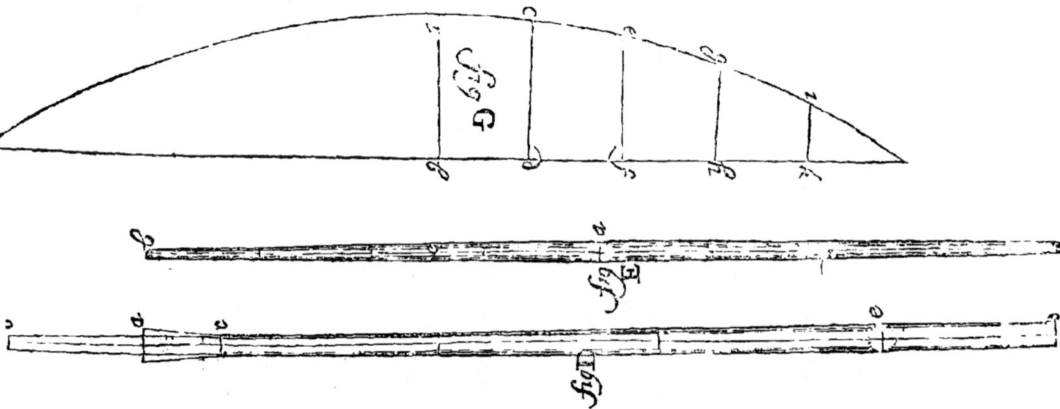

Figure D. is a standing Mast, *d.* is the Heel or Step, and the Partners, or biggest part; *c. a.* the Hounds, and *a. b.* the Head or Scarph, for the Top-mast.

At

At *a* you may obſerve a projecting part, or Shoulders for the Treſle-trees to bear on, and alſo for the Heel of the Top-maſt to ſet. At *b* there's a Cap for the Top-maſt to go through.

Figure E. is a Yard ; *a.* is the Slings or biggeſt part where he is ſlung to hoiſt him up ; and hanging there by the middle, it may be obſerved that he is each ways equally of a Bigneſs, and ought to be in Equilibro ; *e. d.* is the Quarters the part ſets off between the Slings and Yard Arms, *b* and *c.* the Yard Arms.

In the next Place I ſhall ſhew the particular Shape and Dimenſions of the Anchors, obſerving that it's general, for the length of the Shank of the biggeſt Anchor, in any Ship, to be $\frac{2}{5}$ of the Ships extream breadth

Tunnage of the Six Sizes	1677 Tuns		1488 Tuns		969 Tuns		625 Tuns		364 Tuns		225 Tuns	
	C qr l		C qr l		C qr l		C qr l		C qr l		C qr l	
Weight of the biggeſt Anchor	71 2 0		64 0 0		45 0 0		30 0 0		18 3 6		11 2 1	
Cube Root of the Weight	4—[illegible]		4		3—53/100		3—1/10		2—6/10		2—26/100	
	feet	Inch	feet	Inch	feet	Inch	feet	Inch	feet	Inch	feet	Inch
Length of the Shank as aforeſaid	18	6	18	2	16	1	14	2	12	2	10	8
Bigneſs of the great End of ditto	0	11 1/3	0	11 1/10	0	10 1/10	0	8 8/10	0	7 1/2		6 1/2
Ditto at the ſmall end	0	8 1/2	0	8 1/10	0	7 1/2	0	6	0	5 1/2	0	4 1/10
Length of the Square	2	11	2	10 4/10	2	6 4/10	2	3	1	11	1	8
Length to the Nut	1	11	1	10 6/10	1	8 8/10	1	5 6/10	1	3 1/5	1	1 4/10
Bigneſs of the Nut Square	0	2 1/5	0	2 26/100	0	2	0	1 26/100	0	1 61/100	0	1 14/50
Diameter of the Rings inſide clear	2	1 1/2	2	1	1	10	1	7 5/[illegible]	1	3	1	2
Bigneſs of the Ring	0	4	0	3 64/100	0	3 48/100	0	3 6/10	0	3	0	2 7/[illegible]
Diameter of the Hole for the Ring	0	4 6/10	0	4 1/10	0	3 98/100	0	3 5/10	0	3	0	2 66/100
Length of the Crown	1	2	1	1 1/10	0	11 1/10	0	9 3/4	0	8 1/2	0	7 7/10
Length of the Arm	7	0	6	9	6	1	5	0 7/10	4	0 6/10	4	0 1/5
Breadth of the Flook	2	8	2	7 5/10	2	3 8/10	2	0 4/10	1	9	1	6
Length of ditto	3	9	3	8 1/3	3	3 1/2	2	10 4/10	2	5 5/10	2	2
Thickneſs of ditto	0	2 9/10	0	2 95/100	0	2 51/[illegible]	0	2 32/100	0	1 9/10	0	1 68/100
Square of the Arm at the Flook	0	7	0	6 8/10	0	6 1/10	0	5 7/10	0	4 6/10	0	4 1/25
Length of the Bill	0	10 1/2	0	10 3/10	0	9 1/10	0	8 0	0	6 8/10	0	6 1/10
Rounding of the Flook	0	1 16/100	0	1 14/100	0	1 1/10	0	0 8/100	0	0 76/100	0	0 66/100
Clutching of the Arm	3	6	3	5 1/3	3	0 4/10	2	6	2	4 5/10	2	1 2/10
Inſide meeting	6	6										
Outſide meeting	6	6										
Middle meeting	6	6										

And after ſuch a manner may every part of any Anchor (from the biggeſt to the leaſt) be ſhap'd and proportion'd exact and genuine ; I having obſerved that the ſetting of the Flook or Arm is the greateſt Point, which is done by the Meaſuring the length from the Pit of *c* to the Bill *x*, and ſetting of that length ſome will have it to *z.* which is called the inſide meeting, and ſome to *y* which is the middle meeting, and ſome to 2 which is the outſide meeting, ſo that the ſaid Angle to any of thoſe places ſhall make an Equilateral Triangle. Of which I ſhall make an Index.

Length of the Shank, Figure *A. m b*
Bigneſs of the great end, *c d*
Ditto of the ſmall end, *E. f*
Length of the Square, *g b*
Ditto to the Nut, *g. b*
Bigneſs of the Nut Square, *g.*
Diameter of the Ring's inſide clear, *K l* in Figure *B.*
Bigneſs of the Ring, Figure *B. l* 2
Diameter of the Ring's Hole, Figure *A.* 1 3.
Length of the Crown, *m b*
Length of the Arm, *c. x* or *c. n.* Figure *C.*
Breadth of the Flook, *p. q* Figure *B.*
Length of Ditto *R* 4. in either *A.* or *C*
Thickneſs of Ditto 6 5 Figure *A*
Square of the Arm at the Flook, *R.* Figure *A.*
Length of the Bill, 4 *n.* in *A* or *C.*
Rounding of the Flook, 2 4. in *B.*
Clutching of the Arm, *e m.* in *A.*
Inſide meeting, *z x. c* in Figure *A.*
Outſide Ditto *x.* 2. *c* ditto
Middle Ditto, *x y. c.* ditto.

The

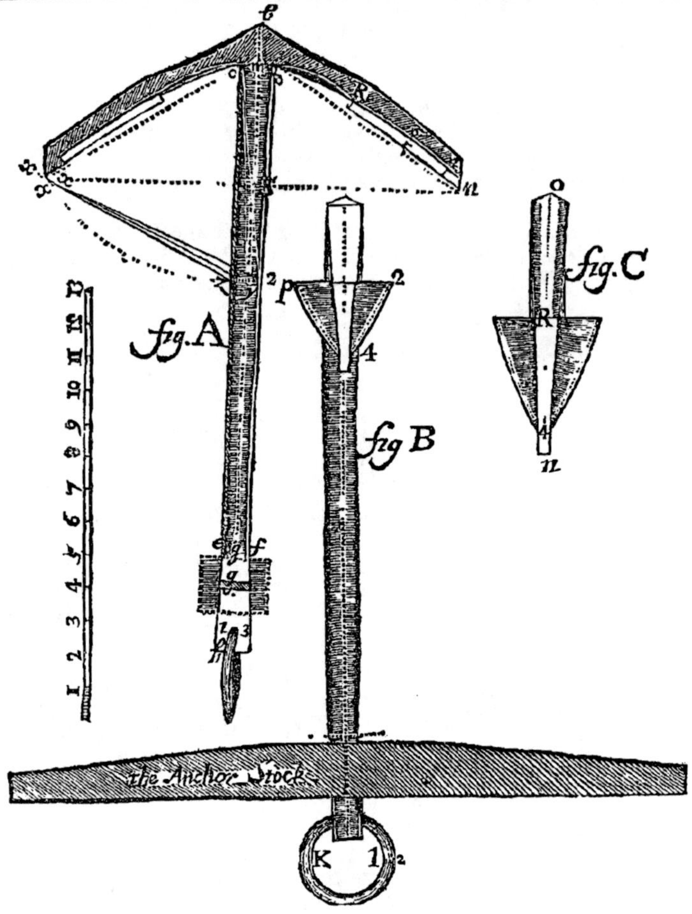

The Opinions in ſetting the Arm of an Anchor, has been always various, ſome ſetting it of by the Outſide Meeting, and ſome by the middle Meeting and others by the Inſide Meeting: *It may be obſerv'd, that ſetting it of by* the Outſide Meeting, will make the Angle more obtuſe with the Shank, and the Crown ought to be the better fortified, for that part will have a greater Strain; and in ſetting it of by an inſide Meeting, will cauſe the Anchor not to hold ſo well in the Ground, by reaſon it ſhortens the Arm This Anchor is ſet by the middle Meeting.

I ſhall end this Obſervation with drawing a Parallel between the largeſt Anchor of a Ship of 1677 Tuns, and a Ship of 225 Tuns, and alſo of the biggeſt Cables

A Ship of 1677 Tuns Cable is 22 Inches and ¾ Circumference.

A Ship of 225 Tuns Cable is 12 Inches Circumference.

The great Anchor is 71 *C* and ¼, and the ſmall Anchor is 11 *C.* and ¼.

Their Shanks are 18 Foot 6 Inches long, and 10 Foot 8 Inches long

Their bigneſs in the middle of the Shanks are, 9 Inches $\frac{2}{10}$, and 5 Inches $\frac{6}{10}$.

The Area's of the Cables are one to another, as 11 to 3.

The Areas of the Anchors in the middle of the Shanks, which is their Proportion of Strength, is one to another, as 19 to 6.

Their Lengths are one to another as 12 to 7.

N Then

Then to make their Lengths suitable to their Areas, and so to be equally strong, one must be 18 6, and the other 5 '-, or else they must be 10 8 and 24

To make the Areas equal to their Lengths, the Areas must be 98 01 and 56 25, or else 31.36 and 53 29, and then the sides will be either 9 9 and 7.5, or 5 6 and 7.3

The Areas of the Anchor Shanks are near as 3 to 1, and if they were of equal Length, they would be strong accordingly, but being in Length as 12 to 7 or near as 2 to 1, their Strength one to another is according to the mixt Fraction -' of -- then × -- by -- is -- : By which Reducement it would appear, that the Proportion of Strength will be as 217 is to 1176, which would be near -; and by that it would appear, that the small Anchor's Strength is reduced, which is contrary, since it is the great Anchor which is lessene' i' Strength, and therefore instead of multiplying the Fractions, they must be divided Then divide -- by -- its --, so that the Proportion of Strength in the Anchors is as 372 is to 686, which is as 6 to 11, and therefore it appears, that according to the Strength requisite in weighing or proving of such Materials, their Strengths will not be found as 2 to 1, although the Weight of the Ships that they are adapted for, is as 8 to 1, and the Strain that they ride, of consequence, near that Proportion.

I now proceed to lay down the other Five Figures, or Sizes of Shipping: And also make an *Index* to each, to lead to their several Parts

An Index to the Parts of the Second Size

a. 2 Length of the Keel from the back of the main Post to the touch of the Stem

f 1 Ditto from the back of the false Post to the extream fore-part of the Keel or Tread.

10, 11 From the fore-part of the Rabbit of the Post, to the aft side of the Rabbit of the Stem, for the length on the Lower Gun-deck, and measur'd there.

Fig B 12, 13 Breadth of the Ship's Timber from Out to Out, in the Midships, (term'd) Moulded

14, 15 Extream breadth of the Ship from Out to Out, of Plank, or Thick-stuff

4 *e* From the Limber-board to the upper Edge of the Gun-deck beam, in the Midships, term'd the Depth in Hold, and formerly the Custom in measuring.

3 1 Half breadth of Floor in the Mid-ships

L I K Narrowing of the Floor Line.

L ⌣ K. Narrowing of the Breadth Line

D C ⌣. Rising Line, being Similar thereto.

B C D. Rising of the Breadth Line.

H E Narrowing of the Breadth aft with a broad Stern.

H L. Breadth of the Transum within the Plank

N H The Narrowing of the Floor Line with a broad Stern, breadthens as the Line, N H. And in such a Position the Narrowing of the breadth Line may be prolong'd to H.

w a ' of the Breadth set back from *w* to *a* for the Rake of the Stem allowed in measuring the Tunnage of the Ship

C 16 15. Sheering-line, or the Hanging-line, of the breadth, from whence the sweep of the Top-timber commences

Lower Gun Deck 41, middle ditto 51, upper ditto 61, Quarter Deck 81, Forecastle Deck 100, Poop Deck 91; all which Decks ought to lye Parallel one from another, and the greatest Perpendicular height between any two of them need not be above Seven Feet at the side.

R. The Head Figure

Q Knee of the Head.

S. Upper

Second Siz'd Ship

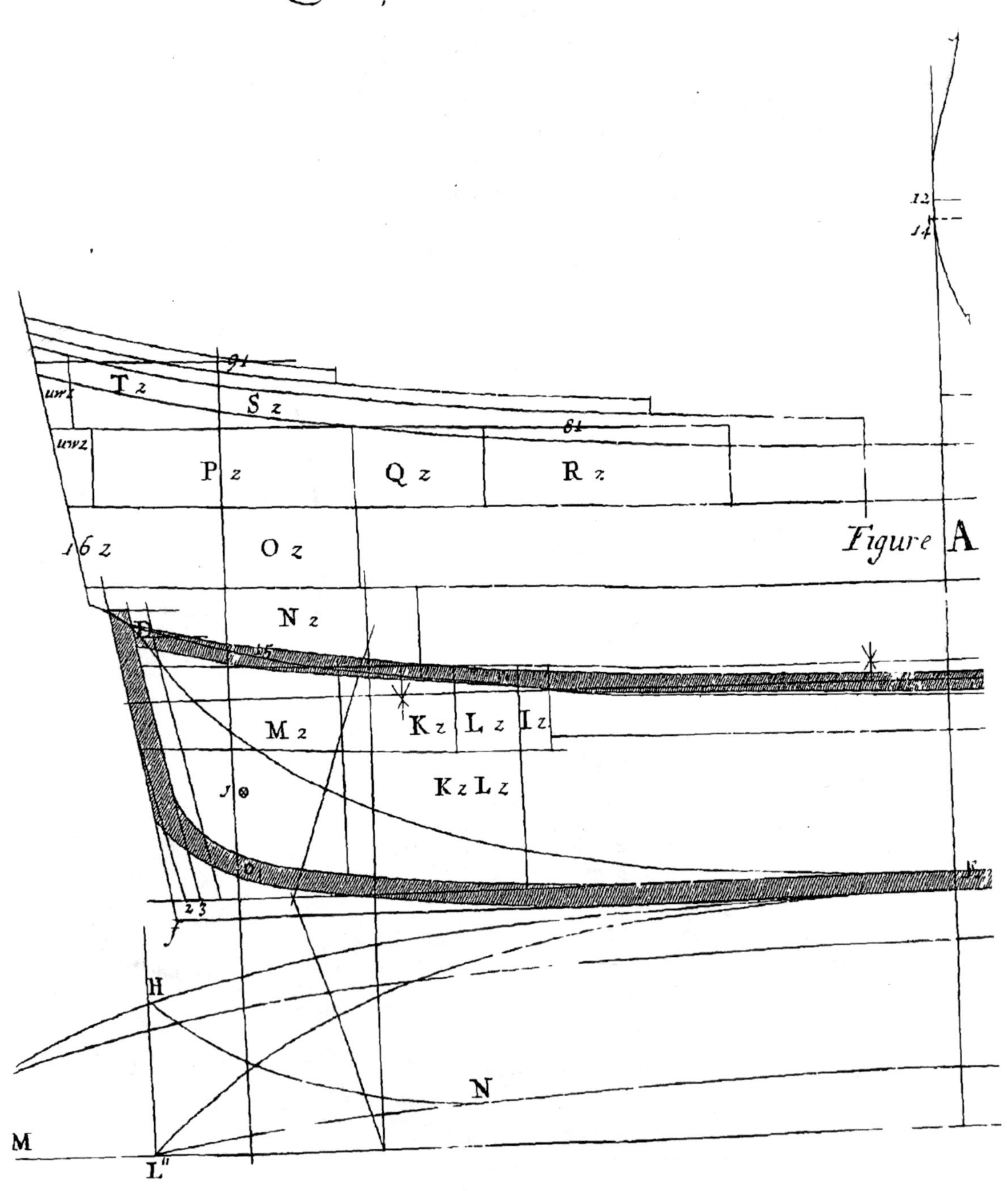

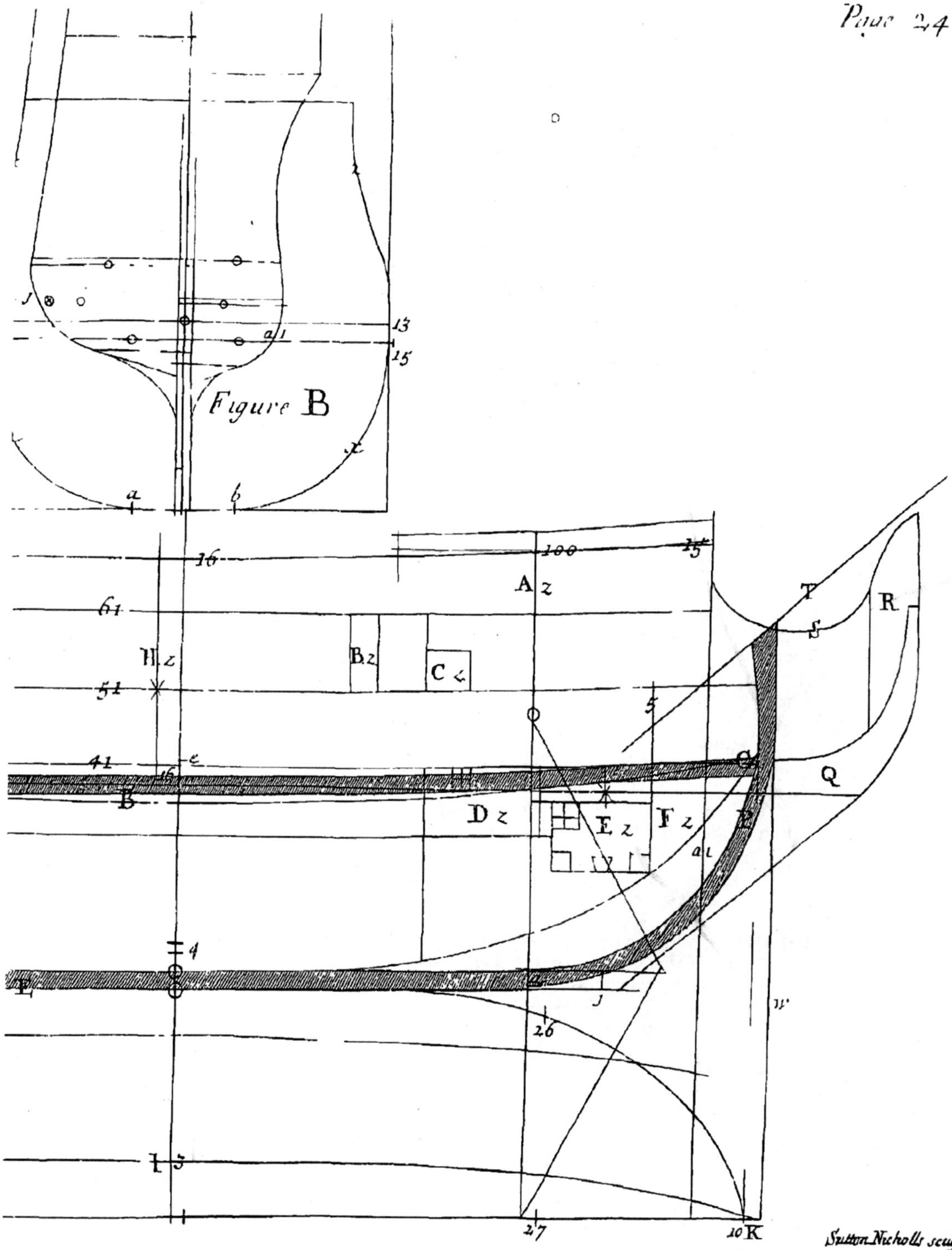

Figure B

Sutton Nicholls sculp

S Upper Rail of the Head.
T. The Steaving, or Angle, the Bowsprit makes with the Stem
5. The Partners, or step of the Bowsprit.
P. The Stem in three Pieces
O 1. Depth of the Keel aft, proposed to raise the Sheer, and to have less Dead Wood, and better fastning.
3. The Foremost part of the Stern-post.
16. z The corner Side Timber of the upright of the Stern.

Figure B. x x x x. The Midship bend of Timbers
A. z. The Forecastle, where there is Lodgings for the Carpenter, Boatswain, *&c.*
B z. A Cook-room, for dressing Victuals for the Commanders, and other Officers.
C z The Furnaces for boiling the Seamens Provisions
D z Apartments for Boatswain's and Carpenters Stores.
F. z. Ditto for Powder, and the Gunners Stores
E. z A filling Room to empty the Powder out of the Barrels into the Cartridges, also Chests and Troughs, and a Lanthorn fix'd to hold a Candle
H z The place of the Jeer, Capstand and treble Jeer on the upper Deck.
I z The Slop Room, to hold Seamens Slop-cloths
K z L z Flag-Officers and Commanders Store Rooms, with Pursers and Surgeons Cabbins.
M z The Bread Room
After Powder Room K. z. L. z Fish Room and Captains Store Room.
N z Gunner, and Gunners Mate's Cabbin in the Gun Room.
O z. The Ward Room and Volunteers Cabbin
P. z The great Cabbin
Q z A Lobby, with some Pantries.
R z The lower Coach.
S z Upper Coach,
T z Round House.
u. w z Balcony's, or Walks in the Stern.

And as to the Lines that shape the Body, they are Similar to the first siz'd Ship, according to the magnitude of the Body

Proportions of the Parts of the Second Size.

	Feet	Inc.
Length of the Keel *a.* 2. from the Touch to the back of the main Post	137	0
Height from the top of the Keel to the Plansheer	38	7
Rake of the main Post to the top of the Plansheer, measur'd to the Stern-side Timber	12	0
Breadth at the Fashion pieces, at the Wing-transum, from inside of the Plank	27	0
Breadth extream afore, at ⅓ of the Load Mark Line } 26, 27 Divided between the inside of the Rabbits,	39	0
Draught of Water loaded { afore	19	0
Draught of Water loaded { abaft	20	6
Rake of the Stem from the touch to the outside aloft, *a w.*	26	0
Figure B Breadth of the Floor	10	6
This Ship may be esteem'd to be worth *per* Tun building 14 *l.* 10 *s.*		
What Guns, as to number according to the Establishment, 90.		
What Men accordingly, 660		
Stern to project and lay Parallel from the main Post aloft Round of the Rail included	2	6

An Index to the Parts of the Third Size.

a. 2 Length of the Keel from the back of the main Post to the touch of the Stem.

f. 1. Ditto from the back of the false Post, to the extream forepart of the Keel or Tread

10, 11 From the fore side of the Rabbit of the Post, to the aft-side of the Rabbit of the Stem, for the length of the Lower Gun-deck measured there.

Fig B 12, 13 Breadth of the Ship's Timber from Out to Out, in the Midships, (term'd) Moulded.

14, 15 Extream breadth from Out to Out of Plank, or Thickstuff, allowed in Measure

4 *e.* From the Limber-board to the upper Edge of the Gundeck beam, in the Midships, term'd the Depth in Hold, and formerly allowed in Measure.

3. 1 Half breadth of Floor in the Midships

L I K Narrowing of the Floor Line

L O K. Narrowing of the Breadth Line.

D C Θ. Rising Line, being Similar thereto.

B C D. Rising of the Breadth Line.

H E Narrowing of the Breadth aft with a broad Stern.

H I Breadth of the Transum within the Plank.

N H Narrowing of the Floor Line with a broad Stern, breadthens as the Line, N H. And in such a Position the Narrowing of the breadth Line may be prolong'd to H

w a ⅐ of the Breadth set back from *w* to *a* for the Rake of the Stem allowed in measuring of the Tunnage of any Ship

C. 16. 15. Sheering-line, or the Hanging-line, of the upper breadth, from whence the back sweep of the Top-timber commences.

Lower Gun Deck 41, upper ditto 61, Quarter Deck 81, Forecastle ditto 101, Poop Deck 91, all which Decks ought to lye Parallel one to another, and the greatest Perpendicular height (need not be) between any two of them, above 6 Foot 11 Inches at the side.

R The Lyon, or other Figure.

Q Knee of the Head or Cut Water.

S Upper Rail of the Head.

T The Steaving, or Angle, the Bowsprit makes with the Stem.

5 The Partners, or step of the Bowsprit.

P The Stem in two Pieces, if possible

O 1. Depth of the Keel aft, proposed to raise the Sheer, and to have less Dead Wood, and better fastning

3 The Foremost part of the Stern-post.

16. z The corner Side Timber of the upright of the Stern.

Figure B. x x x x The Midship Bend of Timbers.

A z. The Fore Castle, where is Lodgings for the Boatswain, Carpenter, and Cooks

C z The Furnaces for boiling Victuals for Seamen; and,

B z Where a small Apartment's made for Officers Provisions.

D. z. Apartments for Carpenters and Boatswains Stores.

F z Ditto for the Powder, and for the Gunners Stores.

E z. A filling Room to empty the Powder out of the Barrels into Cartridges; also Chests and a Trough, and a Lanthorn fix'd to hold a Candle.

H z The place of the Jeer, Capstand, *&c.*

I. z. The Slop Room, to hold Seamens Slop-cloths.

K. z. L. z. Captain's Store Rooms, with the Pursers and the Surgeons Cabbin.

M. z.

Third Size

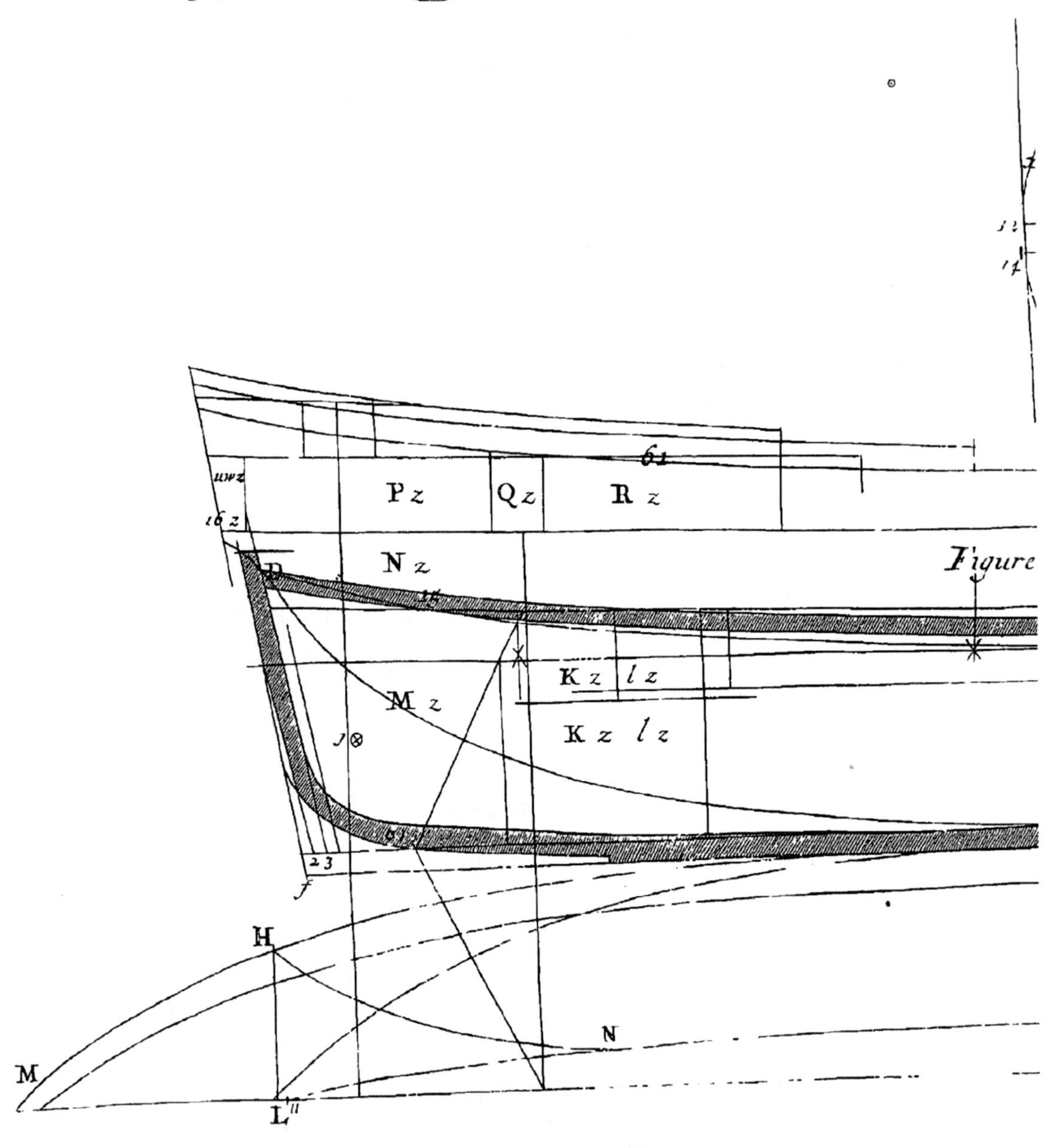

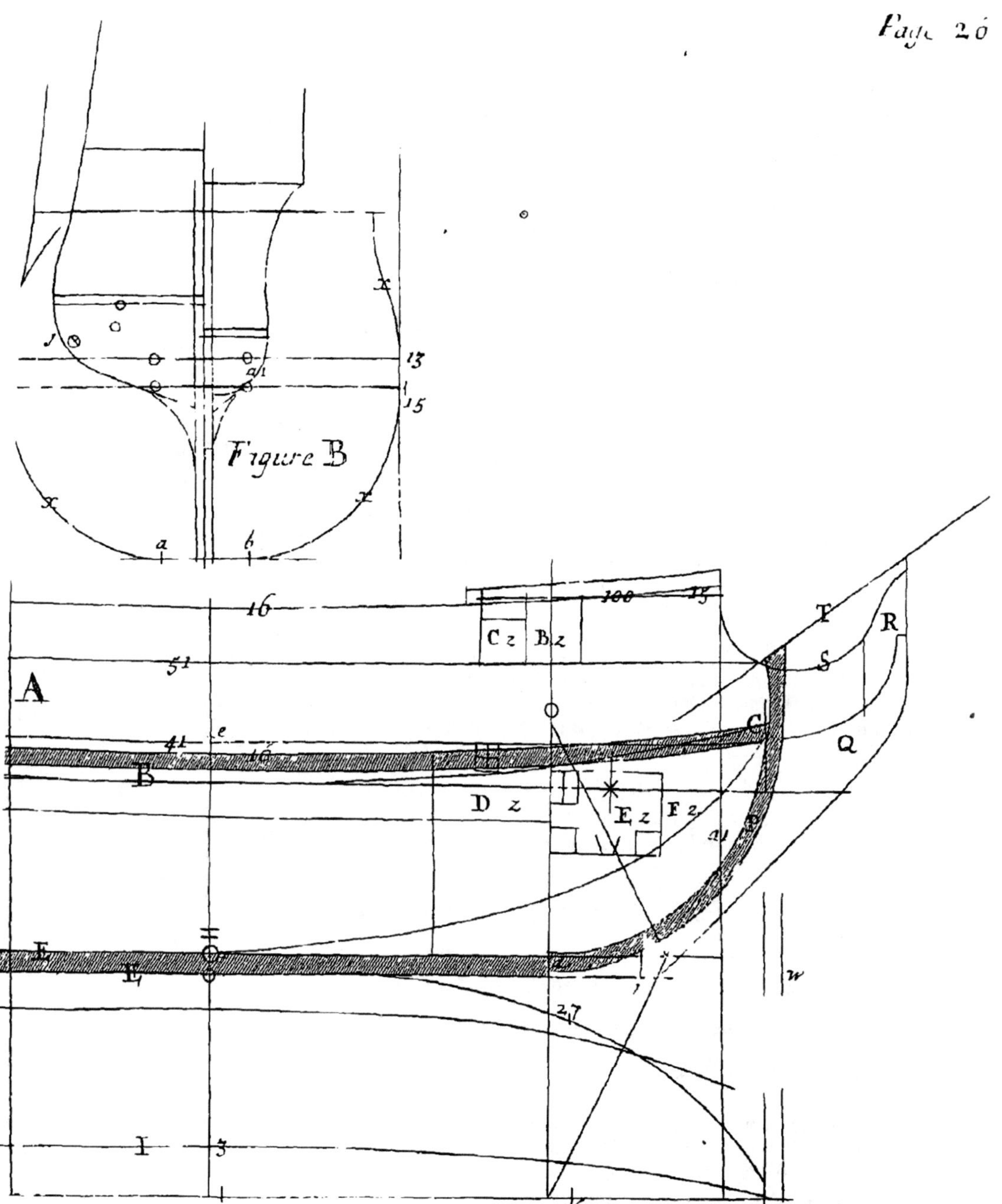

Sutton Nicholls sculp

M z The Bread Room
After Powder Room. K z L z. Fish Room and Captain's Store Room.
N z. Gunners, and Gunners Mate's Cabbins.
P. z. The great Cabbin
Q. z A Lobby, with some Pantries.
R. z The Steeridge.
S z. The Coach.
T. z The Round House.
u. w. z Balcony's, or Walks in the Stern.

A Proportion for the Parts of the Third Size.

	Feet	Inc
Length of the Keel 2. a from the Touch of the Stem to the back of the main Post	124	6
Height from the top of the Keel, to the top of the Plansheer Midship	31	0
Rake of the main Post to the top of the Plansheer, measur'd to the Stern-side Timber	9	0
Stern to project and lay Parallel from the main Post aloft	2	4
Breadth at the Fashion-pieces, at the Wing-transum, from inside of Plank	25	0
Breadth extream afore, at ⅐ of the Load Mark Line, Divided between the inside of the Rabbits, } 26, 27.	31	6
Draught of Water loaded { afore	16	7
Draught of Water loaded { abaft	18	0
Rake of the Stem from the Touch to the outside aloft	23	4
Breadth of the Floor, *Figure* B *a. b*	8	6
This Ship may be esteem'd to be worth *per* Tun building 11 *l.* 18 *s.*		
What Guns, as to number according to the Establishment, 70		
What Men accordingly 460.		

An Index to the Parts of the Fourth Size.

a 2 Length of the Keel from the back of the Post to the touch of the Stem
f 1. Ditto from the back of the false Post to the extream fore-part of the Keel or Tread.
10, 11 From the outside of the Rabbit of the Post, to the fore-side of the Stem, for the length on the Lower Gun-deck, measur'd there.

Fig B 12, 13. Breadth of the Ship's Timber from Out to Out, in the Midships, (term'd) Moulded.
14, 15 Extream breadth from Out to Out, of Plank, or Thickstuff, allow'd in Measure.
e 4 From the Limber-board to the upper Edge of the Gun-deck beam, in the Midships, term'd the Depth in Hold, and formerly allow'd in measure.
3 1 Half breadth of Floor in the Mid-ships.
L I K. Narrowing of the Floor Line.
L ϴ K. Narrowing of the Breadth Line.
D C ϴ. Rising Line, being Similar thereto.
B C D. Rising of the Breadth Line.
H E Narrowing of the Breadth aft with a broad Stern.
H L. Breadth of the Transum within the Plank
N H Narrowing of the Floor Line with a broad Stern, breadthens as the Line, N H. And in such a Position the Narrowing of the breadth Line may be prolong'd to M
w a. ' of the Breadth set back from *w* to *a* for the Rake of the Stem allowed in measuring the Tunnage of any Ship.

C 16 15 Sheering line, or the Line, of the upper breadth, from whence the sweep of the Top timber commences

Lower Gun Deck 41, upper ditto 51, Quarter Deck 61, Forecastle Deck 100, Poop Deck 91, all which Decks ought to lye Parallel one from another, and the greatest Perpendicular height between any two of them need not be above Six Feet Six Inches at the side

R The Lyon, or Figure of the Head.

Q Knee of the Head, or cut Water.

S Upper Rail of the Head

1. The Steeving, or Angle, the Bowsprit makes with the Stem.

5. The Partners, or step of the Bowsprit.

P The Stem in two Pieces

O 1 Depth of the Keel abaft, proposed to raise the Sheer, and to have less Dead Wood, and better fastning.

3 The Foremost part of the Stern-post

16. z The corner Side Timber of the upright of the Stern.

Figure B x x x x The Midship bend of Timbers

A z The Forecastle, where are Cabbins for the Carpenter, Boatswain, and Cook

B z The Furnaces for boiling Seamens Provisions, and a small Apartment

C z For dressing Officers Provisions.

D z Apartments for Boatswain's and Carpenters Stores.

F z Ditto for the Powder, and for Gunners Stores

E z A filling Room to empty the Powder out of the Barrels into the Cartridges; also Chests and Troughs, and a Lanthorn fix'd to hold a Candle.

H z The place of the Jeer, Capstand,

I z The Slop Room, to hold Seamens Slop-cloths.

K z L z Captains Store Rooms, with the Pursers and Surgeons Cabbins.

M z The Bread Room.

K z Fish Room and Captain's Store Rooms

N z Gunners, and Gunners Mate's Cabbins, in the Gun Room.

P. z The great Cabbin.

T z A Round House, or Cabbins for Lieutenant and Master

R z Steeridge.

A Proportion for the Parts of the Fourth Size

	Feet	Inc.
Length of the Keel 2. a from the Touch of the Stem to the back of the main Post	109	1
Height from the top of the Keel to the top of Plansheer Midships	27	0
Rake of the main Post to the top of the Plansheer,	7	0
Stern to project and lay Parallel from the main Post aloft	2	1
Breadth at the Fashion-pieces, at the Wing-transom, from inside of the Plank	20	10
Breadth extream afore, at ÷ of the Load-Mark Line Divided between the inside of the Rabbits, 26, 27	25	2
Draught of Water loaded { afore	14	4
Draught of Water loaded { abaft	15	4
Rake of the Stem from the touch to the outside aloft,	21	0
Figure B Breadth of the Floor *a b.*	7	0

This Ship may be esteem'd to be worth *per* Tun building 9 *l* 4 *s*.

What Guns, as to number according to the Establishment, 50

What Men accordingly, 380

An

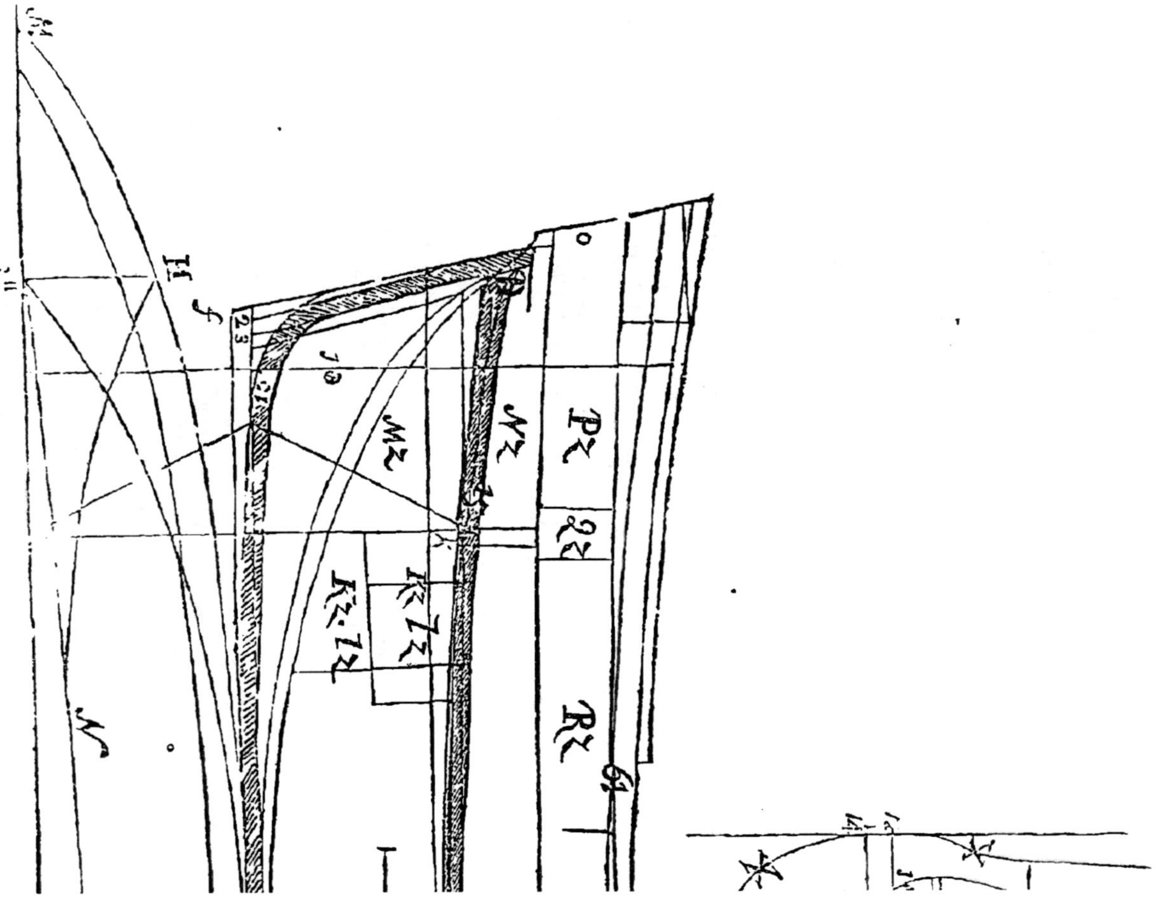

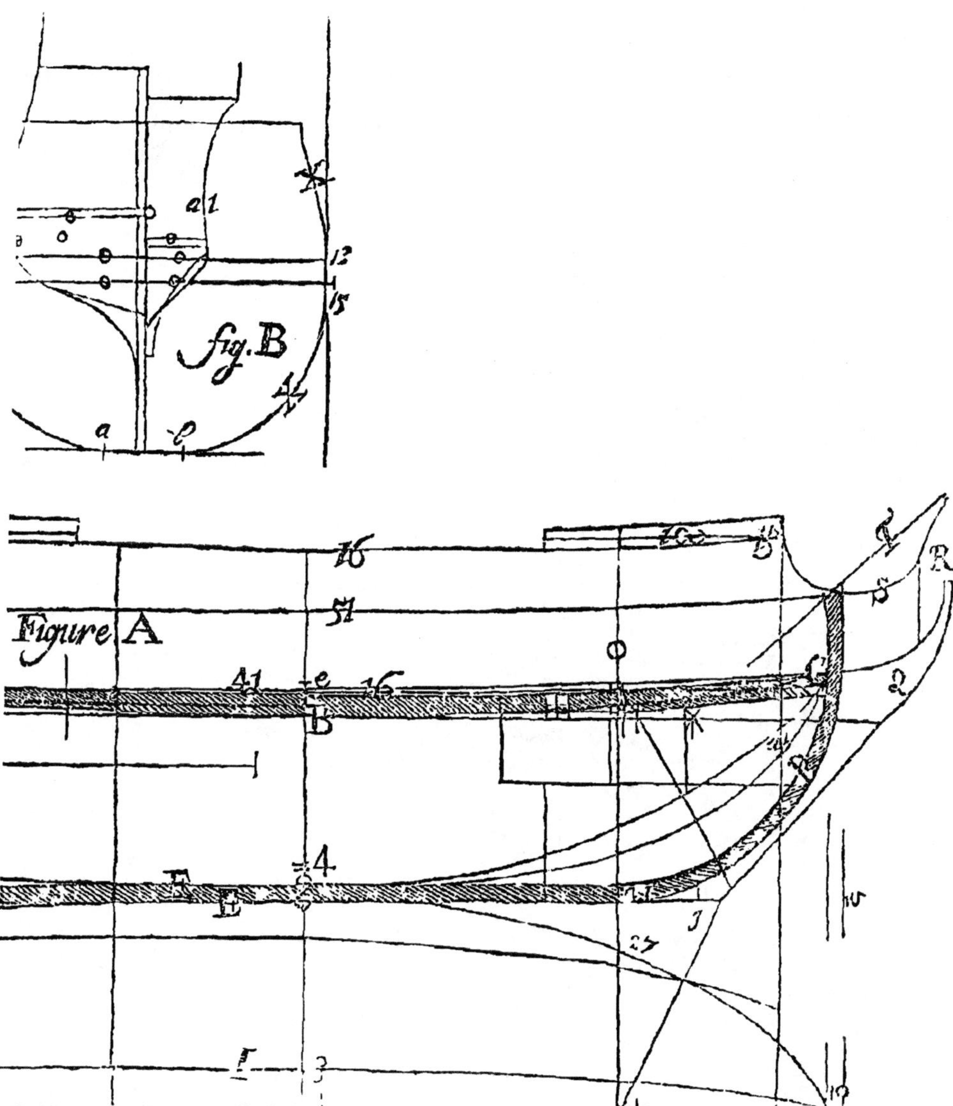
fig. B
Figure A

An Index to the Parts of the Fifth Size

a. 2. Length of the Keel from the back of the Post to the touch of the Stem
f 1. Ditto from the back of the false Post, to the extream forepart of the Keel or Tread.
10, 11 From the fore side of the Rabbit of the Post, to the aft-side of the Rabbit of the Stem, for the length on the Gun-deck measured there.

Fig B. 12, 13. Breadth of the Ship's Timber from Out to Out, in the Mid ships, (term'd) Moulded.
14, 15. Extream breadth from Out to Out of Plank, allowed in Measure.
e. 4. From the Limber-board to the upper Edge of the Gundeck beam, in the Midships, term'd the Depth in Hold, and formerly allowed in Measure.
3. 1. Half breadth of Floor in the Midships
L I K Narrowing of the Floor Line
L ϴ K. Narrowing of the Breadth Line.
D C ϴ. Rising Line, being Similar thereto
B C D. Rising of the Breadth Line.
H E. Narrowing of the Breadth aft with a broad Stern.
H L. Breadth of the Transum within the Plank
N H. Narrowing of the Floor Line with a broad Stern, breadthens as the Line, N H And in such a Position the Narrowing of the breadth Line may be prolong'd to M.
w a ⅓ of the Breadth set back from w to a for the Rake of the Stem allowed in measuring the Tunnage of any Ship
C. 16. 15. Sheering-line, or the Line, of the upper breadth, from whence the sweep of the Top-timber commences
Lower Gun Deck 41, upper ditto 61, Quarter Deck 81, Forecastle ditto 10…, all which Decks ought to lye Parallel one from another, and the greatest Perpendicular height (need not be) between any two of them, above 5 Foot 8 Inches at the side.
R The Lyon, or Figure of the Head.
Q Knee of the Head or Cut Water
S. Upper Rail of the Head
T. The Steaving of the Bowsprit or Angle makes with the Stem.
5 The Partners, or step of the Bowsprit
P. The Stem in two Pieces
O 1. Depth of the Keel abaft, proposed to raise the Sheer, and to have less Dead Wood, and better fastning
3 The Foremost part of the Stern-post
16. z. The corner Side Timber of the upright of the Stern.

Figure B x x x x. The Middle Bend of Timbers
A z. The Fore Castle, where are Cabbins for the Carpenter, Boatswain, and Cook.
B z The Furnaces for boiling Seamens Provisions, and, a small Apartment
C z. For dressing Officers Provisions.
D. z Apartments for Boatswains and Carpenters Stores.
F. z Ditto for the Powder, and for the Gunners Stores.
E. z. A filling Room to empty the Powder out of the Barrels into Cartridges; also Chests and Troughs, and Lanthorn fix'd to hold a Candle.
H. z The place of the Jeer, Capstand
I z. The Slop Room, to hold Seamens Slop-cloths
K z L z. Captain's Store Rooms, with the Purser's and the Surgeon's Cabbins.

M. 7.

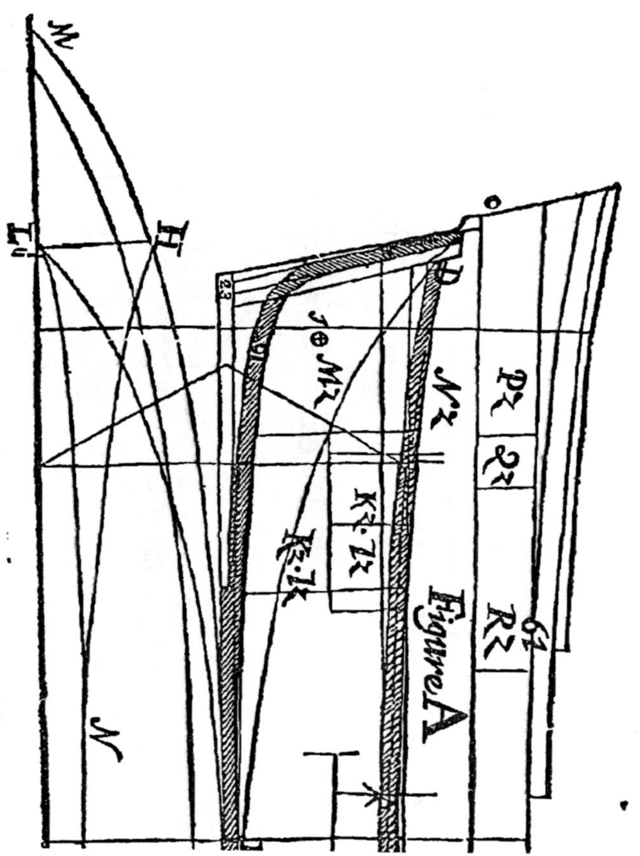
Figure A
P
Q
R
N
M
K·L
H
N
M
L
D
61
23

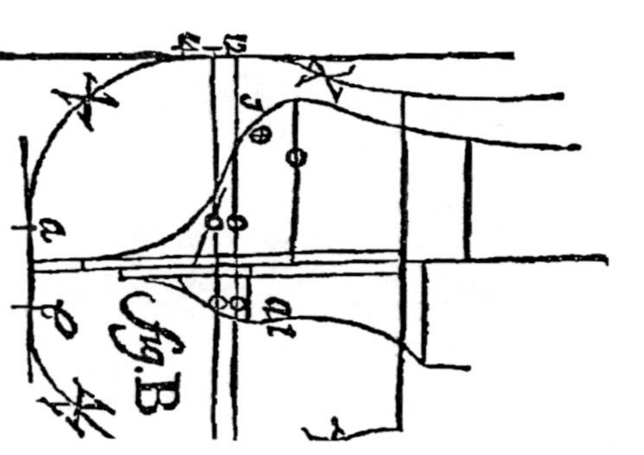
fig. B
a
e
12
14

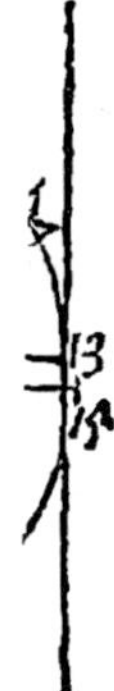

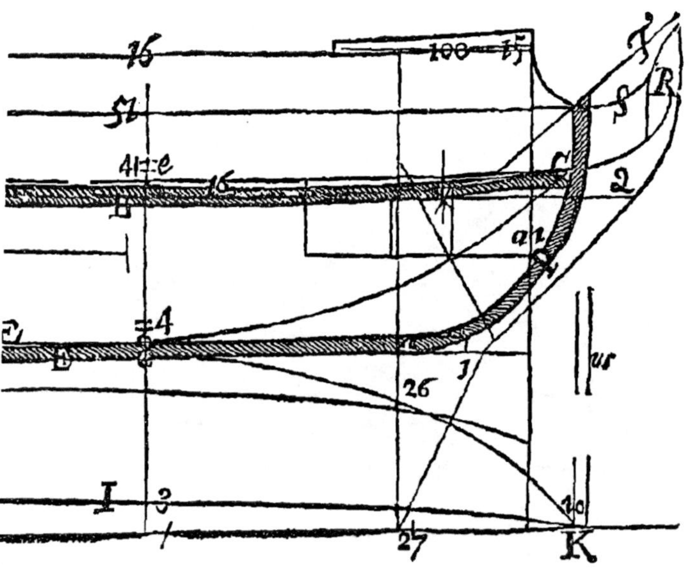
16
100
15
52
41=e
C
2
Q
4
26
10
I
3
27
K

M. z The Bread Room.
K. z Fish Room and Captain's Store Room, if any
N. z Gunners, and Gunners Mate's Cabbin. Gun Room.
P. z The great Cabbin.
R. z. Steeridge.

A Proportion for the Parts of the Fifth Size

	Feet	Inc.
Length of the Keel 2 *a* from the Touch of the Stem to the back of the main Post	89	0
Height from the top of the Keel to the top of the Plansheer in the Midships	23	0
Rake of the main Post to the top of the Plansheer aft,	6	5
Stern to project and lay Parallel from the main Post aloft	1	2
Breadth at the Fashion pieces, at the Wing-transum, from inside of Plank	16	8
Breadth extream afore, at ½ of the Load Mark Line Divided between the inside of the Rabbits, 27, 26.	19	4
Draught of Water loaded { aft	12	10
Draught of Water loaded { afore	12	0
Rake of the Stem from the touch to the outside aloft,	17	0
Figure B. Breadth of the Floor *a b*.	5	0

This Ship may be esteem'd to be worth *per* Tun building 6 *l.* 19 *s.*
What Guns, as to number according to the Establishment, 34
What Men accordingly, 135.

An Index to the Parts of the Sixth Size.

a. 2 Length of the Keel from the back of the Post to the touch of the Stem.

f. 1 Ditto from the back of the false Post, to the extream forepart of the Keel or Tread

10, 11 From the fore side of the Rabbit of the Post, to the aft side of the Rabbit of the Stem, for the length on the lower Gun-deck measured there.

Fig B 12, 13 Breadth of the Ship's Timber from Out to Out, in the Midship, (term'd) Moulded

14, 15. Extream breadth from Out to Out of Plank, allowed in Measure.

e. 4. From the Limber-board to the upper Edge of the Deck beam, in the Midships, term'd the Depth in Hold, and formerly allowed in Measure

3. 1 Half breadth of Floor in the Midships

L I K Narrowing of the Floor Line

L ⊖ K Narrowing of the Breadth Line.

D C ⊖ Rising Line, being Similar thereto.

B C D Rising of the Breadth Line.

H E. Narrowing of the Breadth aft with a broad Stern

H L Breadth of the Transum within the Plank.

N H. Narrowing of the Floor Line with a broad Stern, breadthens as the Line, N H And in such a Position the Narrowing of the breadth Line may be prolong'd to M

w a. ½ of the Breadth set back from *w* to *a* for the Rake of the Stem allowed in measuring the Tunnage of a Ship

C. 16. 15 Sheering-line, or the Line, of the upper breadth, from whence the sweep of the Top-timber commences

Main Deck 41, Quarter Deck 61, Forecastle Deck 71, all which Decks ought to lay Parallel to each another, and the greatest Perpendicular height need not be above 5 Foot 6 Inches at the side, between any two of them.

R. The Lyon, or Figure of the Head.

Q. Knee

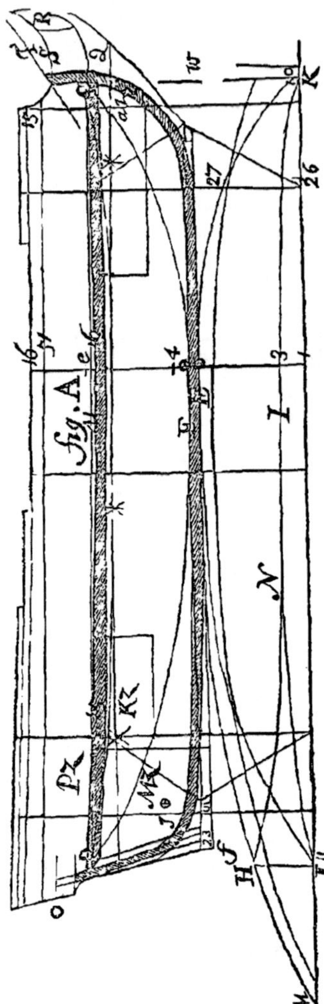

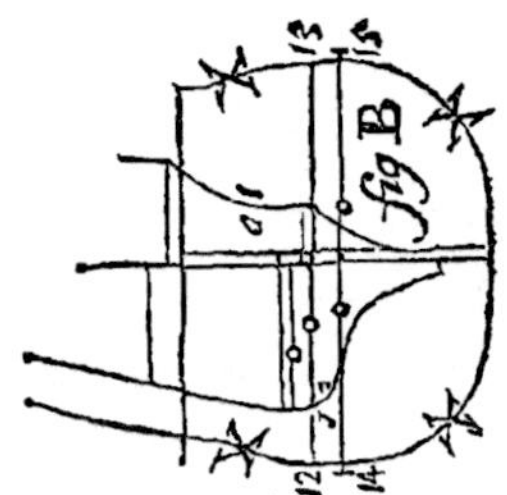

Q Knee of the Head or Cut Water.

S. Upper Rail of the Head.

T The Steaving, or the Angle, the Bowſprit makes with the Stem.

5. The Partners, or ſtirrup, for the Heel of the Bowſprit.

P. The Stem in two Pieces.

O 1. Depth of the Keel abaft, propoſed to raiſe the Sheer, and to have leſs Dead Wood, and better faſtning

3 The Foremoſt part of the Stern-poſt.

16 z The corner Side Timber of the upright of the Stern.

Figure B x x x x. The Midſhip Bend of Timbers

A z. The Fore Caſtle, where are Cabbins for the Cooks, and Proviſion to dreſs Victuals, or between Decks in this Ship.

B z Apartments for the Carpenters and Boatſwains Stores, as alſo for their Lodgings

C z An Apartment for the Gunners Stores and Powder, with all Conveniencies to empty and fill the Cartridges

H. z Place of the Capſtand

I z. Captain's Store Room, Purſer's Cabbin and Slop Room, Surgeon's Cabbin.

M z The Bread Room.

K z Fiſh Room, Gunner's Cabbin.

P. z Great Cabbin, Lieutenant's Cabbin.

A Proportion for the Parts of the Sixth Size.

	Feet	Inc.
Length of the Keel 2. *a* from the Touch of the Stem to the back of the main Post	79	0
Height from the top of the Keel, to the top of the Plansheer in the Midships.	18	0
Rake of the main Post to the top of the Plansheer	5	10
Stern to project and lay Parallel from the main Post aloft	1	0
Breadth at the Fashion-pieces, at the Wing-transum, from the inside of Plank	13	0
Breadth extream afore, at $\frac{1}{7}$ of the Load Mark Line Divided between the Rabbit of the Stem and Post. } 27, 26	16	10
Draught of Water loaded { afore	9	6
Draught of Water loaded { abaft	10	0
Rake of the Stem from the Touch to the outside aloft	10	5
Breadth of the Floor	4	
This Ship may be esteem'd to be worth *per* Tun building 6 *l.* 4 *s.*		
What Guns, as to number according to the Establishment, 24.		
What Men accordingly, 85.		

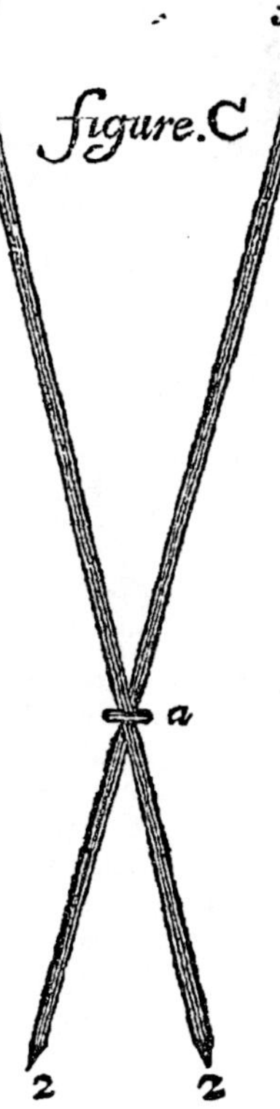

Figure C. is the form of an Instrument called Proportional Compasses, by the help of which you may draw the Draught of any of these Ships mentioned in this Book, to any Size you please. At *a.* is a sliding Collar, by moving of which you extend the Legs 1 2, 1 2, to any Distance. This Instrument, and all others of the finest Sort, are Made and Sold by Mr. *John Rowley*, His Majesty's Master of Mechanicks, and Instrument Maker, Living in *Johnson's Court* in *Fleet-street, London.*

The next Consideration is to the scantling of the Parts, or a general Proportion, for every particular Ship, may be found from the Cube of the Tunnage, provided they were to be proportion'd as 8 to 1. But if, as Sir *William Petty* says, as 16 to 1, then the Square Root of the Tunnage will gain a Proportion.

However

However, I shall proceed in the following Method, that is to say, to draw a Proportion from the Cube of the Tunnage, only with such a Caution from a long Experience in the Practick part, that several Over-launching, Scarphing parts will not be of sufficient strength to be so reduc'd, and several other pieces in the Ship will not require such strength. According to a Cubical Proportion I shall therefore shew, what will, and what will not, with such a Distinction as may be proper to shew the difference, C standing for what is reduc'd by the Cube Root, and E for what is done by Experience

Tun	*Cube Root*		*Square Root*	
1814	12	[illegible]	42	$\frac{6}{10}$
1338	11	3	38	
1064	10	[illegible]	32	3
677	8	8	26	
392	7	[illegible]	19	8
250	6	3	15	8

Then first I shall draw a Parallel between the biggest and the smallest Ship, and say, As the Cube of one is to Cube of the other, so is the Scantling of one to the Scantling of the other, observing that the great Ship's Scantling is sufficiently strong

Inches — *Feet*

Great Ship's / Small Ship's } Floor Timber is { 16 and 14 / 8 and 6 $\frac{1}{2}$ } Bigness { 24 / 12 } Long { 224 / 50 }

Square Root of { 224 / 50 } is { 15 [illegible] / 7 [illegible] } = 1728 by { 224 / 50 } is { 7 & [illegible] / 34 & [illegible] } makes a Foot { 24 / 12 } multiply

by { 12 / 12 } is { 68 / 144 } *Inches* Divide by { 77 / 345 } it's { 374 / 42 } Each Content in Feet

So that such a large Ship is to a small one near as 8 to 1 Now to try the Proportion by the Square Root, and make it as 1 to 16, proceed thus

Square Root { of the large Ship is 42 [illegible] / of the small one is 15 [illegible] } Floor Timber 15 Inches square

Then say if 44 [illegible] gives 15, what shall 15 8 give? And it gives 5 $\frac{6}{10}$ Divide 1728 by 31 2, its 55 Inches [illegible], goes to make 1 Foot, which divide 144, its 2 Feet $\frac{6}{10}$, the Content of the small Ships Floor Timber, according to the Square Root of the Tunnage, which is near as 1 to 16, and may be a general Rule

The Number of Rooms and Spaces in the large Ship is 50, that is 50 Floor Timbers, and 50 Foot-hooks, and in a small Ship, there is 40 of each

	Feet	*Inch*		
Great Ships Room and Space is	2	10	Length of Keel is	142
Small Ships Room and Space is	2	0		80

Now if a Small Ship was to have an equal Number of Timbers to a Great Ship, which is 100, and to be of the abovesaid Scantling, then they would be in a Proportion as 1 to 16. Now 100 multiplied by 12 is 1200, and divided by 56 is 21 $\frac{4}{10}$, for Room and Space But since Timber over small, cannot have sufficient fastning, it may be reasonable to allow, that in the room of 100 of 5 Inches [illegible] Square, there may be 80 of 7 Inches $\frac{1}{10}$ Square, which will be near equal, so that then the Room and Space will be 3 Feet $\frac{3}{10}$ of an Inch, which will be 8 Inches Timber fore and aft, and 10 Inches $\frac{1}{10}$ Space between every Timber, and the Proportion will then be near as 1 to 16 to a great Ship: But to proceed to the general Scantling, from as aforesaid

Scantling, Mould, *or* Meaſure *of the Parts (either as to Le*
what has been ſaid) any other

Keel To be of Elm, not in more pieces than 5
Squar'd in the Midſhips
Each Scarph to be in Length
And bolted with a Bolt of the Diameter of 8
Falſe Keel And to be Sheath'd with a Falſe Keel of Elm in thickneſs
Taper'd at the after-end Thwart-ſhips
Stem To be of Oak, not in more pieces than 3
Breadth fore and aft
Thwartſhips
Length
Falſe Stem, Breadth
Thickneſs
Stern Poſt To be of Oak, in Length
Fore and aft } at the Head
Thwartſhips } at the Head
Fore and aft upon the Keel
Falſe Stern Poſts, { that within ſide, fore and aft allow
{ that without ſide ditto
Faſhion Pieces, Sided
Tranſums, the Wing, and that under the Deck to be ſided
thoſe below the Deck ſided
Space common between them is
Knees, of every Whole Tranſum to be ſided
The Wing Tranſum to have a long Arm fore and aft
Space, of Timber and Room
Floor, Timbers ſided
Up and down on the Keel
In and out at the Floor Head
Length
Foot-Hooks, number of Tires 4
Thickneſs in and out at the Breadth
Scarph at leaſt
Length
To be ſhort of the Keel
Top-timbers Length
Fore and aft } at the Head
In and out } at the Head
Every other Floor Timber to be bolted through the Keel with a Bolt of Diameter
Hawſe pieces, to be in number 4, in breadth
In the Hold { *Keelſon* of Oak, ſcor'd on the Floor Timbers
Thwartſhips
Up and down
Number of thick Strakes on each ſide the Wrung Heads, 9
Thick Strakes, or by ſome term'd Sleepers, middle one in thickneſs
Extreams in thickneſs
Each in Breadth
Two Strakes of middle Bands in thickneſs, (or Orlop Clamps)
One Strake next the Limber boards
Clamps of the Lower Gun-deck, two Strakes in thickneſs

B.

…adth, or Depth) *of Six several Siz'd Ships, by which (only observing* …*ell's Scantling may be found.*

…nage of the …Siz'd Ship is 800 Tuns		Tunnage of the Second Siz'd Ship is 1400 Tuns			Tunnage of the Third Siz'd Ship is 1000 Tuns			Tunnage of the Fourth Siz'd Ship is 600 Tuns			Tunnage of the Fifth Siz'd Ship is 400 Tuns			Tunnage of the Sixth Siz'd Ship is 250 Tuns		
Feet	Inches	Character	Feet	Inches	Character	Feet	Inches	Character	Feet	Inches	Character	Feet	Inches	Character	Feet	Inches
all		E 5			E 4			E 3			E 3			E 3		
1	7 1/2	C	1	6 8/10	C	1	4 7/10	C	1	2	E	1	0	E	0	11
5	8	C	5	3	C	4	9	C	4	1	E	3	10	E	3	4
0	1 1/4	C	0	1 1/10	E	0	1 1/8	E	0	1	F	0	0 1/8	E	0	[illegible]
0	4 1/2	C	0	4 7/10	E	0	4	C	0	3 3/8	E	0	3	F	0	3
1	1	C	1	0 [illegible]	C	0	10 7/10	C	0	9 9/10	E	0	8 1/2	E	0	7 1/2
		E 3			E 3			E 2			E 2			E 2		
1	9	C	1	8	C	1	5 2/[illegible]	C	1	2 8/10	C	1	4/10	E	0	11
1	7 1/2	E	1	6 2/[illegible]	E	1	4 3/10	E	1	2	E	1	0	E	0	11
47	6		45	6		36	3		32	6		27	0		22	0
2	8	C	2	7	C	2	2 5/10	C	1	10 9/10	C	1	7 1/10	C	1	4 1/10
1	0	C	0	11 5/10	C	0	9 [illegible]	C	0	8 3/10	C	0	7 [illegible]	C	0	6 1/10
31	0		29	2		27	0		22	6		20	0		17	0
2	0 1/[illegible]	C	1	11	C	1	7 8/10	C	1	5 [illegible]	C	1	2 4/10	C	1	3/10
2	2 1/2	C	2	1	E	1	10 1/[illegible]	F	1	7	C	1	2 1/[illegible]	C	1	1/10
2	10	C	2	8	C	2	4	C	2	1 8/[illegible]	C	1	9 5/10	C	1	6 4/10
1	8	C	1	7	C	1	4 4/10	C	1	2	C	0	11 8/[illegible]	C	0	10
1	3	C	1	2 4/10	C	1	0 4/10	C	0	10 [illegible]	C	0	8 9/10	C	0	7 [illegible]
1	0	C	0	11 1/2	C	0	10	E	0	9	F	0	8	E	0	7
1	4	C	1	3 4/[illegible]	C	1	1 2/10	C	0	11 5/10	C	0	9 5/[illegible]	C	0	8 2/[illegible]
1	2	C	1	1 5/10	C	0	11 [illegible]	C	0	10	C	0	8 [illegible]	C	0	7 1/10
1	6	C	1	5 1/10	C	1	3	C	1	0 9/10	C	0	10 9/10	C	0	9 3/[illegible]
1	1	C	1	0 [illegible]	C	0	10 [illegible]	C	0	9 9/10	C	0	8 1/2	C	0	7 1/2
17	6	C	16	9	C	14	6	C	12	6	C	10	4	C	8	10
2	10	E	2	7	E	2	4 6/10	E	2	3	E	2	1	E	2	0
1	3	C	1	2 4/10	C	1	1 2/[illegible]	C	0	11 4/10	C	0	9 1/10	C	0	8 2/10
1	7 1/[illegible]	C	1	6 9/10	C	1	4 2/10	C	1	2 1/[illegible]	C	0	11 8/10	C	0	10
1	2	C	1	1 5/10	C	0	11 [illegible]	C	0	10 1/8	E	0	8	F	0	6
24	0	C	23	0	E	21	0	F	18	0	E	14	4	E	12	0
		E 4			E 3			E 3			E 3			E 2		
0	11	C	0	10 6/10	C	0	9 2/[illegible]	C	0	7 [illegible]	C	0	6 [illegible]	C	0	5 [illegible]
7	11	C	7	6	C	6	5	E	6	1	E	5	2	E	4	7
18	6	C	17	9	E	16	0	F	14	9	E	12	0	F	11	0
1	4	C	1	3 4/10	E	1	3	E	1	2	E	1	1	E	1	0
17	10	C	17	2	E	15	10	E	13	10	E	11	4	E	10	6
1	0	C	0	11 6/10	C	0	9 9/10	C	0	8 4/10	C	0	7 [illegible]	C	0	6 1/10
0	4 1/[illegible]	C	0	4 [illegible]	E	0	3 1/[illegible]	E	0	3	E	0	2	E	0	1 [illegible]
0	1 9/[illegible]	C	0	1 4/10	E	0	1 1/8	E	0	1 1/4	E	0	1 1/[illegible]	F	0	[illegible]
2	10	E 4 C	2	8	E 4 C	2	4	E 4 C	2	1 [illegible]	E 4 C	1	9 5/10	E 4 C	1	6 4/10
0	1 [illegible]	C	0	1 4/10	E	0	1 2/10	E	0	1 1/10	E	0	1	E	0	1
1	9	C	1	8	C	1	5 [illegible]	C	1	3	C	1	0 1/10	C	0	10 [illegible]
1	7	C	1	6 [illegible]	C	1	4 1/[illegible]	C	1	2	C	0	11 [illegible]	C	0	10
		E 8			E 7			E 6			E 5			E 4		
0	9	C	0	8 1/10	C	0	7 5/10	E	0	6	C	0	5 [illegible]	C	0	4 3/[illegible]
0	7	C	0	6 1/2	C	0	5 8/[illegible]	E		4	F	0	4	E	0	2 [illegible]
1	5 1/2	C	1	4	C	1	1 [illegible]	C	1	8/10	E	1	0	E	1	0
0	8	C	0	7 [illegible]	C	0	6 [illegible]	C	0	5 [illegible]	C	0	4 [illegible]	C	0	4
0	8	C	0	7 [illegible]	C	0	6 [illegible]	C	0	5 7/10	C	0	4 1/[illegible]	C	0	4
0	9	C	0	9	C	0	8 [illegible]	E	0	6 [illegible]	C	0	5 [illegible]	C	0	4 [illegible]

I

All the rest of the Foot waleing in thickness — — Breadth — — Breadth — —

Notwithstanding, it's my Opinion (although it has been approved of to have the waleing of divers Scantlings, as to thickness, and the chiefest reason is to have some pro- ing parts for Scoring the Riders, to ease the Bolts in the working of the Ship at Sea, or in a Dock) that the Work will be much Stronger to have every Strake of equal breadth thickness, that the Joints may bear equal one against another, and then one projecting Stra the Wake of a Rider will be sufficient to the Use as aforesaid Only at the Heads and Fe the Timbers to have the Inboard Stuff thicker than in other Places, in consideration of the kening caused by half the Timbers being parted, which may be thicc, and those to ser Joggles for the Riders

Orlope Beams, to be in Number 12 — —
Fore and [illegible] — —
Up and d[illegible] — —
Those Beams under the Store Rooms sided
Up and down — —

Riders, Number of Bends — —
Floor Riders fore and aft — —
On the Kelson up and down — —
In and out at the Extreams — —
Length — —
Bolted in every two Foot or twenty Inches with Bolts in bigness — —

Fookhook Riders, Length of the Scarph upwards and downwards — —
To be fore and aft — —
Up and down — —

Top Riders, — — Fore and aft — —
In and out — —

Crutches aft, in Number 2 — —
Sided — —
Each Arm to be in Length — —

Step of the Main-Mast, — — fore and aft — —
Of the Fore-Mast, Ditto — —
Of the Mizon-Mast, Ditto — —

Breast-hooks to be in Length — —
Depth up and down — —
To fay one under each Deck, and one under the Hawse-holes, and also to fay between the Step of the Fore-mast and lower-deck Breast-hook, 5 — —
To be bolted in every eighteen Inches, with Bolts of Diameter — —

Well, to be built from the Cieling or Foot-walling, to the Orlope, with *English* Oak Plank —

Pillars, under each Beam of the Gun-deck and Orlope squar'd — —
Cross Pillars squar'd — —

Gun-deck Beams to round upwards — —
Fore and aft — —
Up and down — —
Every Beam to be Dove-tail'd into the Clamps two Inches, and double knee'd at each end, each Knee sided — —

Gun-deck Knees, the up and down Arm to be in Length — —
And the other not less than in Length — —
And to be bolted in every sixteen or eighteen Inches space with Bolts of Diameter — —
All the Beams ought to lay one under, and one between each Port, except in the Wake of the Main-hatch-way and Main-mast, where the clear of the Hatch-way shall be Fore and aft —
Hatchway Thwartships — —

Carlings, Number of Tires on each side the middle line 3 — —
In some Places more or less, according to the various tapering of the S
Depth up and down — —
Thwartships — —

Ledges, to lye nine Inches asunder, and to be in Depth — —
Breadth — —

Tunnage of the [fir]st Siz'd Ship [is] 1800 Tun[s]			*Tunnage of the Second Siz'd Ship is 1400 Tuns*			*Tunnage of the Third Siz'd Ship is 1000 Tuns*			*Tunnage of the Fourth Siz'd Ship is 600 Tuns*			*Tunnage of the Fifth Siz'd Ship is 400 Tuns*			*Tunnage of the Sixth Siz'd Ship is 250 Tuns*		
[Charact]ers	Feet	Inches	Character	Feet	Inches	Character	Feet	Inches	Character	Feet	Inches	Character	Feet	Inches	Character	Feet	Inches
E all	1	8	C	1	6	C	1	$3\frac{8}{10}$	E	1	3	E	1	2	E	1	1
	0	6	C	5	$\frac{3}{4}$	E	0	4	E	0	4	E	0	3	E	0	2
	1	4	C	1	$3\frac{1}{2}$	C	1	$1\frac{3}{8}$	C	1	0	E	1	0	E	1	0

First Siz'd Ship (continued)

Feet	Inches
1	6
1	4
1	1
1	0
	9
1	$8\frac{1}{2}$
1	3
1	$4\frac{1}{2}$
23	0
0	$1\frac{9}{10}$
9	0
1	6
1	4
1	3
1	$2\frac{1}{2}$
	2
1	3
7	6
3	1
2	10
1	10
16	0
1	4
	$1\frac{9}{10}$
0	4
0	10
1	1
0	6
1	$6\frac{1}{2}$
1	4
1	0
6	0
4	0
0	$1\frac{3}{4}$
9	3
7	6
0	11
1	2
0	$5\frac{3}{4}$
0	7

Second Siz'd Ship (continued)

Character	Feet	Inches
E 12		
C	1	$5\frac{4}{10}$
C	1	$3\frac{1}{10}$
E	1	0
E	0	11
E 7		
C	1	$7\frac{8}{10}$
C	1	$2\frac{4}{10}$
C	1	$3\frac{9}{10}$
C	22	3
C	0	$1\frac{5}{10}$
C	8	8
C	1	$5\frac{4}{10}$
C	1	$3\frac{1}{10}$
C	1	$2\frac{1}{10}$
C	1	$1\frac{9}{10}$
E 2		
C	1	$2\frac{4}{10}$
C	7	3
C	2	$11\frac{3}{4}$
E	2	8
E	1	$8\frac{1}{2}$
C	15	5
E	1	4
E 4		
C	0	$1\frac{5}{10}$
E	0	4
E	0	$9\frac{1}{10}$
C	1	$\frac{6}{10}$
C	0	$5\frac{3}{4}$
C	1	$5\frac{9}{10}$
C	1	$3\frac{4}{10}$
E	0	11
C	5	10
E	4	0
C	0	$1\frac{3}{10}$
E	8	9
C	7	3
E 3		
C	0	$10\frac{1}{2}$
C	1	$1\frac{5}{10}$
C	0	5
C	0	$6\frac{3}{4}$

Third Siz'd Ship (continued)

Character	Feet	Inches
F 11		
C	1	3
C	1	$1\frac{3}{10}$
E	0	11
E	0	10
E 6		
C	1	$5\frac{1}{10}$
C	1	$\frac{4}{10}$
C	1	$1\frac{7}{10}$
E	20	6
C	0	$1\frac{3}{10}$
E	8	0
C	1	3
C	1	$1\frac{3}{10}$
E 2		
C	1	$\frac{4}{10}$
C	6	3
E {	2	$6\frac{1}{2}$
	2	2
	1	7
E	14	0
C	1	$2\frac{1}{10}$
E 4		
C	0	$1\frac{3}{10}$
E	0	$3\frac{1}{2}$
C	0	$8\frac{1}{10}$
C	0	$10\frac{9}{10}$
C	0	$5\frac{1}{4}$
C	1	$3\frac{4}{10}$
C	1	1
E	0	10
C	5	8
C	3	9
C	0	$1\frac{1}{10}$
E	8	3
E	6	6
E 2		
C	0	9
C	0	$11\frac{6}{10}$
C	0	$4\frac{7}{10}$
C	0	$5\frac{8}{10}$

Fourth Siz'd Ship (continued)

Character	Feet	Inches
E 8		
C	1	1
C	0	11
E	0	9
E	0	8
E 5		
C	1	$2\frac{9}{10}$
C	0	$10\frac{7}{10}$
C	0	$11\frac{6}{10}$
E	17	6
E	0	$1\frac{3}{10}$
E	7	6
C	1	1
C	0	$11\frac{5}{10}$
E 2		
C	0	$10\frac{7}{10}$
C	5	5
C E {	2	$2\frac{1}{4}$
	2	
	1	$4\frac{1}{4}$
E	13	0
C	1	$\frac{3}{10}$
E 4		
C	0	$1\frac{3}{10}$
C	0	$2\frac{15}{40}$
C	0	$7\frac{2}{10}$
C	0	5
C	1	$1\frac{1}{10}$
C	0	$11\frac{5}{10}$
E	0	9
E	5	4
F	3	9
E	0	$1\frac{1}{10}$
E	7	9
E	6	0
E 2		
C	0	$7\frac{8}{10}$
C	0	10
C	0	$4\frac{3}{4}$
C	0	5

Fifth Siz'd Ship (continued)

Character	Feet	Inches
E 5		
C	0	$10\frac{9}{10}$
C	0	$9\frac{6}{10}$
E	0	8
E	0	7
E 4		
C	1	$\frac{4}{10}$
C	0	$8\frac{9}{10}$
C	0	10
C	13	11
E	0	$1\frac{1}{10}$
E	7	0
C	0	11
C	0	$9\frac{6}{10}$
E 2		
C	0	$9\frac{1}{10}$
E	4	10
E {	1	$9\frac{1}{2}$
	1	$6\frac{1}{2}$
	1	$1\frac{1}{2}$
E	12	0
C	0	$10\frac{3}{10}$
E 3		
C	0	$1\frac{1}{10}$
C	0	$2\frac{4}{10}$
C	0	6
C	0	$4\frac{7}{10}$
C	0	$11\frac{2}{10}$
C	0	$9\frac{6}{10}$
E	0	$7\frac{1}{2}$
E	4	10
E	3	8
F	0	1
E	7	3
E	5	6
E 2		
C	0	$6\frac{5}{10}$
C	0	$8\frac{4}{10}$
C	0	$3\frac{15}{40}$
C	0	$4\frac{2}{10}$

Sixth Siz'd Ship (continued)

Character	Feet	Inches
E 4		
C	0	$9\frac{6}{10}$
E	0	7
E	0	$6\frac{1}{2}$
E	0	$5\frac{1}{2}$
E 3		
C	0	$10\frac{4}{10}$
C	0	$7\frac{6}{10}$
C	0	$8\frac{4}{10}$
E	13	0
E	0	$\frac{7}{10}$
E 2		
	0	$7\frac{1}{10}$
E	4	6
E {	1	6
	1	3
	0	11
E	11	0
C	0	$8\frac{5}{10}$
E 3		
C	0	$\frac{7}{10}$
C	0	2
C	0	5
E	0	$5\frac{1}{2}$
C	0	$9\frac{4}{10}$
C	0	8
E	0	$6\frac{1}{2}$
E	4	6
E	3	7
E	0	1
E	6	9
E	5	0
E 2 Fur		
C	0	$5\frac{5}{10}$
C	0	7
C	0	$2\frac{33}{40}$
C	0	$4\frac{4}{10}$

Flat of the Deck to be Oak Plank, in thickness
Ports to be in Number 14
Fore and aft
Up and down
Distance from the upper part of the lower Cell to the Gun-deck Plank
Cable Bit-Pins, the aftermost square at the Head
Foremost pair square at the Head
And to continue that Substance as much below the Deck, as above, for Length
Cross Pieces to be 1 Inch deeper than the square of the Pins here
And to be fore and aft

Partners of the	Main Mast	Thickness
	Fore Mast	
	Mizon Mast	
	Capstan's	

Lead Scuppers, according to conveniency, 28
Of such Lead as goes to the Foot square, 13 pound
Standers, Number on each side 10, — sided
Spirkit-rising, to be in Thickness
Lining between the Spirkit-risings and Clamps of the other Deck, Thickness
Partners of the Bowsprit or Step, Thickness
Main Capstan, Diameter of the Barrel

Middle Deck *Clamps* — Thickness
Beams the Longest to Round
Fore and aft
Up and down
Carlings, — Depth
Thwart-ships
Ledges, — Depth
Fore and aft
Knees sided
Bolts in Bigness
Standers, Number on each side 7 — sided
Plank in Thickness
Ports, — Fore and aft
Up and down
Distance between the Deck, Plank and the Cell
Spirkit-rising in Thickness
Pillars squar'd

Upper Deck. *Clamps*, in Thickness
Beams, the Longest to Round
Fore and aft
Up and down
Carlings, — Depth
Breadth
Ledges, — Depth
Breadth
Knees sided
And Bolted in every 16 Inch space with Bolts, in Diameter
Standers, in Number of each side 3 — sided

Ports	Fore and aft
	Up and down
	Distance, as aforesaid

Plank for the flat Part of Firr, in Thickness
Spirkit-rising, — Thickness
String in the Waste, under the Ports prick'd home to the side, and be in Thickness
And to be left 1 Inch without the *Spirkit-rising*
String above the Ports to be in Thickness
And prick'd ¼ of an Inch about the Timber, or the Timber let into him
Bits for the Topsail Sheets, and Main Jeers, about the Main Mast, squar'd at the He[ad]

Tunnage of the First Siz'd Ship 1800 T.			Tunnage of the Second Siz'd Ship [illegible] 00 Tuns			Tunnage of the Third Sized Ship is 1000 Tuns			Tunnage of the Fourth Siz'd Ship is 600 Tuns			Tunnage of the Fifth Siz'd Ship is 450 Tuns			Tunnage of the Sixth Siz'd Ship is 250 Tuns		
[illegible]	[illegible]	Inch	Character	Feet	Inch	Character	Feet	Inches	Character	Feet	Inches	Character	Feet	Inches	Character	Feet	Inch
E all	0	4	E	0	4	F	0	3	E	0	3	First C	0	2 [illegible]	First C	0	2 [illegible]
			E 13			E 13			E 12			E 6			E 11		
	3	7	C	3	5 1/2	E	3	3	E	2	10	E	2	7	E	2	5
	2	8	C	2	7		2	6		2	4		2	2		2	1
	2	6	C	2	5		2	4		2	1		1	10		1	8 1/2
	1	9	C	1	8 [illegible]	C	1	5 [illegible]	E	1	4	E	1	2	E	1	0
	1	6	C	1	5 [illegible]	C	1	3	C	1	1	C	0	10 [illegible]	C	0	9 [illegible]
	24	6		23	2		22			19	6		15	4		13	6
	2	0	C	1	11 [illegible]	C	1	8	C	1	5 [illegible]	E	1	3	E	1	2
	0	11	C	0	10 [illegible]	C	0	9 [illegible]	C	0	7 [illegible]	E	0	7	E	0	6
	0	10	C	0	9 [illegible]	C	0	8 1/8	C	8	7 [illegible]	E	0	6 [illegible]	E	0	5 [illegible]
	0	8	C	0	7 1/4	C	0	6 [illegible]	C	0	5 [illegible]	C	0	4 [illegible]	C	0	4 1/2
			E 28			E 26			E 20			F 12			E 18		
			Po 12			11 Pou			10 Pou			9 Pou			Wood		
	1	4	L 8 C	1	3 [illegible]	E 6 C	1	1 [illegible]	E 4 C	0	11 [illegible]	E 3 C	0	9 [illegible]	E 2 E	0	8 [illegible]
	0	8	C	0	7 1/4	C	0	6 [illegible]	E	0	4 1/4	E	0	3 1/2	E	0	3
	0	4 [illegible]	C	0	4 [illegible]	C	0	3 [illegible]	C	0	3 1/4	C	0	2 [illegible]		0	2 [illegible]
	0	8 1/2	C	0	8 [illegible]	C	0	7 [illegible]	C	0	6 [illegible]	C	0	5 [illegible]			
	2	10	E	2	7	C	2	4	C	2	[illegible]	E	1	10	E	1	8
	0	8	C	0	7 [illegible]												
	0	9 [illegible]	C	0	9 [illegible]												
	1	3	C	1	3												
	1	1 [illegible]	C	1	1												
	0	9	C	0	8 [illegible]												
	0	10	C	0	9 [illegible]												
	0	5	C	0	4 [illegible]												
	0	5 [illegible]	C	0	5 [illegible]												
	0	9 [illegible]	C	0	[illegible]												
	0	1 [illegible]	C	0	1 [illegible]												
	1	1	E 6 C	1	[illegible]												
	0	3 1/2	C	0	3 [illegible]												
	3	2	C	3	[illegible]												
	2	7	C	2	6												
	2	3	C	2	2												
	0	6 1/2	E	0	5 1/2												
	0	8	E	0	7												
	0	6 1/2	C	0	6	C	0	5 [illegible]	F	0	4	C	0	3 [illegible]	C	0	2 [illegible]
	0	10 1/2	E	0	9 [illegible]	C	0	8 [illegible]	C	0	7 [illegible]	E	0	6 [illegible]	C	0	5 [illegible]
	1	1	C	1	[illegible]	C	0	10 [illegible]	E	0	10 [illegible]	E	0	8 [illegible]	C	0	6 [illegible]
	0	11	C	0	10 [illegible]	C	0	9 [illegible]	E	0	8 [illegible]	C	0	6 [illegible]	C	0	5 [illegible]
	0	7	C	0	6 3/4	C	0	6	C	0	5 [illegible]	C	0	4	C	0	3 [illegible]
	0	8 [illegible]	C	0	8 [illegible]	C	0	7 [illegible]	C	0	6 [illegible]	C	0	5 [illegible]	C	0	4 [illegible]
	0	4	C	0	3 [illegible]	C	0	3 [illegible]	C	0	2 [illegible]	C	0	2 [illegible]	C	0	2 [illegible]
	0	5	C	0	4 [illegible]	C	0	4 [illegible]	C	0	3 [illegible]	C	0	3	C	0	2 [illegible]
	0	7	E	0	6 [illegible]	C	0	6 [illegible]	E	0	6	E	0	5	C	0	3
	0	1 [illegible]	C	0	1	F	0	1	E	0	[illegible]	E	0		C	0	[illegible]
	0	10	E 3 E	0	9	E 3 E	0	9	E 2 C	0	7 [illegible]	E 2 C	0	6 [illegible]	C	0	5 [illegible]
	2	9	C	2	8	E	2	7	E	2	3	E	2	0	F	1	3
	2	6	C	2	5		2	4		2	0		1	10			3
	2	1	C	2	0		1	10		1	6		1	3			0
	0	3	C	0	2 [illegible]	C	0	2 [illegible]	C	0	2 [illegible]	C	0	2	E	0	2
	0	4	C	0	3 [illegible]	E	0	3 [illegible]	E	0	3	E	0	2	E	0	2
	0	8	C	0	7 [illegible]	C	0	6 [illegible]	C	0	5 [illegible]	C	0	4 [illegible]		0	4 [illegible]
	0	4	C	0	3 [illegible]	C	0	3 [illegible]	C	0	2 [illegible]	C	0	2 [illegible]		0	2 [illegible]
	1	0	C	0	11 [illegible]	C	0	10	C	0	8 [illegible]	E	0	8 [illegible]	E	0	7 [illegible]

If the Sixth Rate has any Upper Deck

Tunnage

Long combing *Carlings* — Breadth —
Depth —
Bulkhead *Brackets* of the Steerage and Forecastle Bulkhead — sided —

Forecastle and Quarter-deck *Clamps* of Oak — Thickness —
Breadth according to the Distance between the Deck and the Ports
String in the Wake of the Great Cabbin of Elm, into which the Beams are to be Dove-tail'd, and the *String* Bolted in every 16 Inches space, with Bolts, in Diameter —
String { Thickness —
Depth —
Beams, the Longest to Round —
Fore and aft } to lay 2 Foot, or 2 Foot 6 Inches asunder { —
Up and down } —
Knees — sided —
Bolts in Diameter —
Plank of the Deck, in Thickness —
Ports { Up and down —
Fore and aft —
Distance from the Deck to the Cell —
Spirket-rising, in Thickness —
Bits for the Fore Topsail Sheets, and Fore Jeers, about the Fore Mast, squar'd —
Cat-heads squar'd, or 2 Inches bigger fore and aft, for the Shivers, up and down —
To steave in every Foot —
Length without the Side, according to the various Flairing of the Bow, but as custo[m]

Poop *Beams* to lay asunder, 2 Foot the Longest to Round —
Fore and aft —
Up and down —
Ports, Fore and aft, and up and down, equal —
Distance from the Deck to the Cell —

Out-Board Work *Plank* wrought in the Bottom — Thickness —
To well fasten with Trenels of the Diameter
Plank wrought at the Breadth, about the Wales —
At the Top-timber Head —
Lower Wale, to be in Breadth up and down —
Thickness in and out —
Upper Wale, to be in Breadth up and down —
Thickness in and out —
Chain Wale, Lower — Depth —
Thickness —
Chain Wale, Upper — Depth —
Thickness —

Channels { *Main* { Length —
Breadth { at the after end —
at the foremost end —
Thickness —
Number of Shrouds, 9 —
Fore { Length —
Breadth { at the after end —
at the foremost end —
Thickness —
Number of Shrouds, 8 —
Mizon { Length —
Breadth { at the after end —
at the foremost end —
Thickness —
Number of Shrouds, 6 —

Sheering Rail, at the Gunnel, Depth —
The *Tire of Brackets* next above the Counter, sided —
Quarter Piece —

…nage of the …t Siz'd Ship is …800 Tuns			Tunnage of the Second Siz'd Ship is 1400 Tuns			Tunnage of the Third Sized Ship is 1000 Tuns			Tunnage of the Fourth Siz'd Ship is 600 Tuns			Tunnage of the Fifth Siz'd Ship is 400 Tuns			Tunnage of the Sixth Siz'd Ship is 250 Tuns		
…cter	Feet	Inches	Character	Feet	Inches	Character	Feet	Inches	Character	Feet	Inches	Character	Feet	Inches	Character	Feet	Inches
all	1	2	C	1	1 5/8	C	0	11 7/8	C	0	10 1/2	C	0	8 5/8	E	0	8
	1	0	C	0	11 6/8	C	0	10	C	0	8 1/8	C	0	7 5/8	F	0	7
	0	11	C	0	10 6/8	C	0	9 2/8	C	0	7 [illegible]	C	0	6 [illegible]	C	0	5 1/2
	0	4	E	0	4	E	0	3 1/4	E	0	3	I	0	2 1/4	E	0	2
	0	1 1/8	E	0	1	E	0	1	E	0	5/8	E	0	[illegible]	E	0	[illegible]
	0	8 1/2	C	0	8 2/8	C	0	7 [illegible]	E	0	6 1/2	E	0	6	E	0	5
	1	0	C	0	11 [illegible]	C	0	10	E	0	10	E	0	10	E	0	10
	1	0	C	0	11 6/8	E	0	9 1/2	E	0	8 1/4	E	0	7 1/4	L	0	6
	0	10	I	0	9	C	0	8 3/8	C	0	7 2/8	C	0	6	(	0	5 1/4
	0	8	E	0	7	C	0	6 [illegible]	C	0	5 [illegible]	C	0	4 [illegible]	C	0	4
	0	6 [illegible]	C	0	6 2/8	E	0	6 2/8	F	0	5	C	0	4 5/8	(	0	3 [illegible]
	0	0 [illegible]	C	0	[illegible]	F	0	[illegible]	E	0	[illegible]	F	0	0 [illegible]	E	0	[illegible]
	0	2 [illegible]	E	0	2 1/2	E	0	2	F	0	2	E	0	2	E	0	2
	2	1	C	2	0	C	1	8 1/4	E	1	6 1/2	E	1	4		1	3
	2	3	C	2	2	C	1	10	E	1	6 1/2	F	1	4	E	1	3
	1	4	C	1	3 4/8	E	1	3 1/4	E	1	2 1/2	E	1	1 1/2	(	1	0
	0	3	E	0	3	E	0	3	Firr C	0	2 [illegible]	Firr C	0	2 4/8	Firr (	0	2
	0	10	L	0	10	C	0	9 4/8	C	0	8 1/2	C	0	6 [illegible]	C	0	5 [illegible]
	1	3 [illegible]	C	1	3	C	1	1 [illegible]	C	0	11 [illegible]	C	0	10	(	0	8 [illegible]
	0	2 [illegible]	E	0	2 1/2	F	0	2 [illegible]	E	0	2 1/2	F	0	2 1/2	E	0	2 [illegible]
	6	0	E	5	9	E	5	0	E	4	4	E	3	8	E	3	0
	1	2	C	1	1	C	0	10 [illegible]	C	0	8 [illegible]	C	0	7 [illegible]			
	0	7	C	0	6 3/4	C	0	6 [illegible]	C	0	5 [illegible]	C	0	3 4/8			
	0	5 [illegible]	C	0	5 3/8	C	0	5 1/8	C	0	3 [illegible]	C	0	3 5/8			
	1	9	C	1	8	C	1	7									
	1	1	C	1	[illegible]	C	1	0									
	0	4	C	0	4 3/8	C	0	4	C	0	3 1/2	C	0	2 5/8	C	0	2
		2			1 [illegible]			1 7/8			1 [illegible]			1 5/8			1 [illegible]
	0	8	C	0	8 [illegible]	C	0	7 [illegible]	E	0	4	E	0	4	E	0	3 [illegible]
	0	3	C	0	2 [illegible]	C	0	2 [illegible]	E	0	2	C	0	1 3/4	C	0	1 [illegible]
	1	7	C	1	6 [illegible]	C	1	4 [illegible]	C	1	2	C	0	11 [illegible]	C	0	10
	1	[illegible]	C	1	0	C	0	10	E	0	8	C	0	7 [illegible]	F	0	5 [illegible]
	1	4 [illegible]	C	1	3 [illegible]	C	1	1 [illegible]	C	0	11 [illegible]	C	0	10	C	0	8 [illegible]
	0	11	C	0	11 [illegible]	C	0	9 [illegible]	E	0	7 1/4	F	0	6 [illegible]	I	0	5 [illegible]
	1	0	C	0	11 [illegible]	C	0	10 [illegible]	E	0	9	E	0	8 [illegible]	E	0	7 [illegible]
	0	6	C	0	6 [illegible]	C	0	5 [illegible]		0	4		0	4		0	3 [illegible]
	0	11	C	0	10 [illegible]	C	0	9 [illegible]	E	0	8	E	0	8	E	0	7
	0	6 [illegible]	C	0	5 [illegible]	C	0	5		0	4 [illegible]		0	3 [illegible]		0	3 1/2
	34	0	C	33		C	28	6	C	24	6	C	20	6	E	0	17
	2	8		2	6		2	1	E	1	11	E	1	8	E	1	4
	2	6 [illegible]		2	4 [illegible]		2	0	F	1	10	E	1	7	E	1	4
	0	7	C	0	6 [illegible]	C	0	5 [illegible]	C	0	5 [illegible]	C	0	4 [illegible]	C	0	3 [illegible]
			No 9			No 8			No. 7			No 6			No 5		
	26	0	C	25	0	C	21	9	C	18	10	C	15	10	C	14	0
	2	6 1/2		2	4		2	0	E	1	10	E	1	6	E	1	2
	3	1 [illegible]		2	10		2	4	E	2	2	F	1	10	E	1	7
	0	6	C	0	5 [illegible]	C	0	4 [illegible]	C	0	4 [illegible]	C	0	3 [illegible]	C	0	3 [illegible]
			No. 8			No 7			No 6			No 5			No 4		
	16	0	C	15	6	C	13	6	C	11	8	C	9	9 1/2	C	8	4
	1	7		1	6		1	3 1/4	E	1	2	E	1	0	E	0	10
	1	7		1	6		1	3 [illegible]	F	1	2	E	1	0	E	0	10
	0	4	C	0	3 [illegible]	C	0	3	C	0	2 [illegible]	C	0	2 [illegible]	C	0	2 [illegible]
			No 6			No 5			No 4			No 3			No 3		
	0	7	(	0	6	(	0	5	C	0	5 [illegible]	F	0	5	E	0	4 [illegible]
	1	5	C	1	4 [illegible]	(	1	2 [illegible]	C	1		C	0	10 [illegible]	C	0	8
	2	0	C	1	11	(	1	8 [illegible]	C	1	6	C	1	3	C	1	[illegible]

Gallery Brackets, sided at the lower Tire of Lights ———
Rudder { fore and aft at the Head ———
{ Thwart-ships ditto ———
Fore and aft allow ———
Number of *Braces*, or *Rudder Irons*, 8 ———
Term Pieces, or *Drift Pieces*, ——— sided ———
Counter Rail to Round Upwards, on the flat of the Stern ———
Outward Rounding ———
Depth ———
Head Length afore the Stem ———
Lower Check, sided ———
Great or *Upper Rail*, at the after end, besides the Plansheer, fore and aft———
Bracket against the *Stem*——— sided———

Tunnage of the First Siz'd Ship is 1800 Tuns			*Tunnage of the Second Siz'd Ship is 1400 Tuns*			*Tunnage of the Third Siz'd Ship is 1000 Tuns*			*Tunnage of the Fourth Siz'd Ship is 600 Tuns*			*Tunnage of the Fifth Siz'd Ship is 400 Tuns*			*Tunnage of the Sixth Siz'd Ship is 250 Tuns*		
Character	Feet	Inches	Character	Feet	Inches	Character	Feet	Inches	Character	Feet	Inches	Character	Feet	Inches	Character	Feet	Inches
E all	1	0	C	0	11 7/10	C	0	10 [illegible]	C	0	8 [illegible]	C	0	7 7/10			
	2	3	C	2	2	C	1	10 1/2	C	1	7 1/10	C	1	4 [illegible]	C	1	1 9/10
	1	11	C	1	9 1/10	C	1	6 6/10	C	1	4	C	1	1 3/10	C	0	11 4/8
	5	9	E	5	4 3/4		4	9 1/2		4	1		3	4 3/4		3	1/2
			E 7			E 6			E 6			E 5			E 5		
	1	1 1/2	C	1	1	C	0	11 3/10	C	0	9 8/10	C	0	8 [illegible]	C	0	6 9/10
	1	1	C	1	[illegible]	C	0	10 8/10	C	0	9 1/10	C	0	7 8/10	C	0	6 1/2 3/10
	0	10	C	0	9 13/20	C	0	8 7/10	C	0	7 5/10	C	0	6 5/20	C	0	5 11/20
	1	3	C	1	2 5/10	C	1	5/10	C	0	10 8/10	C	0	9	C	0	7 7/10
	17	2	E	16	1	E	12	3	E	10	7	E	8	10	E	6	5
	1	1	C	1	5/10	C	0	10 8/10	C	0	9 7/20	C	0	7 8/10	C	0	6 1/2 3/10
	1	3	C	1	2 5/10	C	1	5/10	C	0	10 8/10	C	0	9	C	0	7 7/10
	1	4	C	1	3 5/10	C	1	1 4/10	C	0	11 6/10	C	0	9 7/10	C	0	8 1/4

In the next Place, I ſhall ſet down the Meaſure of the *Maſts*, *Yards*, *Tops*, *Caps*, *Truſletrees* and *Stumps*, proper and ſizable, for any Ship from 46 Foot broad to 20 Foot broad: And ſhall alſo diſtinguiſh what will bear to be Reduc'd by a Cubical Proportion, and what is drawn from Experience: Obſerving, That whatever Member is Mark'd with a C. (for Cubical), either in the preceeding Scantling of *Ships Frames*, or in the following Table of *Maſting*, comes ſo near to the Experimental Rules, that it will be very hard to define, whether they are alter'd for the better, or for the worſe.

A TABLE

A TABLE of Masting, &c. for Fourteen Sizes of Shipping, of those

Breadth	46 Foot broad		44 Foot broad		42 Foot broad		40 Foot broad	
	Foot	Inches	Foot	Inches	Foot	Inches	Foot	Inches
Length Gun-deck	170	0	165	0	156	6	150	0
Breadth Extream	46	0	44	0	42	0	40	0
Depth in Hold	18	6	18	0	17	8	16	10
Height Gun-deck	6	10	6	10	6	10	6	10
Height Middle Deck	7	0	7	0	6	10		
Height in the Waste	4	9	4	8½	4	8	5	2

		Chara.	Masts Long Feet Inc	Masts Dia Inches	Yards Long Feet Inc	Yards Dia Inches	Chara.	Masts Long Feet Inc	Masts Dia Inches	Yards Long Feet Inc	Yards Dia Inches	Chara.	Masts Long Feet Inc	Masts Dia Inches	Yards Long Feet Inc	Yards Dia Inches	Chara.	Masts Long Feet Inc	Masts Dia Inches	Yards Long Feet Inc
Bowsprit	Mast	C	75	35	63	14		71	34	60	13½		68	31	57	12½	C	64 6	30	5[illegible]
	Head		6 2	8				5 8	7½				5 2	7				5 0	6½	
	Trussle-trees		6 6	6'				6 0	6				5 6	5½				5 2	5	
	Top			10 foot				9 8	Diameter				9 2	Diameter				8 9	Diameter	
	Cap		3 1	18	Breadth			2 10	17	ditto			2 7	16	ditto			2 6	15	ditto
	Top-mast	C	28	8	31 6	8		24	7	30	7½		22	7½	28	6½	C	20	6½	27
	Head		2 6	4				1 10	3				1 9½	3½				1 9½	3¼	
	Trussle-trees		2 6	3½				1 10	3				1 9½	2½				1 9½	2¼	
	Cap		1 4	8	Breadth			1 2	7	ditto			1 1	6½	ditto			1 1	6¼	ditto
	Staff		2[illegible]	4				20	3½				18 6	3¼				18	3	
Fore	Mast	C	99 8	33	91	22		94 4	31	87	21		91 0	30	85	19	C	87	28	78
	Head		11 0	23				10 6	20½				10 1	20½				9 8	19	
	Trussle-trees		14 0	13¾				13 6	12				13 0	11½				12	10	
	Top			18 ft 6 inc Dia				17	8 Diam				16 10	Diam.				16	Diam	
	Cap		5 8	34				5 4	32				5 2	31				4 10	29	
	Top-mast	C	59 6	17 3	51	12		56	16½	51	11½		53 9	16	46 6	11¼	C	52 6	15	43
	Head		5 8	8½				5 6	8¾				5 3	8				5 1	7½	
	Trussle-trees		5 4	5¼				4 11	5				4 8	4½				4 4	4	
	Cap		3 2	19				2 11	17				2 10	17				2 8	16	
	Topgall Mast	C	28	8	25 8	6½		24	7	21 3	5½		22 6	6¾	20 6	5½	C	22	5½	20
	Head		2 6½	4				2 4	3½				2 2	3½				2 1½	3¼	
	Trussle-trees		2 6½	2½				2 4	2¾				2 2	2½				2 1½	2½	
	Cap		1 6	9				1 4	7				1 1½	6¾				1 1	6½	
	Stump		17	3¾				16	3				14 8	3¼				13	3	
Main	Mast	C	112	37	106	24		106	35	100	23½		101 6	33	96	21½	C	97	32	91
	Head		12 6	24½				11 8	23				11 2	22				10 8	21½	
	Trussle-trees		16	14				15	13				14 6	12½				13	12	
	Top		20 Foot Diameter					19 Foot 4 Inc Diam					18 Foot 4 Inc Diam					17 Foot 6 Inc		
	Cap		6 2½	37				6	36				5 8	34				5 5	32	
	Top-mast	C	67	20	58 6	13¾		63 2	19¼	55 6	13		60 6	18	53 0	12¼	C	58 6	17	51
	Head		6 ½	10				6 3	9½				6 0	9				5 7	8½	
	Trussle-trees		5 10	5½				5 6	5				5 2	4½				5 0	5	
	Cap		3 6	21				3 3	20				3 2	19				3 0	18	
	Topgall Mast	C	29 0	9	29 0	7		26 6	8	28 4	6½		25 6	7½	26 6	6	C	25	7¼	24
	Head		2 9	4½				2 7	4				2 6	3¾				2 5	3½	
	Trussle-trees		2 9	3¼				2 7	3				2 6	2½				2 5	2½	
	Cap		1 8	10				1 4	8				1 3	7½				1 3	6¼	
	Stump		18 6	4¼				17 6	4				16 6	3¾				16	3½	
Mizon	Mast	C	96	22	90	14½		93 0	20½	87	14		89	19½	85	13½	C	85	18½	78
	Head		7 5	11½				7	10½				6 8	9¾				6 6	9¼	
	Trussle-trees		7 0	7				6 7	6½				6 4	6				6 3	6	
	Top		10 Foot Diameter					9 Foot 8 Inc Diam					9 Foot 2 Inc Diam					8 Foot 9 In.		
	Cap		4 0	24				3 6	21				3 4	20				3 2	19	
	Top-mast	C	37 0	11	30 6	[illegible]		35	10½	30	7		33 8	9½	28	6½	C	32	9¼	26
	Head		3 8	5½				3 4	5¼				3 3	4¾				3 1	4¼	
	Trussle-trees		3 8	3½				3 4	3				3 3	3				3 1	2½	
	Cap		2 3	13½				2	12				1 8	10				1 7	9½	
	Stump		24 3	5½				23	5¼				22 6	5				20	4½	
Ensign-Staff			40	9				38	8				26	7½				34	7	

Three Masts ; from which any Three Masted Ship's Members may be found.

8 Foot broad

Foot

0 / 0 / 8 / 9 / 0 / 0 Inches

Masts Long Inc	Masts Dia Inches	Yards Long Feet.Inc	Yards Dia Inches
	28½	53	11½
10	6		
2	4¼		
3	Diameter		
4½	14	ditto	
6	6	26 6	5¼
9¼	3		
9½	2¼		
½	6	ditto	
6	2¾		
6	26	76	17½
3	17¼		
6	9½		
4	Diameter.		
6	27		
	14½	42 10	10
0½	7¼		
3	4		
6	15		
0	5⅝	19 6	5¼
1	3		
0	2¾		
0	6		
0	3		
6	30	86 6	19½
3	20½		
6	11½		
Foot 6 Inc Diam			
2	31		
	16½	49 6	11
6	8		
8	4½		
9	16¼		
½	7	24	5¾
4	3½		
4	2¼		
2	6		
6	3¼		
6	18½	76	12½
4	9		
2	5½		
Foot 3 Inc Diam			
	18		
0	8½	25	5¼
0	4½		
0	2⅛		
5	8½		
	4½		
	6½		
		52	8½

36 Foot broad

132 / 36 / 14 / 6 / 0 / 4 Foot — 0 / 0 / 10 / 7 / 0 / 11 Inches

Charac	Masts Long Feet Inc	Masts Dia Inches	Yards Long Feet.Inc	Yards Dia Inches
	58 6	26½	51	11¼
	4 6	5½		
	5 0	4½		
	7 11	Diameter		
	2 2	13	ditto	
	18	5½	25 6	5½
	1 9	2¾		
	1 9	2¼		
	0 11	5¾	ditto	
	16	2¾		
	79 6	25	73 ½	16⅓
	8 8	16¾		
	11	9		
	14 6	Diameter		
	4 4	26		
	47 6	14	41 6	9½
	4 7	7		
	3 11	3½		
	2 4	14		
	20 6	5	19	5
	2	2¾		
	2	2		
	11	5½		
	11 6	2⅞		
	88	28½	83	18½
	9 6	18¾		
	12	11¼		
	15 Foot 6 In. Diam			
	4 10	29		
	53	15½	47	10¾
	5 2	7½		
	4 4	3½		
	2 6	15		
	22 6	6¼	22 6	5½
	2 2½	3		
	2 2½	2¼		
	1	6		
	13 6	2¼		
	77	16½	69 11	11½
	5 10	8¼		
	5 10	5¼		
	7 Foot 11 Inc Dia			
	2 10	17		
	29 0	8	24 6	5½
	2 8	4		
	2 8	2¼		
	1 4	8		
	18 0	4⅛		
	32 6	6¼		
			48 6	8¾

34 Foot broad

130 / 34 / 14 / 6 / 0 / 4 Foot — 0 / 0 / 0 / 5 / 0 / 8 Inches

Charac	Masts Long Feet Inc	Masts Dia Inches	Yards Long Feet Inc	Yards Dia Inches
C	56	24	48	11
	4 0	5		
	Bees			
	2 1	12¼	ditto	
C	16 0	5¼	24	5
	1 8	2½		
	1 8	2		
	0 11	5½	ditto	
	14 6	2½		
C	74 6	22¾	68	15¾
	8 4	15½		
	10 6	8¾		
	13 8	Diameter		
	3 9	23		
C	44 6	12½	37 6	9
	4 3	6¼		
	3 6	3		
	2 1	12½		
C	18 3	5	18 9	4¾
	1 10	2½		
	1 10	2		
	10½	5¾		
	10	2½		
C	83	25¼	78 6	17½
	9 2	16		
	11 9	10½		
	14 Foot 10 In. Diam			
	4 4	26		
C	50 6	14½	43 6	10
	5 1	7½		
	4 0	3½		
	2 5	14½		
C	21 6	6	21 6	5
	2 1	2½		
	2 1	2⅛		
	1 0	6		
	12 6	2¼		
C	72 6	16	65	11
	5 6	8		
	5 6	4½		
	7 Foot 5 Inc Diam			
	2 6	15		
C	27	7½	22 6	5¼
	2 7	3¾		
	2 7	2		
	1 3	7½		
	17	3¼		
	30 6	6		
			45	7½

32 Foot broad

122 / 32 / 13 / 6 / 0 / 4 Foot — 0 / 0 / 2 / 2 / 0 / 6 Inches

Charac	Masts Long Feet Inc	Masts Dia Inches	Yards Long Fe Inc	Yards Dia Inches
	52	22½	45	9½
	3 10	4½		
	Bees			
	1 11	11½		
	14 6	4½	22 6	5
	1 6	2¼		
	1 6	1⅞		
	0 10	5		
	12 6	2¼		
	70 6	21½	63	14½
	7 9	14½		
	10 3	8		
	12 Foot 8 Inc Diam			
	3 8	22		
	42 6	12	35	8½
	4 2	6		
	3 4	2¾		
	2 0	12		
	17 6	4⅛	17 6	4½
	1 9	2¼		
	1 9	2		
	10	5		
	10	2½		
	78	24	73	16½
	8 8	16		
	11 6	10¼		
	14 Foot Diameter			
	4 1	24½		
	47	14	40 6	9½
	4 6	7		
	3 10	3		
	2 4	14		
	20	5	20	4½
	1 11	2½		
	1 11	2		
	0 11	5½		
	12 0	2¼		
	68 6	14½	60 6	10½
	5 2	7¼		
	5 2	4¾		
	7 Foot Diameter			
	2 3	13½		
	26	6½	21 5	5
	2 6	3½		
	2 6	2		
	1 1	6½		
	16	3½		
	29	5½		
			42	7

30 Foot broad

114 / 30 / 12 / 5 / 0 / 4 Foot — 0 / 0 / 4 / 7 / 0 / 0 Inches

Charac	Masts Long Feet Inc	Masts Dia Inches	Yards Long Feet Inc	Yards Dia Inches
	48 6	21	40 6	9
	3 7	4½		
	Bees			
	1 10	11		
	13 0	4½	20 6	4½
	1 3	2⅛		
	1 3	1⅞		
	9½	4¾		
	12	2½		
	66	20	61 6	14
	7 0	13¾		
	10	8		
	12 Foot 2 Inc Diam			
	3 5	20½		
	39 6	11¾	34 8	8
	3 10	5½		
	3 2	2½		
	1 11	11½		
	16 6	4½	17	4
	1 6	2¼		
	1 6	2		
	10	5		
	9 6	2¼		
	73 6	22	70	15½
	8 2	15		
	11	9		
	13 Foot 3 In. Diam			
	3 8	22		
	43 6	12½	38 9	9
	4 3	6½		
	3 8	2½		
	2 2	13		
	18 6	4¾	18 6	4½
	1 9	2¼		
	1 9	2		
	10	5		
	12 0	2¼		
	64 3	14	58	10
	4 10	7		
	4 10	4		
	6 Foot 8 Inc. Diam			
	2 2	13		
	25	6	20	4¾
	2 4	3		
	2 4	2		
	1	6		
	15 6	3		
	27 6	5½		
			40	6¾

A Continuation of the Mast Table.

Breadth	28 Foot broad (Foot)	(Inches)	26 Foot broad (Foot)	(Inches)	24 Foot broad (Foot)	(Inches)	22 Foot bro[ad] (Foot)	(Inches)
Length Gun-deck	106	0	98	0	91	0	84	0
Breadth Extream	28	0	26	0	24	0	22	0
Depth in Hold	11	4	10	5	9	11	9	2
Height Gun-deck	5	2	4	10	4	6	4	1
Height Middle Deck	0	0	0	0	0	0	0	0
Height in the Waste	3	10	3	9	3	6	3	4

28 Foot broad

		Chain	Masts Long (Feet Inc)	Masts Dia (Inches)	Yards Long (Feet Inc)	Yards Dia (Inches)
Bowsprit	Mast	C	45	19	38	8½
	Head		3 4	4½		
	Trusle-trees		Bees			
	Top					
	Cap		1 8	10		
	Top-mast	C	12	4¼	19	4½
	Head		1 2	2		
	Trusle-trees		1 3	2		
	Cap		9	4½		
	Staff		10 10	2¼		
Fore	Mast	C	61 6	18½	56 6	12¼
	Head		6 9	12		
	Trusle-trees		9 3	7½		
	Top		11 Foot 5 Inc Diam			
	Cap		3 1	18½		
	Top-mast	C	36 6	10½	31 6	7
	Head		3 6	5		
	Trusle-trees		2 8	2¼		
	Cap		1 10	11		
	Topgall Mast	C	15 3	4½	15 3	3¾
	Head		1 5½	2⅛		
	Trusle-trees		1 6	2		
	Cap		10	5		
	Stump		9	2¼		
Main	Mast	C	68 6	20½	65	14½
	Head		7 6	13¾		
	Trusle-trees		10	9		
	Top		12 Foot 4 Inc Diam			
	Cap		3 5	20½		
	Top-mast	C	41	11½	36	8½
	Head		3 11	6		
	Trusle-trees		3 4	3		
	Cap		1 11	11½		
	Topgall Mast	C	17	4½	17	4
	Head		1 7	2½		
	Trusle-trees		1 8	2¼		
	Cap		10	5		
	Stump		11	2¼		
Mizon	Mast	C	60	13½	54 6	8½
	Head		4 6	6⅔		
	Trusle-trees		5 5	5		
	Top		6 Foot 2 Inc Diam			
	Cap		2 3	13½		
	Top-mast	C	22 9	5½	18 6	4½
	Head		2 2	2¾		
	Trusle-trees		1 11	2		
	Cap		1	6		
	Stump		15	2¼		
	Ensign-Staff		26	5⅛		
	Cross-Jack Yard				37 6	6¼

26 Foot broad

		Chain	Masts Long (Feet Inc)	Masts Dia (Inches)	Yards Long (Feet Inc)	Yards Dia (Inches)
Bowsprit	Mast		43	18	36	8
	Head		3	4¼		
	Trusle-trees		Bees			
	Top					
	Cap		1 6	9		
	Top-mast		11 4	4	18	3¾
	Head		1 1	2		
	Trusle-trees		1 2½	1¾		
	Cap		8	4		
	Staff		10	2		
Fore	Mast		57 6	17	52 6	11¼
	Head		6 4	11¾		
	Trusle-trees		9	7½		
	Top		10 Foot Diam			
	Cap		2 8	16		
	Top-mast		34 4	9¼	29	6¼
	Head		3 3½	4¾		
	Trusle-trees		2 6	2⅜		
	Cap		1 7	9½		
	Topgall Mast		14 4	3¾	14 4	3½
	Head		1 3	2		
	Trusle-trees		1 3	1¾		
	Cap		8	4		
	Stump		8 6	2⅛		
Main	Mast		64	19	60 6	13½
	Head		7 1	12⅔		
	Trusle-trees		9 6	8½		
	Top		11 Foot 6 Inc Diam			
	Cap		3 3	19½		
	Top-mast		38 6	10½	33 6	7½
	Head		3 8	5⅜		
	Trusle-trees		3 1	2½		
	Cap		1 10	11		
	Topgall Mast		16	4	16	4¼
	Head		1 6	2¼		
	Trusle-trees		1 6	2⅛		
	Cap		9½	4¾		
	Stump		10	2¼		
Mizon	Mast		56 10	12¼	50	8¼
	Head		4 3	6⅛		
	Trusle-trees		5 1	4½		
	Top		5 Foot 9 Inc Diam			
	Cap		2 2	13		
	Top-mast		21 4	5	17 4	4
	Head		2 2	2½		
	Trusle-trees		1 7	2		
	Cap		11	5½		
	Stump		14	2½		
	Ensign-Staff		24	4½		
	Cross-Jack Yard				34	5½

24 Foot broad

		Chain	Masts Long (Feet Inc)	Masts Dia (Inches)	Yards Long (Feet Inc)	Yards Dia (Inches)
Bowsprit	Mast	C	39 6	16	34	7½
	Head		2 10	4		
	Trusle-trees		Bees			
	Top					
	Cap		1 4	8		
	Top-mast	C	10 8	3½	17	3½
	Head		1	1¾		
	Trusle-trees		1 2	1½		
	Cap		8	4		
	Staff		8 6	1⅞		
Fore	Mast	C	53 6	15½	48 6	11
	Head		5 8	10		
	Trusle-trees		8 6	6½		
	Top		9 Foot 8 Inc Diam			
	Cap		2 7	15½		
	Top-mast	C	32	8¼	26 9	6
	Head		3 ½	4½		
	Trusle-trees		2 4	2		
	Cap		1 5	8½		
	Topgall Mast	C	13 3	3½	13 4	3¼
	Head		1 2	1¾		
	Trusle-trees		1 2	1½		
	Cap		7½	3¾		
	Stump		8	2		
Main	Mast	C	59	17	55 6	12
	Head		6 6	10		
	Trusle-trees		9 3	8		
	Top		10 Foot 8 Inc Diam			
	Cap		2 10	17		
	Top-mast	C	35 6	9¼	31 6	7¼
	Head		3 5	4¾		
	Trusle-trees		2 9	2¼		
	Cap		1 9	10½		
	Topgall Mast	C	14 ¾	4¼	14 ½	3¾
	Head		1 5	2		
	Trusle-trees		1 5	2		
	Cap		9	4½		
	Stump		9	2⅛		
Mizon	Mast	C	51 8	11	46 9	8
	Head		3 10	5½		
	Trusle-trees		4 7	3½		
	Top		5 Foot 4 Inc Diam			
	Cap		2	12		
	Top-mast	C	19 6	4¾	16	3¾
	Head		1 11	2¼		
	Trusle-trees		1 5	2		
	Cap		9	4½		
	Stump		11	2⅛		
	Ensign-Staff		22	4½		
	Cross-Jack Yard				32 6	5¼

22 Foot bro[ad]

		Chain	Masts Long (Feet Inc)	Masts Dia (Inches)	Yards Long (Feet Inc)
Bowsprit	Mast		35 6	14½	33
	Head		2 6	3½	
	Trusle-trees		Bees		
	Top				
	Cap		1 3	7½	
	Top-mast		9 8	3¼	16
	Head		11	1¼	
	Trusle-trees		1 1	1½	
	Cap		7	3½	
	Staff		7 6	1¾	
Fore	Mast		48	14	43
	Head		5 4	9½	
	Trusle-trees		8	5½	
	Top		8 Foot 9 In D[iam]		
	Cap		2 5	14½	
	Top-mast		29	[illegible]	24
	Head		2 10	3¾	
	Trusle-trees		2	2	
	Cap		1 3	7½	
	Topgall Mast		12	3½	12
	Head		1 1	1½	
	Trusle-trees		1 1	1½	
	Cap		7¼	3½	
	Stump		7 6	1⅞	
Main	Mast		53 6	15¼	50
	Head		5 8	10	
	Trusle-trees		8	6½	
	Top		9 Foot 8 Inc D[iam]		
	Cap		2 7	15½	
	Top-mast		32	8¼	30
	Head		3 1	4¼	
	Trusle-trees		2 6	2⅛	
	Cap		1 5	8½	
	Topgall Mast		13 6	4½	13
	Head		1 3	2	
	Trusle-trees		1 3	2	
	Cap		8½	4¼	
	Stump		8	2	
Mizon	Mast		47 8	10½	43
	Head		3 6	5¼	
	Trusle-trees		4 2	3	
	Top		4 Foot 10 Inc D[iam]		
	Cap		1 10	11	
	Top-mast		17 8	4½	16
	Head		1 8	2⅛	
	Trusle-trees		1 4	2	
	Cap		8	4	
	Stump		10	2⅛	
	Ensign-Staff		20 8	4½	
	Cross-Jack Yard				32

A Continuation of the Mast Table

20 Foot Broad					
76 Feet		0 Inches			
20		0			
8		5			
3		10			
0		0			
3		1			
Masts			*Yards*		
Long Feet	Inc	Dia Inches	Long Feet	Inc	Dia Inches
32		13	28	6	6
2	2	3			
Bees					
1	1	$6\frac{1}{2}$			
8	6	$2\frac{3}{4}$	14		$3\frac{1}{2}$
	9	$1\frac{1}{4}$			
1		$1\frac{1}{2}$			
	$6\frac{1}{2}$	$3\frac{1}{4}$			
6	6	$1\frac{1}{2}$			
44.		12	40.		10
5		8			
7		5			
8 Foot Diameter					
2	3	$13\frac{1}{2}$			
26	8	$6\frac{1}{2}$	22.	3	$4\frac{1}{2}$
2	6	$3\frac{1}{4}$			
1	8	2			
1	$1\frac{1}{2}$	$6\frac{3}{4}$			
11		3	11		$2\frac{3}{4}$
1		$1\frac{1}{2}$			
1		$1\frac{1}{2}$			
	7	$3\frac{1}{2}$			
7		$1\frac{1}{2}$			
49.		14	46		$10\frac{1}{4}$
5	5	$9\frac{1}{2}$			
8		$6\frac{1}{4}$			
8 Foot 9 Inc Diam					
2	5	$14\frac{1}{2}$			
29	6	$7\frac{1}{2}$	25	6	$5\frac{1}{2}$
2	10	$3\frac{1}{2}$			
2	6	$2\frac{1}{8}$			
1	3	$7\frac{1}{2}$			
12	3	$3\frac{1}{2}$	12	3	$3\frac{1}{4}$
1	2	2			
1	2	2			
	8	4			
7	6	2			
42	11	$9\frac{1}{4}$	38	6	$6\frac{3}{4}$
3	2	$4\frac{1}{2}$			
3	9	$2\frac{3}{4}$			
4 Foot 4 Inc Diam					
1	8	10			
16	6	4	13	10	$3\frac{1}{2}$
1	5	2			
1	3	2			
	8	4			
8	6	2			
19		4			
			28		$4\frac{3}{4}$

This *Calculation* was performed by a most concise *Shipwright*: One that, for his Knowledge in *Ship-Building*, and his Industry and Diligence in the said Affairs, may, without Vanity, be number'd amongst the Best of our Practical *English Shipwrights*.

How the Opinions of other Men vary from his, I cannot say: However, I shall set down the *Calculation* of Six several Sizes of *Masting*, &c. made by an Able *Mast-maker*; who, by a continual Series of Years in his particular Function had observed the Opinions, and Fashions of divers other *Mast-makers*, as well as his own

And here you will have the Charge of making a Suit of *Masts* and *Yards*, with the Time, and Number of Men, requisite to perform such a Service: Also what other Materials will be wanting to perform and finish the Work.

Observing, That in the first Column towards the Left-hand, you have the Names of the Places of each *Mast*, as *Main*, *Fore*, *Mizon*, *Bowsprit*; and in the second and third Columns, you have the Distinguishment upwards, whether *Masts* or *Yards*, under that you have in four Columns, the Length of the *Masts* and *Yards* in Yards, and their Diameter in Inches; in the 6th and 7th Columns, you have the Nature and Quality of Hands, or Inches, that will make such *Masts* and *Yards*; in the 8th, 9th, 10th and 11th, you have the Number of Men and Days which will be required to make such *Masts* and *Yards*; in the 12th and 13th, you have the Price and Value of the *Rough Mast*; in the 14th and 15th, you have the Mens Wages for Finishing each *Mast* or *Yard*, in the 16th, the Quantity and Value of the *Iron-work* from the Forge, in the 17th, the Quantity and Value of the *Oak Timber* Rough for Cheeks, Heel of the Mizon Mast, and Knee of the Bowsprit; in the 18th, 19th, 20th, 21st, 22d and 23d, the Dimensions of the Cross and Trussle-trees for each Mast, and the whole Quantity and Value by its self, in the 24th, 25th and 26th, you have the Dimensions of the *Caps*; in the 27th, the Value of all the *Elm* used in making them; in the 28th, the *Nails* of divers sorts, in the 29th, the *Tallow*; in the 30th, the *Rozin*; in the 31st, the *Tar*; and in the 32d, the *Thrums*. All which Particulars being what is only necessary in Performing and Finishing the *Masts*, *Yards*, and every Material proper for Compleating them. Which several and respective Sums being put together, you have an Account of the whole Charge, for making such Suits of *Masts*. All which are drawn from Practical and respective Rules, as aforesaid.

Here follows the Dimensions and Value of making

A Ship of 49 Foot broad, & other Proportions agreeable to the preceeding Proportions	Masts		Yards		Number of Hands		Num of Men		Number of Days		Price of the Rough Tree				Mens Wages for making such						Weight of Work f the For requisite Hoops, Bolts
	Length in Yards	Diam in Inches	Length in Yards	Diam in Inches	To make a Mast	To make a Yard	To make a Mast	To make a Yard	To make a Mast	To make a Yard	To make a Mast		To make a Yard		A Mast			A Yard			
											l	s	l	s	l	s	d	l	s	d	C qr
Main	38¾	39	34½	24	New England 2	20	9	9	19½	4½	242	10	66	0	17	16	3	4	4	4½	6—2—
Top-mast	22¾	20	19[illegible]	13[illegible]	21	14	7	5	4½	2	38	5	5	0	3	5	7½	1	0	10	Val 9l
Topgal Mast	9¾	8½	9½	7	8	7	3	3	2	1	1	2	0	15	0	12	6	0	6	3	
Fore	33[illegible]	34	30¾	21¼	New England	24	9	9	16½	4	130	14	71	10	15	9	4½	3	15	0	5—0—
Top-mast	20	17½	16 8/10	11⅕	17	11	6	4	5	2½	13	7	3	0	3	2	6	1	0	10	Val 7l 13
Topgal Mast	8¼	7¼	8½	6¼	7½	6½	3	3	2	1	1	0	0	12	0	12	6	0	6	3	
Mizon	32½	22	30	16	22	16	7	7	4½	3	58	0	10	5	3	5	7½	2	3	9	0—2—
Top-mast	12½	10¾	9[illegible]	7¼	10¾	7½	5	3	2	1	2	10	1	0	1	0	10	0	6	3	Val 17s
Bowsprit	27	36[illegible]	21¼	15	New England	16	9	7	6	2	107	17	10	5	5	12	6	1	9	2	1—1—
Sprits Topm	7¼	7½	11	8¼	7½	8½	3	3	2	1	1	0	1	8	0	12	6	0	6	3	Val 2l 7
Crofs Jack Yd			19⅞	9⅔		10		5		2	0	0	2	0	0	0	0	1	0	10	
										Total—	596	5	171	15	51	10	2½	15	19	9½	20l 13s 1

A Ship of 45 Foot broad, & other Proportions, as afore-mentioned	Masts		Yards		Number of Hands		Num of Men		Number of Days		Price of the Rough Tree				Mens Wages for making such						Weight of Work f the For requisite Hoops, Bolts
	Length in Yards	Diam. in Inches	Length in Yards	Diam in Inches	To make a Mast	To make a Yard	To make a Mast	To make a Yard	To make a Mast	To make a Yard	To make a Mast		To make a Yard		A Mast			A Yard			
											l	s	l	s	l	s	d	l	s	d	C qr
Main	36½	36½	32½	22½	New England	23	9	9	18½	4	181	6	61	10	17	6	10½	3	15	0	5—2—
Top-mast	22½	19	18	12⅔	19	13	7	5	4½	2	23	0	5	0	3	5	7½	1	0	10	Val 8l
Topgal Mast	9¼	7¾	9	6¾	8½	6½	3	3	2	1	1	8	0	12	0	12	6	0	6	3	
Fore	31½	31½	28¼	19¾	New England	21	9	9	16	3½	94	0	38	5	15	0	0	3	5	7½	4—2—
Top-mast	19½	16½	15⅔	11⅜	15½	11	6	4	4½	2½	9	7	3	0	2	16	3	1	0	10	Val 6l
Topgal Mast	8	6¼	7[illegible]	5⅞	6½	6	3	3	2	1	1	2	0	10	0	12	6	0	6	3	
Mizon	30	20½	28	14¾	21	16	7	7	4½	3	38	5	10	5	3	5	7½	2	3	9	0—2—
Top-mast	11½	9¾	9	7	10	7	5	3	2	1	2	0	0	15	1	0	10	0	6	3	Val 15
Crofs Jack Yd			18¾	9		11		5		2			3	0	0	0	0	1	0	10	
Bowsprit	25	33¾	19⅘	14	New England	15½	9	7	6	2	78	11	9	7	5	12	6	1	9	2	1—0—
Sprits Topm	6⅞	6⅞	10	7½	6½	6½	3	3	2	1	0	12	0	12	0	12	6	0	6	3	Val 1l
										Total—	429	11	132	16	50	5	2½	15	1	0½	17l 7s

Mafs

Masts, Yards, &c for Six several Sizes of Shipping.

Oak Timber for Cheeks, and Heel of the Mizon-mast	Length of the Cross-trees	Length of the Trussle-trees	Breadth of the Cross-trees	Breadth of the Trussle-trees	Depth of the Cross-trees	Depth of the Trussle-trees	Elm Cap Length	Elm Cap Breadth	Elm Cap Depth	Quantity and Value of the Cap	Thrums	Weight & Value of the Nails of every sort	Weight and Value of the Tallow	Ditto of the Rozin	Ditto of the Tar
Feet	Feet	Feet	Inch	Inch	Inch	Inch	Feet	Inch	Inch	Feet					
195	17 6	17 6	10⅓	10⅕	6	12⅗	6 9	40	18						
l s d	7 0	7 0	4	4	3	6¼	3 3	19	9						
14 0 0	3 0	3 0	2	2¼	1⅛	3⅛	1 8	10	5						
175 Value	16 3	16 3	9¼	9	6	12⅛	6 4	38	16¾		lb	C	C qr	C qr	Bar
12 5 0	6 9	6 9	4	4⅗	3⅜	6	3 0	18	8	550	3½	3	1 1	1 1	2¾
	2 9	2 9	1	1	1	3	1 5	8½	4½	l s	s d	l s	l s d	l	l s
31 Value	9 0	9 0	5	5	3	6	3 4	19	9	38 15	2 11	6 6	2 0 3	1	15
1 13 6	3 5	3 5	2	2	1	3⅜	1 9	10	5¼						
20 Value	9 0	9 0	4	4	3	6	3 0	18	9						
2 10 6	2 9	2 9	2	2	1½	3	1 8	10	5						
Tot Val 30 9 0	*Oak-Timber* 143 *Feet* for Cross and Trussle-trees at 13 *d per Foot* is 7 *l* 14 *s* 11 *d*														

	l	s	d
Rough Tree for *Masts*	59[illegible]	5	[illegible]
Ditto for *Yards*	171	15	0
Oak Timber for Cheeks	30	9	0
Ditto for Cross & *Trussle trees*	7	14	11
Elm for *Caps*	38	15	0
Iron from the Forge	20	1[illegible]	11½
Nails of divers sorts	6	6	0
Tallow	2	6	3
Rozin	1	0	0
Tar	2	15	0
Thrums	0	2	11
Mens Wages	67	10	0
Total	945	13	0½

Oak Timber for Cheeks and Heel of the Mizon-Mast	Length of the Cross-trees	Length of the Trussle-trees	Breadth of the Cross-trees	Breadth of the Trussle-trees	Depth of the Cross-trees	Depth of the Trussle-trees	Elm Cap Length	Elm Cap Breadth	Elm Cap Depth	Quantity and Value of the Cap	Thrums	Weight & Value of the Nails of every sort	Weight and Value of the Tallow	Ditto of the Rozin	Ditto of the Tar
Feet	Feet	Feet	Inch	Inch	Inch	Inch	Feet	Inch	Inch	Feet					
180	17 0	17 0	10	10	6½	12½	6 6	39	17						
l s / 12 18	6 10	6 10	4¾	4¾	3½	6⅛	3 0	18	8						
	2 11	2 11	2	2	1	3	1 6	9	4½						
160 Value	15 0	15 0	9½	9½	5	10½	5 8	34	15		lb	C qr	C	C	Bar
9 12	6 0	6 0	4½	4½	2	5	2 6	15	8	490	3	2 3	1	1	2
29	2½	2½	1½	1¾	1¼	2¼	1 2	7	4½	l s	s d	l s d	l s	s	l s
Value	8 6	8 6	5¼	5	3½	6½	3 2	19	9	34 6	2 6	5 15 6	1 17	16	2 10
1 11	3 4	3 4	2½	2	1¾	3	1 8	10	5						
Ke. 18 value	8 6	8 6	4½	4	2⅞	5¾	2 6	15	8						
2 5	2	2¾	1½	2	1¼	2	1 6	9	4½						
Tot Val 25 6	*Oak Timber* 127 *Feet* for Cross and Trussle-trees, at 13 *d per Foot* is 6 *l* 17 *s* 7 *d*														

	l	s	d
Rough Trees for *Masts*	429	11	0
Ditto to make *Yards*	132	16	0
Oak Timber for Cheeks	26	6	0
Ditto for the Cross and Trussle-trees	6	17	7
Elm for *Caps*	34	6	0
Iron from the Forge	17	7	0
Nails of divers sorts	5	15	6
Tallow	1	17	0
Rozin	0	16	0
Tar	2	10	0
Thrums	0	2	6
Mens Wages	65	6	3
Total	72[illegible]	1[illegible]	10

A Continuation of the Mast Table.

A Ship of 40 Foot broad, & other Proportions agreeable	*Masts.*		*Yards*		*Number of Hands*		*Num of Men*		*Number of Days*		*Price of the Rough Tree*				*Mens Wages for making such*						*Weight of Work the F[…] requisit Hoops, Bolts*
	Length in Yards	*Diam in Inches*	*Length in Yards.*	*Diam. in Inches*	*To make a Mast*	*To make a Yard*	*To make a Mast*	*To make a Yard*	*To make a Mast*	*To make a Yard*	*To make a Mast*		*To make a Yard.*		*A Mast*			*A Yard*			
											l	*s*	*l*	*s*	*l*	*s*	*d*	*l*	*s*	*d*	*C qr*
Main ——	32	30½	30	20½	New England 12		8	8	16	3	88	11	54	0	13	6	0	2	10	0	4—0—
Top-mast —	20	17¾	17	11¼	17½	12	6	4	4	2	14	15	4	0	2	10	0	0	16	8	Val 6*l* 11
Topgal. Mast	8⅓	7½	8⅔	6¼	8	6	2	2	2	1	1	2	0	10	0	8	4	0	4	2	
Fore ——	29	27½	26	18	N w England 20		8	8	14	3	77	1	33	0	11	13	4	2	10	0	3—1—
Top-mast —	17⅓	15	15	11	15	10	6	4	4	2	8	9	2	0	2	10	0	0	16	8	Val 5*l* 3
Topgal Mast	7⅓	6⅓	8	5½	7½	6	2	2	2	1	1	0	0	10	0	8	4	0	4	2	
Mizon ——	28¼	18	26½	13½	20	15	6	6	4	3	33	0	8	9	2	10	0	1	17	6	0—1—
Top-mast —	10½	9	9	6¾	9	6½	4	2	2	1	1	14	0	12	0	16	8	0	4	2	Val 10
Crofs Jack Yd			18	9½		11½		4		2	0	0	3	10	0	0	0	0	16	8	
Bowfprit —	21⅓	30	18	12½	New England 13		8	6	6	2	59	0	5	0	5	0	0	1	5	4	0—3—
Spritf Topm	6⅓	6½	9½	6	6	6	2	2	2	1	1	0	0	10	0	16	8	0	4	2	Val 1*l* 1
										Total—	285	12	112	1	39	19	4	11	9	6	13*l* 11*s*

A Ship of 34 Foot broad, & other Proportions agreeable	*Masts*		*Yards.*		*Number of Hands*		*Num of Men*		*Number of Days*		*Price of the Rough Tree*				*Mens Wages for making such*						*Weight of Iron Work from the Forge requisite for Hoops, and Bolts*
	Length in Yards	*Diam in Inches*	*Length in Yards.*	*Diam in Inches*	*To make a Mast*	*To make a Yard*	*To make a Mast.*	*To make a Yard*	*To make a Mast*	*To make a Yard*	*To make a Mast*		*To make a Yard*		*A Mast*			*A Yard.*			
											l	*s*	*l*	*s*	*l.*	*s*	*d.*	*l.*	*s*	*d*	*C qr lb*
Main ——	28	24	25	16½	22	18¼	8	6	12	3	54	0	16	0	10	0	0	1	17	6	2—2—7
Top-mast —	17	14½	14⅓	10½	13	11	6	4	3	2	5	0	3	0	1	17	6	0	16	8	Val 4*l* 3*s* 6*d*
Topgal Mast	7	5½	7⅔	4½	6	Can't spare	2	2	2	1	0	10	0	3	0	8	4	0	4	2	
Fore——	24⅔	21½	22	14	19	16	8	6	10	2	23	0	10	5	9	7	6	1	5	0	2—1—8
Top-mast —	15⅓	12½	12⅔	9	12	9	4	2	4	2	4	0	1	14	1	13	4	0	8	4	val 3*l* 15*s* 10*d*
Topgal Mast	6½	5	6½	4	6	Can't spare	2	2	2	1	0	10	0	3	0	8	4	0	4	2	
Mizon ——	24	14½	20	10	15½	11	6	6	3	2	9	7	3	0	1	17	6	1	5	0	0—1—0
Top-mast —	8	6½	8	4½	6½	Can't spare	2	2	3	1	0	12	0	3	0	12	6	0	4	0	Val 7*s* 6*d*
Crofs Jack Yd			14	1		8		2		2	0	0	1	2	0	0	0	0	8	4	
Bowfprit —	17½	22	15	10½	19	10	6	6	4	2	23	0	2	0	2	10	0	1	5	0	0—0—20
Spritf Topm	5	5	8	5½	6	6	1	1	1	1	0	10	0	10	0	2	1	0	2	1	Val 5*s* 10*d*
										Total—	120	9	38	0	28	17	1	8	0	3	8*l* 12*s* 8*d*

A Continuation of the Mast Table.

Oak Timber for Cheeks and Heel of the Mizon Mast	Length of the Cross-trees	Length of the Trusle-trees	Breadth of the Cross-trees	Breadth of the Trusle-trees	Depth of the Cross-trees	Depth of the Trusle-trees	Elm Cap Length	Elm Cap Breadth	Elm Cap Depth	Quantity and Value of Oak Timber	Weight & Value of the Nails of every sort	Weight and Value of the Tallow	Ditto of the Rozin	Ditto of the Tar	Quantity and Value of the Cap
Feet	Feet	Feet	Inch	Inch	Inch	Inch	Feet	Inch	Inch	Feet					Fe.
158	15	15	9½	9½	5½	10½	5 8	34	15						
l s d	6	6	4½	4½	2¾	5	2 6	15	8						
9 12 0	2½	2½	1½	1¾	1¼	2¼	1 2	7	4½						
146	13½	13½	8½	8½	5	9½	5 0	30	14		C q. lb	qr	qr	Bar	
Value	5	5	3½	3½	4½	4	2 2	14	6	344	1 3 13	3	3	2	225
5 03 13	2½	2	1¼	1½	1¼	2	1 1	6½	4	l s	l s d	l s d	s	l	l s
25 Value	8	8	5	5	3¼	6	3 0	18	9	21 7	3 18 4	1 8 6	12	2	1 5
1 05 0	2¼	2¾	2	2	1¾	2½	1 4	8	4¼						
Knee 15 Value	8	8	4½	4½	2¼	5½	2 2	14	6						
1 16 0	2½	2	1½	1¾	1¼	2¼	1 2	6¾	4½						

	l.	s.	d.
Oak Timber	21	07	00
Nails	3	18	04
Tallow	1	08	06
Rozin	0	12	00
Tar	2	00	00
Forge Iron	13	11	06
Mens Wages	51	08	10
Cap	11	05	00
Rough Trees for *Masts*	285	12	00
Ditto for *Yards*	112	01	00
Ditto for the Cross and Trusle-trees	4	09	00
Total	507	13	02

Rough Timber to make the Trusle and Cross-trees 89 *Feet* at 12 *d per Foot*, is 4 *l* 9 *s* the Waste allowed for Sawing.

Oak Timber for Cheeks and Heel of the Mizon-Mast	Length of the Cross-trees	Length of the Trusle-trees	Breadth of the Cross-trees	Breadth of the Trusle-trees	Depth of the Cross-trees	Depth of the Trusle-trees	Elm Cap. Length	Elm Cap. Breadth	Elm Cap. Depth	Quantity and Value of Oak Timber.	Weight & Value of the Nails of every sort	Weight and Value of the Tallow	Ditto of the Rozin	Ditto of the Tar	Thrums Quan. & Value	Quantity and Value of the Cap
Feet	Feet	Feet	Inch	Inch	Inch	Inch	Feet	Inch	Inch	Feet						Feet
130	12½	12½	7¼	7¼	4½	8½	4 10	29	12							
l. s. d	5	5	3¼	2¼	2¼	4	1 10	11	5½							
[illegible] 16 0	2	2	1½	1½	1¼	2	1 6	9	4½							
110 Value	11	11	6½	6½	3¾	7½	4 2	25	10¾		C qr	qr	qr	Bar.	lb	
6 14 0	3¾	3¾	3½	3	2	3½	1 8	10	5	259	1 : 1	2	2	1	2	168
10	2	2	1¼	1¾	1¼	2	1 4	8	4	l s d	l s d	s d	s	l	s d	l s
Value	7	7	3½	3¾	2	3¾	2 2	13	6½	15 11 1½	2 12 6	18 6	8	1	1 8	8 16
0 12 0	2½	2	1½	1¾	1¼	2¼	1 2	7	3½							
9 Value							1 8	10	5							
11. 1½	1½	1½	1½	1½	1¼	2	1 2	7	3½							

	l	s.	d
Oak Timber	15	11	01½
Nails	2	12	06
Tallow	0	18	06
Rozin	0	08	00
Tar	1	00	00
Forge Iron	8	12	08
Mens Wages	36	17	04
Cap	8	16	00
Rough Trees for *Masts*	120	09	00
Ditto for *Yards*	38	00	00
Ditto for Cross and Trusle-trees	3	07	00
Total	236	12	01½

Rough Timber for Trusle and Cross-trees 68 *Feet*, at 12 *d per Foot* is 3 *l* 7 *s*.

A Continuation of the Mast Table

A Ship of 28 Foot broad, & other Proportions agreeable	Mast		Yard		Number of Hands		Num of Men		Num of Days		Price of the Rough Tree				Mens Wages for making such						Weight of the Work for the requisite Hoops, Bolts
	Length in Yards	Diam in Inches	Length in Yards	Diam in Inches	To make a Mast	To make a Yard	To make a Mast	To make a Yard	To make a Mast	To make a Yard	To make a Mast		To make a Yard		A Mast			A Yard			
											l	s	l	s	l	s	d	l	s	d	C q.
Main	23	19	20 5/7	14	18	15	6	6	[illegible]	2	16	0	8	9	6	5	0	1	5	0	1—0
Top-mast	14 5/8	11	11 3/7	8	11	8	4	2	4	2	3	0	1	8	1	13	4	0	8	4	val 1
Topgal Mast	5	4 1/2	5 3/7	4	can't spare		2	2	2	1	0	4	0	4	0	8	4	0	4	2	
Fore	20	17	17 5/7	12	15	12	6	6	Ch[illegible]	2	9	7	4	0	5	0	0	1	5	0	1—0
Top-mast	12 2/3	10	9 2/7	6 7/8	10	7	4	2	3	2	2	0	0	15	1	5	0	0	8	4	Val 1l
Topgal Mast	4	4	4 3/7	3 1/2	can't spare		2	1	2	1	0	4	0	4	0	8	4	0	2	1	
Mizon	18 5/8	12 1/4	17 2/7	9 1/2	13	11	4	4	4	2	5	0	3	0	1	13	4	0	16	8	0—0
Top-mast	7	5 1/2	5 5/6	4 1/2	Can't spare		2	1	2	1	0	10	0	4	0	8	4	0	2	1	Val 5
Cross Jack Yd			11 1/7	6 1/4	0	7		2	0	2	0	0	0	15	0	0	0	0	8	4	
Bowsprit	15 4/5	1[illegible]	12	8	16	8	6	4	3	1	10	5	1	2	1	17	6	0	8	4	0—0
Sprit Topm	3 2/3	4	5 1/6	4 1/2	can't spare		1	1	1	1	0	2	0	2	0	2	1	0	2	1	Val 3
									Total		46	12	20	3	9	1	3	5	10	5	4 l 4

A Ship of 24 Foot bread, & other Proportions agreeable	Mast		Yard		Number of Hands		Num of Men		Num of Days		Price of the Rough Tree				Mens Wages for making such						Weight of the Work for the requisite Hoops, Bolts
	Length in Yards	Diam in Inches	Length in Yards	Diam in Inches	To make a Mast	To make a Yard	To make a Mast	To make a Yard	To make a Mast	To make a Yard	To make a Mast.		To make a Yard		A Mast			A Yard			
											l	s.	l	s	l	s	d	l	s	d	C qr
Main	20 1/3	16 1/8	17 5/7	12 3/4	15	12 1/2	6	6	4	2	8	9	4	10	2	10	0	1	5	0	0—0—1
Top-mast	12 2/3	10 1/8	9 3/8	7 1/8	9	8	3	2	2	1	1	14	1	2	0	12	6	0	4	2	Val 5 s 9
Topgal Mast	4 5/8	4 3/8	4 1/3	3 1/2	1/2 Can't spare		2	1	1 1/2	1	0	2	0	2	0	5	2	0	2	1	
Fore	17 1/3	14 1/6	15 1/7	11	14	11	4	4	5	2	5	0	3	0	2	1	4	0	16	8	0—0—1
Top-mast	10 2/3	8 1/2	8 1/2	6 1/2	8	6	3	2	2	1	1	2	0	10	0	12	6	0	4	2	Val 5 s 9
Topgal Mast	4 2/3	4 1/8	4 1/2	3 1/6	1/2 Can't spare		2	1	1 1/2	1	0	2	0	2	0	5	2	0	2	1	
Mizon	16 1/7	10 1/4	15	7 3/8	11	9	3	2	4	1	3	0	1	14	1	5	0	0	8	4	0—0—1
Top-mast	6 3/4	4 7/8	5 1/2	3 3/4	1/2 Can't spare		2	1	2	1	0	2	0	2	0	8	4	0	2	1	Val 4
Cross Jack Yd			10	5 1/8		6		1		1	0	0	0	10	0	0	0	0	2	1	
Bowsprit	13	15	10 1/3	7	14	7	4	2	4	1	7	0	0	15	1	13	4	0	4	2	0—0—1
Sprit Topm	3 1/3	3 3	5 1/8	3 3/7	1/2 Can't spare		1	1	1	1	0	2	0	2	0	2	1	0	2	1	Val 3 s 6
									Total		26	13	12	9	9	15	5	3	12	11	19 s 1

Oak Timber for Cheeks and Heel of the Mizon-mast	Length of the Crosstrees	Length of the Trussletrees	Breadth of the Crosstrees	Breadth of the Trussletrees	Depth of the Crosstrees	Depth of the Trussletrees	Elm Cap Length	Elm Cap Breadth	Elm Cap Depth	Quantity and Value of the Cap	Value of ditto	Weight and Value of the Nails of every sort	Weight and Value of the Tallow	Ditto of the Rozin	Ditto Price of the Tar	Ditto Thrums
Feet	Feet	Feet	Inch	Inch	Inch	Inch	Feet	Inch	Inch	Feet						
	10⅓	10	5½	5½	3¾	6½	3 10	23	9½							
95	4	4	2¾	2¾	2	3½	1 6	9	4⅛							
value	1½	1½	1¼	1¼	1	1¼	1 2	6½	3¼							
4l 15	9	9	5	5	3	6	3 4	20	8½							
	3½	3½	2	2	1¼	2½	1 5	8	4							Pounds
85	1⅓	1⅓	1¼	1¼	1¼	1	0 11	5½	3	84		29	2 9	2 qrs	¾ bar	2
value	4	4	2¾	2¾	2¾	2	1 10	11	5¾	4l 8s		1l 1s	18 s	8 s	15 s	1s 8d
4l 5s	1¼	1¼	1¾	1¼	1¾	1	1 0	6	3				6 d			
Knee 7f							1 4	8	4							
value	1½	1¾	1¼	1¼	1¼	1¾	1 0	5¾	3							
14s																
9l 14s																

	l	s.	d
Oak Timber	9	14	0
Cap of Elm	4	8	0
Nails	1	1	0
Rozin	0.	8	0
Tallow	0	18	6
Tar	0	15	0
Thrums	0	1	8
Iron-work from Forge	4	0	4
Mens Wages	24	11	8
Rough Trees for Masts	47	8	0
Rough Trees for Yards	20	3	0
Total Sum to make each a Sett of Masts is	112	19	2

Rough Timber to make the Cross and Trussle-trees, 23 Feet, at 9 d per Foot is 17 s 3 d add to 112 l 19 s 2 d is the total charge 113 16 5

Oak Timber for Cheeks and Heel of the Mizon-mast	Length of the Crosstrees	Length of the Trussletrees	Breadth of the Crosstrees	Breadth of the Trussletrees	Depth of the Crosstrees	Depth of the Trussletrees	Elm Cap Length	Elm Cap Breadth	Elm Cap Depth	Quantity and Value of the Cap	Value of ditto	Weight and Value of the Nails of every sort	Weight and Value of the Tallow	Ditto of the Rozin	Ditto Value of Tar	Ditto Value of Thrums
Feet	Feet	Feet	Inch	Inch	Inch	Inch	Feet	Inch	Inch	Feet						
30	8⅔	8⅓	5	5	3	6	3 4	10¼	8⅛							
value	3½	3½	2¼	2¼	2	2¾	1 5	8⅛	4							
1l 10s	1½	1⅓	1¼	1¼	1	1¾	1 0	6	3							
16	8	8	4½	4½	2¾	5¾	2 10	17	8⅝							
	2⅚	2⅚	2	2	1¼	2½	1 4	7½	3½							Pound
value	1½	1⅓	1¼	1¼	1	1¾	0 10	5	2½			Pounds	Pounds	Pound		
16 s	3⅔	3⅔	2½	2½	1½	3	1 5	8⅜	4⅞	42		16	28	28	½ bar	1
6	1¾	1⅔	1¼	1¼	1	1¾	0 10	5	2½	2l 6s		6 s	9s 3d	4 s	10s	d
value																10
6s							1 2	7	3½							
Knee 5f	1½	1¾	1½	1¼	1	1½	0 11	5½	2⅜							
value																
5s																
l 17s																

	l.	s	d
Rough Trees for Masts	20	13	0
Ditto to make Yards	12	9	0
Oak Timber for Cheeks	2.	17	0
Ditto for the Cross and Trussletrees	0	9	4
Elm for Caps	2	6	0
Iron-work from Forge	0	19	8
Nails of divers sorts	0	6	0
Tallow	0	9	3
Rozin	0	4	0
Tar	0	10	0
Thrums	0	0	10
Mens Wages	13	8	4
Total Charge	60	11	10

Oak Timber 14 Feet for Cross and Trussle-trees, at 8 d per Foot, is 0 9 4

Having laid down the Dimenfions of Mafts, and every individual part belonging to them, for three Maft Ships, I fhall briefly fhew fome general Proportions for Mafting other Veffels of different Species, having been more particular in defcribing the nature of Mafting, by reafon it is a thing of moment, and often neglected by Seafaring-Carpenters, for want of Knowledge, although it is the very Rudiment that ought to give them the name of Sea-Carpenters; fince plainly fpeaking, an Examination ought to be made on every Carpenter of a Ship, before that Truft fhould be invefted on him, whether he can make a Suit of Mafts, or a Rudder, or any Capftern, as knowing fuch Materials are oftner wanted, than any other piece of Movables belonging to a Ship.

For a Ketch's Mafts, &c.

TO find the length of the Main-maft, add the breadth from Outfide to Outfide, and the depth in Hold together, and in fome burthenfome Veffels add half the Breadth to that, and for every one of the Feet made by fuch a Product allow three Foot, which will give you the length of Maft and Top-maft together, $\frac{3}{4}$ of the fame allow for the Standing-maft, and $\frac{1}{4}$ for the Top-maft. Obferve, that if they are made in two pieces, the $\frac{3}{4}$ includes the Head of the Lower-maft.

Breadth from Out to Out	18	Foot
Depth in Hold	8	
	26 Foot	

The $\frac{3}{4}$ is 19 $\frac{1}{2}$; and fo many Yards fuch a Ketch's Main-maft muft be, allowing 4 Inches to every Yard the Maft is to be long for the Head, which will be 6 Foot 6 Inches in this; but if you Scarfe a Top-maft, allow 4 Inches $\frac{1}{2}$ for the Head. For the Diameter in the Partners, allow $\frac{3}{4}$ of an Inch to every Yard in length, and $\frac{3}{4}$ of that bignefs allow at the upper part of the Hounds, where the Shrouds fets, befides the Stops, and half of the Partners at the Head, if the Top maft is to be hoifted; but if Scarfed, then fomething lefs.

The Maintop-gallant-maft is to be $\frac{2}{3}$ of the Top-maft in Length, allowing to every Yard in length, one Inch in Diameter.

Bowfprit $\frac{5}{6}$, and in fome the $\frac{5}{7}$ of the breadth, as aforefaid, allowing one Yard to one Foot as in a Ketch of 15 Foot broad, the length of the Bowfprits to be 9 Yards 2 Foot, or 10 Yards 2 Foot, allowing one Inch to a Yard for bignefs.

Main-yard $\frac{2}{3}$ of the Main-maft, Diameter $\frac{2}{3}$ of an Inch to a Yard.

Topfail-yard $\frac{5}{9}$ of the Main-yard, Diameter $\frac{5}{7}$ of an Inch to a Yard.

Maintop-gallant-yard $\frac{5}{9}$ of the Topfail-yard, Diameter $\frac{5}{7}$ of an Inch to a Yard.

Mizon-maft $\frac{3}{4}$ of the length of the Main-mafts length, without Maintop-maft, Diameter $\frac{2}{3}$ of an Inch to a Yard.

Mizon yard $\frac{5}{7}$ of the Main-yard, Diameter $\frac{3}{4}$ of an Inch to a Yard.

For Hoys Mafts.

ADD the breadth and depth together in Feet, gives the length of the Maft Head and all in Yards, as was aforefaid; and this is in full bearing Veffels, but in others abate; you allow $\frac{1}{4}$ of the whole length for Head, the bignefs to be $\frac{}{8}$ of an Inch to a Yard in length; allow $\frac{3}{4}$ of the Partners for the Hounds, and $\frac{}{3}$ of the Partners at the top or head.

Sprit twice the breadth of the Hoy, and Diameter 1 Inch to every Yard at the Crutch, and $\frac{2}{3}$ of that bignefs at the other end.

Bowſprit $\frac{5}{7}$ of the Hoys breadth in Yards as aforeſaid, and Diameter $\frac{1}{4}$ of an Inch to a Yard.

Mizon-maſt, if any, $\frac{5}{8}$ of the length of the Hoy, allowing $\frac{2}{3}$ of an Inch to every Yard.

Mizon-Yard $\frac{1}{2}$ a Yard longer than the Mizon-maſt, from the Deck upwards.

Boats Maſts.

MAin-maſt three times the breadth of the Boat, Fore-maſt $\frac{4}{5}$ of the Main-maſt, allowing $\frac{2}{5}$ or $\frac{1}{4}$ of an Inch to a Yard

Boats Maſt with Croſs Sails, three times the breadth of the Boat, and half the breadth, gives the length in Yards, if the Sails are *Viteroys Canvas*, but if *Noyl's*, two Foot leſs; that is meant of the Yard, which is to be $\frac{2}{3}$ of the Maſt, if the Sails are *Viteroys*, but if *Noyl's*, then two Foot ſhorter; and this is in a Boat of Six or Seven Foot broad, allowing for the bigneſs of Maſt and Yard $\frac{1}{4}$ of an Inch to a Yard.

Sprits of Wherrys Sails, as long as their reſpective Maſts, allowing $\frac{1}{2}$ an Inch (to every Yard in length) for bigneſs.

Shoulder Mutton-Sails, the Maſt muſt be four times the breadth of the Boat, Diameter $\frac{1}{2}$ of an Inch to a Yard in length. Boom $\frac{3}{4}$ of the Maſts length, Diameter $\frac{3}{7}$ of an Inch to a Yard in length, at the biggeſt end, and half the biggeſt, or after end, for the Fore-maſt end, where there is a Rack. Bowſprit the length of the Main-maſt to the Shrouds, and allow $\frac{7}{8}$ of an Inch for bigneſs to a Yard.

Bermoodoes Sail, the Main-maſt three times the breadth of the Boat, and one Foot longer; the Fore-maſt to be one Foot ſhorter than the Main-maſt, Diameter $\frac{5}{8}$ of an Inch to a Yard.

Smack Sails for Boats, Main-maſt three times the breadth of the Boat in Foot length, taking Notice of the ſhape as aforeſaid: Fore-maſt, if any, $\frac{4}{5}$ of the Main-maſt, which is ſometimes leſs than three times the breadth of the Veſſel, Diameter $\frac{7}{10}$ of an Inch to a Yard in length, the Sprit one Foot longer, and allow $\frac{4}{5}$ of an Inch to a Yard in length.

It cannot be very improper to annex to theſe Calculations of Maſting, the Cuſtomary Methods for Importing rough Maſts, and the Promiſcuous Opinions of Maſt-makers in allowing of the Converſions, ſince ſome Maſt-makers will have it, that a rough Tree of twenty Hands will make a Maſt of twenty five Inches Diameter, which is really impoſſible, for the Diameter of 80, the Circumference producted from a twenty handed Maſt, is but 25 Inches and $\frac{1}{2}$ Diameter, that there will be but half an Inch to work upon, and provided there was no Sap in Maſts, which I am apt to believe was never known otherwiſe, and that the Maſt grew as true and regular, as could be expected, it would not be proper to put him out of hand, without ſhaving of him to ſee the defects.

Others are of Opinion, that a Maſt of 20 Hands, will make a converted Maſt fitting for Service of 21 Inches Diameter, which may be variouſly allowed of; but the major part of Maſt-makers allow, that an equal number of Hands in the Circumference of any Maſt rough, will make a Maſt of as many Inches Diameter, and allow him to be even, and fine drawn, and take out the Sap and other Defects, which muſt of conſequence add to the ſtrength of the Maſt, from which I ſhall produce this following Table.

The Length and Number of Hands proper to transport Rough Masts, for the Use of Shipping in general.

Species	Length in Yards	Diameter Inches	Difference	Hands proper	Diameter rough	[illegible]
Main and Fore-mast	33 ½ 29 ½ 24 ½ 21 21 18 [illegible]	30 [illegible] 26 [illegible] 21 18 ½ 16 ½ 14	3 3 3 ½ 2 ½ 4 ½ 3 ½	21 18 16 ½ 14	26 ½ 23 ½ 20 ¾ 7	5 ½ 5 4 ¾ 3 [illegible]
Mizon-mast	32 ½ 17	22 10 [illegible]	10 ½ 6 ½	22 10 ½	28 13	6 2 ½
Bowsprit	14 ½	15	0 [illegible]	15	19	4
Main and Fore-top-masts	22 ½ 12 20 11	20 10 17 ½ 9	2 ½ 2 2 ½ 2	20 10 17 ½ 9	25 12 ½ 22 11 ½	5 2 ½ 4 ½ 2 ½
Mizon-top-masts	12 6	10 5	2 1	10 5	12 [illegible] 6 ½	2 ½ 1 ¾
Spritsail-top-masts	7 4	7 4	0 0	7 4	8 ½ 5 ½	1 ½ 1 ½
Main and Fore-top-gallant masts	9 ½ 8 ½ 5 ½ 4 ½	8 ½ 7 ½ 4 ½ 3 ¾	¾ 1 1 [illegible]	8 ½ 7 ½ 4 ½ 3 ¾	10 ¾ 9 ½ 6 ½ 5 [illegible]	2 [illegible] 2 1 [illegible] 1 [illegible]
Main and Fore yards	34 ½ 30 18 16	24 21 ½ 12 11	10 ½ 8 ½ 6 5	24 21 ½ 12 11	30 27 15 14 ½	6 5 ½ 3 3 ½
Mizon-yards	30 28 26 23 18 16	16 14 13 12 9 8	14 14 13 11 9 8	16 14 13 12 9 8	20 [illegible] 17 ½ 16 ½ 15 11 ½ 10	3 ½ 3 ½ 3 ½ 3 2 ½ 2
Spritsail-yards	21 19 18 16 13 11	15 14 12 11 9 7	6 5 6 5 4 4	15 14 12 11 9 7	19 17 ½ 15 14 [illegible] 11 ½ 8 ½	4 3 ½ 3 3 [illegible] 2 [illegible] 1 [illegible]
Main and Foretop-sail yards	19 10 16 8	17 7 11 6	6 3 5 2	13 7 14 7	16 ½ 8 ½ 16 ½ 7 ½	3 [illegible] 1 [illegible] 3 ½ 1 ½
Mizon-yards	9 5 [illegible]	7 4	2 1 ½	11 6	14 [illegible] 7 ½	3 [illegible] 1 ½
Spritsail Topsail-yards	11 10 9 8 7 5	8 7 7 6 5 4	3 3 2 2 2 1	8 7 7 6 5 4	8 ½ 8 ½ 8 ½ 7 6 5	½ 1 ½ 1 ¼ 1 1 1
Cross-jack yards	19 18 15 14 11 10	9 9 8 7 6 5	10 9 8 7 5 5	9 9 8 7 6 5	11 [illegible] 11 ½ 0 9 8 7	2 ½ 2 ½ 2 2 2 2
Topgallant-yards Main and Fore	9 8 5 ½ 4	7 6 3 ½ 3	2 2 2 1	7 6 5 ½ 4	7 ½ 6 ¾ 7 6	[illegible] [illegible] 1 ½ 2

Since

Since it has been a general Custom in transporting rough Masts to allow, that to the number of Hands each Mast measures, there shall be an Addition of 6 put for the Length in Yards; that is, if any Mast shall measure twelve Hands, then the Length to be 18 Yards; and so on for every Mast so imported.

I have therefore Calculated this Table to shew the Errors, since out of 14 particular parts of Masting, it will appear by this Table, that in 8 of them the difference is but 2 $\frac{3}{4}$, which being Top-masts and Small Yards, and oftnest broke and wore out; and therefore in them particulars, two Yards and three quarters may suffice for Waste in lieu of six Yards.

Several others reach but to 3 and 4, and few to 6 Yards, although there be several other small Vessels, whose parts of Masting falls under divers Denominations. This Table shews you the particulars from a Ship of 1700 Tuns, to one of 200 Tuns, sufficient to guide you to the Transportation of such Materials, Exact and Genuine

Note, that the first Column towards the left hand is the Denominations of the Masts and Yards, where the number affix'd shews you the various Meetings in the six particulars

The second Column shews you the number of Yards contain'd in each. The third is the Diameter in Inches The fourth is the difference between the length and bigness The fifth, the number of Hands proper to make such a Mast or Yard The sixth is the Diameter rough from the number of Hands. The seventh is the Waste made by such Conversions.

Although I have been seemingly very particular in describing the Nature of Masting; notwithstanding there is still three Material Parts remaining, which are not mentioned; and that is, the Cheeking of Masts, the Scarphing of Yards, and making of Masts with divers pieces, what Shipwrights term, *made Masts*.

As to the Cheeking of Masts, it is by adding two Pieces of Oak, one of each side of the Mast, at the Head, and for two Material Reasons, the first of which is, when Masts has not Substance upwards to head themselves, as is generally found in large Masts, that are sparingly reduced, in order to continue the Substance at the Partners; and the other Reason is, that in large Masts they have great Weights of Tops, Caps and Trussetrees: all which requiring more strength, and Security, than what Firr is able to bear

There is some general Observations made in Cheeking of Masts, that the Cheeks ought to be half the length of the Mast, and that the Mast shall be made as big Thwartships, at the Stop of the Trusletrees, with Firr and Oak together, as he is at the Partners, or biggest Place.

As to the length of the Cheeks, I am of Opinion, they need be no longer than to reach as low as the Mast will continue the Substance of such a Mast as you design to make; neither need a Cheek'd Mast be any bigger upwards than a Mast that heads himself, for although several Pieces put together cannot be so strong as an intire Piece, and that Tabling and Coaking (as its term'd) may weaken, yet notwithstanding the different strength between Oak and Firr, will make up for such wants.

And since Cheeking any Mast can be no other than supplying the wants in the rough Tree, therefore there is nothing else required in making them, than to work them as far as they have Substance, as any others Mast is wrought that heads themselves, and from that Place to strike a straight Line to the Head, allowing $\frac{1}{3}$ of the bigness at the Head Firr, the Waste and Tabling included into $\frac{1}{3}$, and let the Oak be $\frac{2}{3}$ wrought, besides making up the Waste made by Joining and Tabling.

And for a more clear Illustration I shall lay down some Figures of the Nature of Cheeking any Mast.

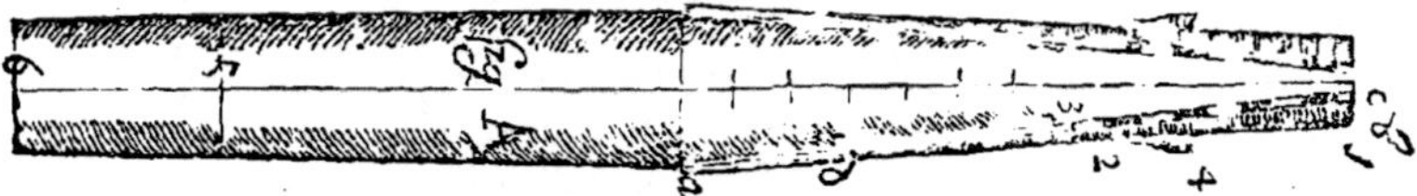

Figure A imitates any ſtanding (or lower) Maſt; not that its drawn in direct Proportion, as exact length to exact bigneſs, but only to ſhew the Nature of fitting the Cheeks, 5 being the Partners or biggeſt part of the Maſt, 6 the Heel, or extream length downwards, and 1 the extream length upwards, called the Head, though all from 1 to 4 is taken for the Head of the Maſt; where may be obſerved a projecting part, which is made for a Reſt, or Shoulder, for the Truſletrees, which Truſletrees make another Step for the Top maſt: from 4 to 2 is the Hounds.

The Cheeks are all from *a.* to *b* which is half the length of the Maſt, tho' I am of Opinion, that if the Cheeks were no longer than from *b* to *d*. it may be as well, and much cheaper, for ſince the lower part is wrought ſo very thin, it can be of no Service, only to ſhape the Maſt, provided the Maſt has his Subſtance to *d*.

The dark Shadow being Oak of each ſide of the Maſt, you are to underſtand that the Oak and Firr (which is the Maſt) is not barely join'd, but one part is let into the other, the Firr always into the Oak; and this is term'd, Coaking or Tabling, ſomewhat imitating Mortiſeing, and Tenoning in Joynery.

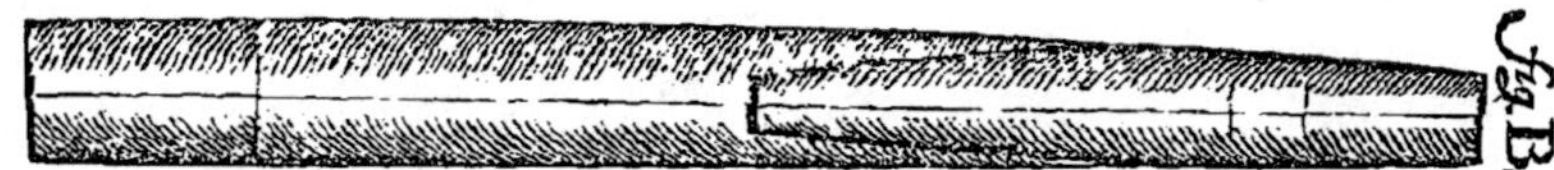

In *Figure* B. you may obſerve the Faſhion of the Cheeks fore and aft.

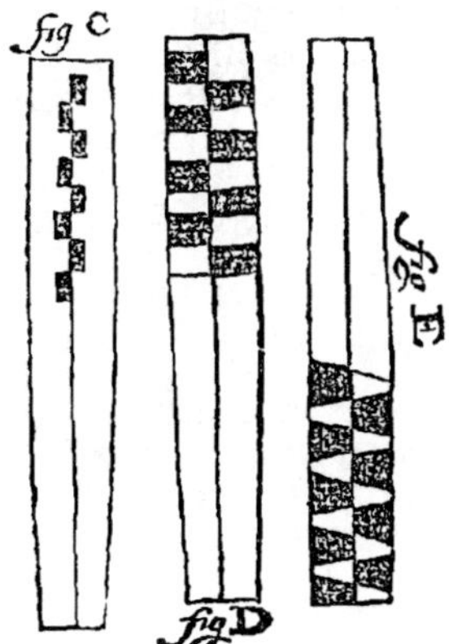

In *Figures* C. D. E. may be ſeen the Nature of Coaking and Tabling, C is Coaking, and its thus; The Wood in the Wake of the dark Shadow is cut in an Inch, or ſomething more or leſs, according to the bigneſs of the Maſt, and ſuch cutting is made up with Firr. The reaſon is very plain; for ſuch working one part into another, ſtops the Maſt where its join'd, that the extraordinary twiſting cauſed by Sailing, ſhall not looſen the Joint.

Notwithſtanding its my Opinion, that leſs Proviſion may ſuffice, than what is at ſometimes uſed. when the Tabling is cut ſo very deep, and eſpecially at the Edges, it doth undeniably cauſe a great Weakneſs, and may endanger the loſing of the Maſts.

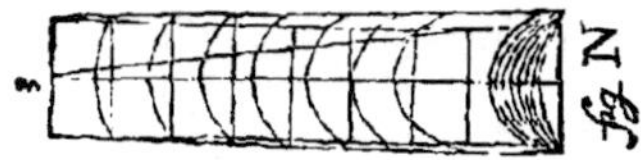

Figure N. ſhews how Cheeks may be fairly wrought from 3, the lower part of ſuch Coaking, ſince the Maſt is flatter at 3 than at the lower end of the Cheeks.

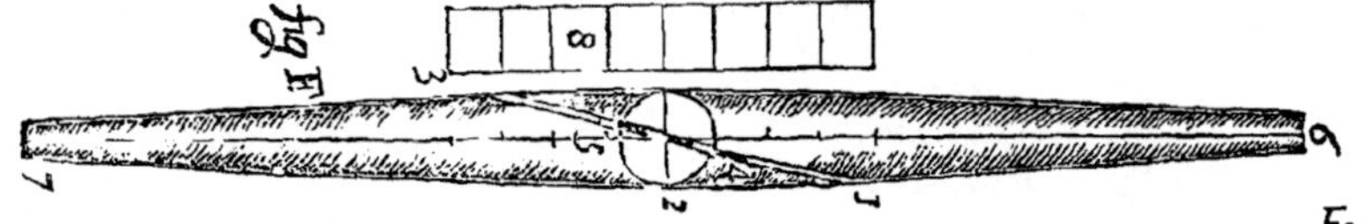

Figure

Figure F is the Figure of a large Yard, when two Trees are put together, 2 being the Slings, and 6, 7, the Yard Armes, the Scarph is generally allowed to be ⅓ of the extream length, which may be considered from what was mentioned in Cheeking of Mast, for it must needs follow, that long Scarphs without a Proportional Substance to bear it, is a weakening to any piece so scarph'd. From 3 to 1 is the length of the Scarph, and from 4 to 5, it is either Coak'd or Tabled; the other part is only worked with hollows and bollows, as its term'd, almost in the Nature of working the lower part of the Cheeks

You are to be very careful in working from a middle Line, each way, that one side of the Mast may have as much Oak as the other, and to make your Mast as straight as possible, for which there is several practical ways, both in working the Cheeks, and in cutting the Heel of the Mast, that will be great helps to make a crooked Tree a straight Mast, chiefly observing one thing in faying the Cheeks, to let your middle Line be Horizontal, and exactly level.

But to proceed in shewing something Material in making large Masts with divers Pieces, of which there be divers Fashions, some using a Spindle, and working several Pieces round that Spindle, others putting four square Pieces together without a Spindle; which I cannot approve of to be good work.

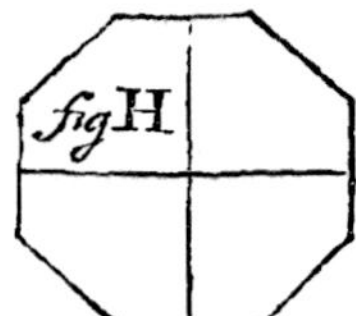

But to proceed to the Spindle Fashion, and that is to prepare a Piece, or several Pieces, by scarphing the length of the Mast you design, and bring such a Spindle into 8 Squares, as the Figure H: And by the way it may not be improper to shew a very plain and Mechanical way of setting of an 8 Square, on any Tree, either Square or Waney.

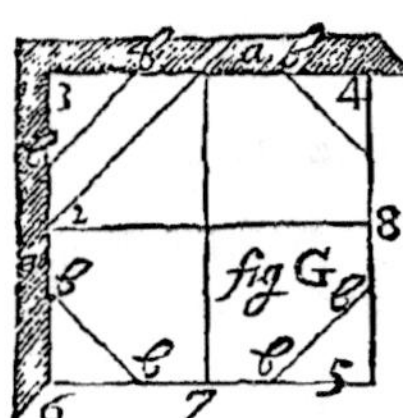

Provided there was a Tree to be wrought into an eight Square, as 3, 4, 6 and 7, then taking any common Square, as *a a* shadow'd, and lay upon such a Tree, marking the middle line in 1 and 2, on the Square; then take the distance from 1 to 2, with any pair of Compasses, and set off from 3. to *b* and the other way from 4 to *b*. so is the distance from *b* to *b*. on the side 3, 4, the exact eight Square.

This Method of setting off eight Squares would be extreamly useful at Sea, when a Mast requires to be overhal'd or lessened 1 Inch, or less.

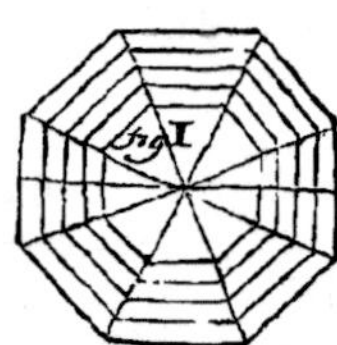

In preparing the Spindle for a made Mast, mind to taper him upwards and downwards, in due proportion according to the Shape of the Mast you design to make, according to such a Method as may be seen in Figure I.

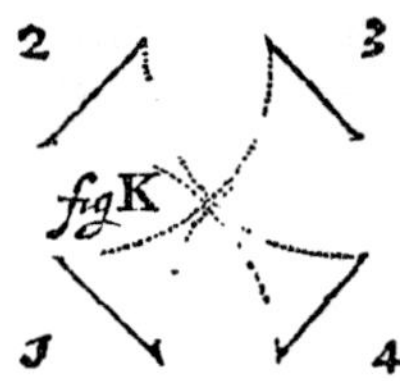

Figure K Shews you another Method of setting off an eight Square on the Flat, as if there was any pieces of board to form into an eight Square, as 1, 2, 3, 4 stick in the Compasses at every one of the Corners, and intersect the Center *a* which shall describe an eight Square on the Lines of Bounding 1, 2. 2, 3. 3, 4 and 1, 4.

Figure L

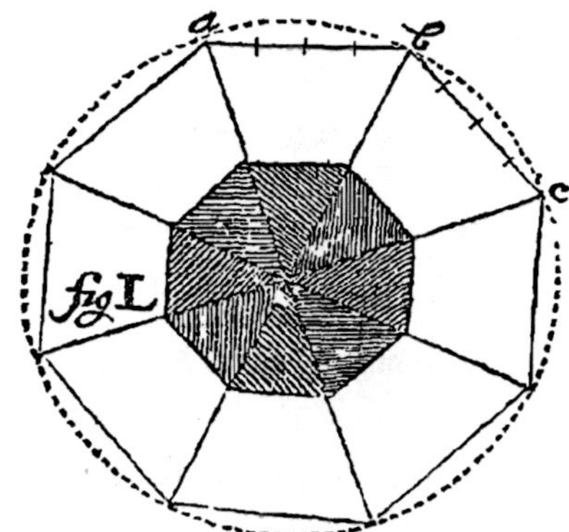

Figure L Shews how the Pieces are brought on upon the Spindle, to make a large Maſt; the Shadows ſhew how eight Pieces are brought on, and ſcarph'd one over another length ways, till the Maſt is made as large as requiſite, according to the magnitude of the Ship; and ſuch Figures ſhould be laid down at every Quarter, as is cuſtomary in ſetting of any other Maſt, obſerving that a 16 Square is ſet off by dividing an eighth Square into four parts, as the Limbs *a b. c.* and ſo is a 32 Square from a 16 Square.

It would be really worth the Trial, or Expence made by ſuch an Obſervation, to ſee whether Elm caſed with Oak, would not make ſuch large Maſts, if they could be found as durable: I cannot ſee any material Objection why it may not be put in Practice; not for what would be ſav'd by doing ſo, but in caſe the large Firr Trees, and ſmall ones too, could not be obtain'd.

Elm is of a tough Nature, and not heavy; its but as 12 to 11, in Gravity to Firr, and Oak is much more durable than either, and ſtronger, and in weight to Fir as 8 to 5; and therefore I am apt to believe, that they need not be made much heavier than a Firr Maſt, Cheek'd with Oak.

And in divers other dry parts of the Ship Elm may be uſed in lieu of Oak and Firr, and it would come much cheaper

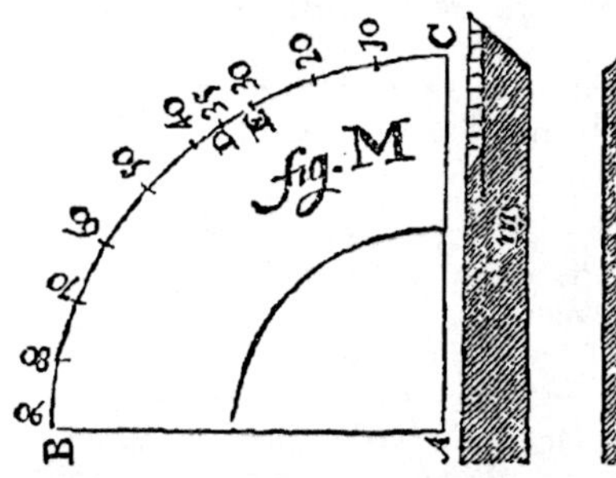

Figure M and N Are two Battons, miter'd at one end; which would be a very good Rule to mark off an eight Square, or 16 Square; for ſuch Rulers having the eight ſquares, and 16 ſquares, from the middle line mark'd on them ſuitable to every four ſquar'd Maſt that you are to make; then by placing the eight or ſixteen Square on your Batton, at the middle line on your Maſt, ſuitable to the four ſquare of the Maſt or Yard you are working, then the end of the Batton, or ſharp part of your Mitre, will ſhew you the eight or ſixteen Square you require; ſince an eight Square is no other than a Mitre from the four Square.

Figure M Shews how to ſet off the Beveling of the Crutch for a Smack Sail; to *E.* the Quadrant *A. B C* dividing the Limb into 90 degrees, ſet off from *C* make 30, and from *C.* to *D.* 35, ſo ſhall them lines *A. D A E.* give you the Beveling of the Crutch.

To ſet off the Quarters of any Maſt or Yard by Gunter's *Line.*

A Standing Maſt { Thwartſhips at the Partners } the [illegible] Firſt Quarter, the [illegible] in the middle, $\frac{5}{6}$ at the Hounds, and $\frac{2}{3}$ at the Head
{ Fore and Aft, } the $\frac{2}{3}$ at the Croſs-trees, and [illegible] at the Head, and $\frac{4}{5}$ at the Heel

The Bowsprit to be of the Bead the $\frac{40}{41}$, the $\frac{9}{10}$, the $\frac{5}{6}$ and $\frac{1}{2}$ at the Head, and $\frac{4}{5}$ at the Heel

Top-masts to be of the Cap first $\frac{14}{15}$, $\frac{7}{8}$, $\frac{3}{4}$, [illegible], Topgallant mast ditto, Spritsail Top-mast to be first $\frac{3}{4}$, the $\frac{11}{12}$, the $\frac{5}{6}$, the $\frac{2}{3}$ and [illegible] at the Head

Yards of the Slings each way the $\frac{30}{31}$, the $\frac{7}{8}$, $\frac{2}{3}$, $\frac{1}{2}$, or otherwise $\frac{1}{2}$ at the Yard Arm

Mizon-yard lower end, $\frac{9}{10}$, $\frac{5}{6}$, $\frac{11}{12}$, $\frac{20}{21}$ Slings, $\frac{24}{25}$, $\frac{13}{15}$, $\frac{4}{5}$, $\frac{1}{2}$ top end

And after all these intricate Methods, the plain Instrument, that I have described, will do the Work exacter and readier.

I shall in the next place mention something concerning the Capsterns or Windless's in Ships, which I shall endeavour to prove in some Measure, not to be suitable to the design'd Service, but will require something of a Theory, as well as altogether the Practick part.

All Ship's Capsterns may properly be called Engines, or Machines in Machines, or a Wheel within a Wheel, since they are reducible to that Mechanick Power called a Wheel in *Peritrochio*, as I shall just mention hereafter, but first shall shew some practical Observations, that are used in making; and using of Ships Capsterns

I shall first mention the Main-capstern, which ought to be first and principally considered, since the chief Use is to heave up the Anchors; for the hardest Service in a Ship may, and is at sundry Times perform'd without the help of the Main-capstern

This Main-capstern is placed something abaft the Main-mast, or where the Pumps stand; not that I shall mention in this place, the great Safeguard that would be made to Shipping in general, if there were one or two large Chain Pumps placed and worked on Necessity by the said Main-capstern, which might undeniably be done without any disadvantage to the other Service, that may be required from the said Main-capstern; neither will it be very Chargeable, considering that it might be a means to save both Ship and the Ship's Crew.

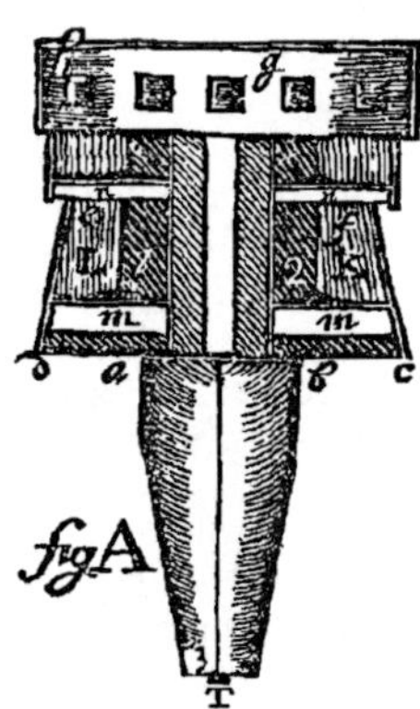

Figure A is the shape of a Main capstern, which is worked upon the lower Gun-deck, and steps under that Deck five or six Foot, this Capstern is seldom used but in Extremity, and then the Cable is brought to the Capstern, or a Hawser, called a Messenger When the Cable is brought too, there is some difficulty in keeping him up from rubbing on the Deck, which is term'd Surgeing · To assist in this Case, there is pieces of Wood call'd Nippers, put into Straps, that are receiv'd in the Whelps of the said Capstern · And this is the reason the Capstern is made tapering upwards, to stop the sliding down of such heavy Ropes, if a Cable may be term'd so.

There are several Practical Rules to proportion the parts of a Capstern, as that the Diameter of the Barrel of a Main-capstern shall be five Diameters of the biggest Cable, though some will have it to be as big as the Main-mast in the Partners.

However, since Experience has taught us, that five Diameters of the biggest Cable will be big enough for a Main-capstern, and that by such a Capstern, the Cable will be the first that breaks, it will be as well against the Rules of good

Husbandry, as the facilitating the Purchase of the Anchor, to have the Main-capstern any bigger.

The bigness of the Spindle *a b* is at some times allowed to be the $\frac{1}{9}$ of the Barrel, which in such a large Capstern will be near three Inches · But why a Capstern should be so reduc'd, is (I must needs confess) a Parodox to me

For since its the Opinion of most Men, that the weakest part of any Mechanick Power will first be broke, and the Spindle of any Capstern being nearer the middle than either of the Barrels, must of Consequence be most materially effected with the strain: Besides, Experience has taught us, that the Spindle of any Capstern complains first; for if the upper Barrel is first sprain'd, its caused by the insufficiency of the workmanship, or otherwise by working green Timber that is shrunk, by which means the Thrum-head of the said Capstern becomes loose, and twists the other parts.

The conveniencies in Joggling a Capstern, or to make such a difference between the Barrel and Spindle are two; the first is, because there be Grooves cut in the Barrel for the Sole of every Whelp, which in the largest Capstern is cut in one Inch, and so proportionally for a lesser sort. The second conveniency is for cutting a Groove close to the Spindle, for to run over an Iron Hoop fix'd in the Partners of the Capstern; which Groove need not be above half an Inch, and would be better supplied with another Iron Hoop fitted to make a Groove, and much better for the ease and wear of the Capstern, since Iron to Iron is more agreeable in working, than Iron with Wood

And therefore it would be much better and stronger for all Capsterns, if the Barrels and the Spindles were (at the largest difference) within one Inch, one as big as the other.

That the Whelps *L K* shall be at the lower end, *b. c. a d* half the Diameter of the Capstern in the Barrel, which large Whelps are only requisite where the extreams of such Capsterns require to be large, for the conveniency of a great Cable to be bent about them.

That the Surge shall be two Inches and $\frac{4}{5}$ in every Foot perpendicularly upwards; or otherwise, that the Whelps being divided into three parts, and at two parts from below, let the Whelps be $\frac{4}{5}$ of what they are at the lower end *f. n.* $\frac{1}{5}$ of *b c.* then the Stop or Joggle to be $\frac{2}{7}$ of the $\frac{4}{5}$, the Heads upwards to taper $\frac{1}{2}$ an Inch in a Foot, or if it was not for a little Comeliness, there would be a Conveniency in working the Heads perpendicular; it would steady the Thrum Head.

To have the Thrum Head as big in Diameter as the Sweep of the Capstern at the lower end of the Whelps, and $\frac{1}{4}$ of the Diameter for the Thickness of him, to divide the Thickness into 13 parts; then let 5 of those parts be left below the Holes, 4 of them for the Bar Holes, and 4 above.

The Chocks in the lower ends $\frac{1}{3}$ of the Whelp's height, and to be placed high enough for to make room for the Pall of the Capstern, which Pall will be various according to the bigness of the Ship, the greatest thickness need not be above 5 Inches · The Chocks in the upper part half the bigness of the Chocks in the lower part, and be plac'd an Inch above the Stops in the upper part of the Whelps.

The Whelps to be cut tapering side ways, each way from a middle line 1 Inch and $\frac{1}{4}$, observing to have convenient fastning to all the Whelps, Chocks, and Thrum Head, but to have no Iron in the Wake of the Wear of your Ropes or Cables; the Bar Holes to be cut half an Inch tapering in one Foot deep, and the Step or Toe of the Capstern, to be half what he is in the Spindle.

And this is what has materially occurr'd in the Practical part of making Main-Capsterns: I shall now proceed to shew what has been the Methods of making of Jeer-capsterns, or Capsterns of a lower Size, with two Tire of Whelps.

Figure B.

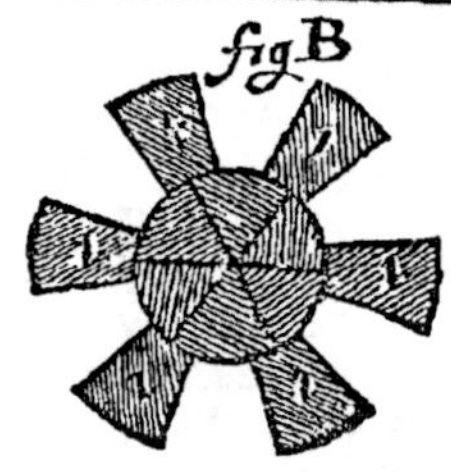

But first observing that there is a conveniency or advantage attends the cutting of the Whelps taper outward, for the less taper the better the Cable or other Rope is held, and the more taper the worse; since if the Capstern was intirely fill'd up between the Whelps, it would not hold an Inch of a Cable. But the Capstern would be forc'd about, without purchasing any thing by such heaving, provided the end was not made fast to the Capstern, and all the Rope, as its hove in, turn'd about the Whelps 1, 1, 1, 1, 1, 1.

Therefore in cutting the Whelps, the Proportion of tapering this way, should be also gain'd from the bigness of the Cable, or other Rope that is materially manag'd by such a Capstern; however that difference being so small, I shall refer it to the Practick part, and proceed to the Jeer Capstern.

The Jeer Capstern is placed between the Main-hatch, and the Bitts, and has two Tire of Whelps, one Tire between the Decks, and the other upon the middle or upper Deck, according to the Size of the Ship

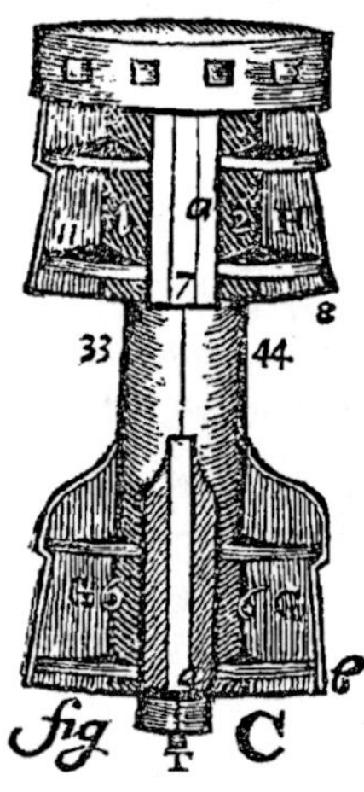

Figure C Imitates the Jeer Capstern · the lower Whelp's C. are placed opposite to the Hawse Holes, and is always used to heave up the Anchor, though the Cable is not brought to this Capstern, but a large Rope, imitating a Cable, of a lower Denomination than the real Cable is.

This large Cabled Rope is call'd a *Vyol*, whose Diameter is to the Diameter of the biggest Cable as 9 to 16, and can be used either way, with the Cable of one side, or the Cable of the other.

The Diameter of the upper barrel of the Jeer Capstern is to the Diameter of the Main-capstern's Barrel, as 6 to 7, and the Spindle of the Capsterns in the same Proportion, the lower Barrel's Diameter to the upper Barrel's Diameter, is as 13 to 14.

The Surge or Tapering of the Whelps in this Capstern are Practically cut less than in the Main-capstern, in every perpendicular height, but all the other Members are proportioned from the preceeding Rules, according as the magnitude of one Capstern is to the magnitude of the other

I shall not at present be absolute in my Opinion, that the Spindle of the Jeer Capstern ought to be as big as the Spindle of the Main-capstern, but am pretty positive, that at some times, the small Capstern heaves as great a Purchase (or a dead Weight) as the Main capstern, and much oftner used, since the Main-capstern is never used without the Jeer, provided the Jeer is not disabled; but the Jeer is used ten times for the others once.

The Sweep of the Whelps in this Capstern, that heaves the *Vyol*, need be no otherways proportioned, than as the Diameter of *Vyol* is to the Diameter of the biggest Cable, so shall the Sweep or Circumference of the lower Whelps in the Jeer Capstern be, to the Circumference of the Whelps in the Main-capstern.

And the Surge may be thus proportion'd; as the weight of one Fathom of the largest Cable, is to the weight of a Fathom of the *Vyol*, so shall the Surge of the Main-capstern be, to the Surge of the Whelps in the lower Tire of the Jeer-capstern

I do really admire, that such an advantagious Faculty is not minded, in making of the upper part of the Jeer-capstern's, especially in Ships of three Decks, since

ſince they can be ſerviceable in heaving no larger Rope than the Jeers or Top-rope, or ſome Hawſer of near the Diameter of the Jeers, which is not much above half the Diameter of the *Vyol*

Not that I would have the Spindle leſs, but rather as aforeſaid; therefore the Reducement ſhall lye wholly in the Whelps, ſince the height of a Whelp is ſo far from adding Strength to the Barrel, that undeniably its rather a weakning, and actually aſſiſting in twiſting the Capſtern to pieces; ſo that Figure D. will be more ſuitable for ſhaping a Jeer-capſtern than Figure C, which is very near the ſhape of all our Practical Jeer-capſterns.

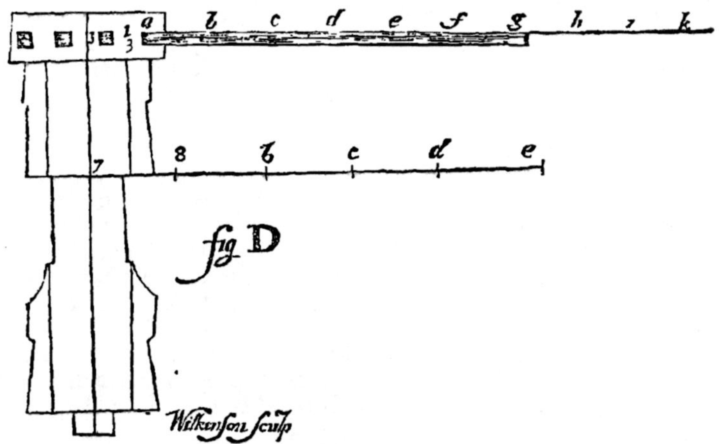

In *Figure* D. you may obſerve, that the lower Whelps are proportioned to *Figure* A. according to my preceeding Demonſtration; but the Whelps in the upper part are much bigger than ſuch a Rule will allow of, whichis allow'd for the advantage of having a large Thrum Head, for the conveniency of fitting in the Capſtern-bars.

All the other Members are particularly fitted by the ſame Rule as is aforementioned, only in conſideration of the facilitating the work that may be required to be done, and leſſening the Number of Men, that may not be in the way, when ſuch Services are required to be done, I have laid down theſe Rules, which may be ſeen farther by the diſproportion between the Semidiameter of the Sweep of the Whelps 1. 3. in Figure D and the Semidiameter of the Whelps in Figure C 7. 8. and the common length of the Capſtern bar 1. *g*. for the diſproportion of theſe Engines lies there.

Now it may be obſerv'd, that in two Capſtern-bars of equal length, one in the Figure C. and another in the Figure D they are as 5 to 7. in this ſmall matter of reducing the Whelps, ſo that the Bar in D. is ſeven Semidiameters of the Sweep of the Whelps from the Center of the Capſtern 7, and the Bar in the Figure C but 5, and that 5 Men at *e*. imitating the Figure C. is but equal to 5 Men at *e*. in Figure D. and 5 Men at the Bar prolong'd to *K*. in Figure D. ſhall be equal to 10 Men at the Bar at *e*. in Figure C. and the Bar only augmented $\frac{3}{7}$ part more.

By which it may appear what the Purchaſe may be increaſed, or Power leſſened, in doing the hardeſt Services that may be required to be done: Alſo that a Bar of the length from 3. to *e* in Figure D will do equal Service to a Bar of the length from 3 to *g*. in Figure C. the bigneſs may be alſo reduced in proportion to the ſhortening; and alſo the Hole in the Thrum Head may be made leſs. The Charge of the Whelps, Thrum Heads, and other Members, will be alſo leſſened as well as the Weight, and the Capſtern ſtronger, and of greater Service.

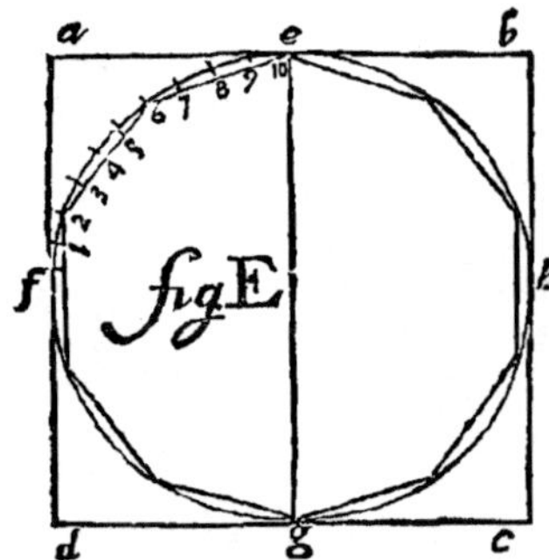

Figure E Shews the Nature of reducing the rough Piece of Timber designed for the Capstern, into any number of Squares. In this Figure it may be observed to be 10 Square, or a regular Polygone, consisting of ten sides.

You are to observe, that a Circle equal in Diameter to what the Barrel of any Capstern is required to be, will not do; for the reducing of it out of a Round into either 12, 10, 8 or 6 Squares, but will lessen the Pieces, although it will not be worth the trouble of calculating such a Table of what the allowance ought to be, in every particular Size of Capsterns, and every particular number of Squares, but shall only hint at present, that any Man may make such easie Trials, when he is placed on such a Service, on his, or any other common Kitchen Floor, or what is nearer, when he has provided a rough piece of Timber, that is designed for such a Service (which cannot be too sound and clear of Defects) get him into some convenient place assigned for such a Use, then cut off the Ends as square or perpendicular to the sides as you can, and on the Ends you may mark the Squares; observing, that after you have sweep'd out a Circle, as *e f. g h* divide it into four Quadrants, as supposing *h e* to be one of the four, then divide this Quadrant from *h* to *e.* into an equal number of parts, as you design to have sides to your Barrel, as let it be 12 or 10, the common number, for they must be even, because of an even number of Whelps; then four of that number shall mark out the exact side of your Squares, as taking in your Compasses the distance from *h.* to 4. that distance will be exactly extended ten times in the Circle *e. h g. f* and so of any other number of Squares whatever.

And here you may observe, that the difference between the first reducing of a rough piece of Timber into four Squares, and bringing of him into a ten Square piece, fitting for the Barrel of a Capstern in 7 Foot 8 Inches, is 4 Inches, since the piece in a 4 Square is 7 Foot 8, and in the 10 Square but 7 Foot 4 And such Demonstrations may produce us exact Methods for reducing several valuable pieces of Timber, observing that in making of Capsterns, the Sap of the Timber ought to be taken wholly out.

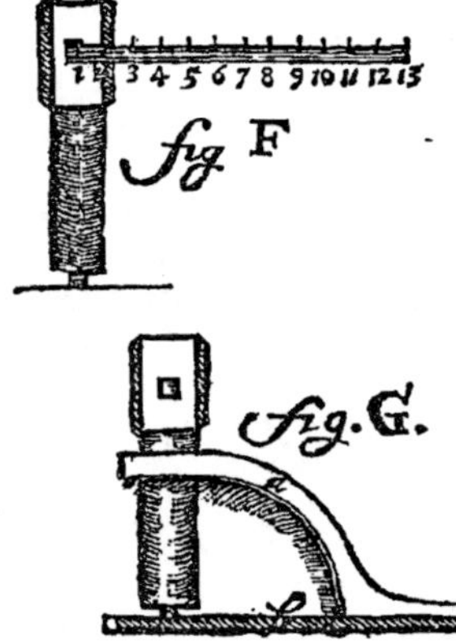

Figure F is term'd a *Crab*, or it may be call'd a Vertical Windless, where may be observ'd the Power is in proportion to the Weight, as 13 to 1. These sorts of Instruments are extreamly serviceable in Ship work, since they may be remov'd from Place to Place, as the Service requires, having a nice Provision made to move with the Windless, as a Frame which is universally useful where-ever the Mechanical Operation is required to be wrought, as may be seen in Figure G That *a.* is part of such a Frame, and having other Members branch'd out Perpendicular from the part *a* stept in a Bed, at *b.* fitted for that Purpose all the whole Frame is intire, and may be shifted at Pleasure, and in divers Cases, far more serviceable than a Horizontal Windless can be made.

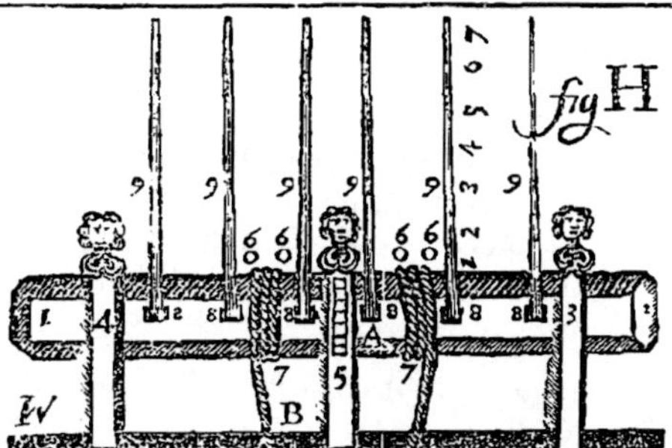

Figure H. imitates a Horizontal Windlefs, a Windlefs or Inftrument in common Ufe Aboard of all fmall Ships and Veffels, efpecially fuch as has but one Deck, or that heaves in their Cables on the upper Deck.

The Conveniencies are, that the Cables may be always brought about the Windlefs in order to purchace, or heave up the Anchor without doing of any Prejudice to any other Service; and farther, the Cables of each fide may be hove (as its term'd) together provided the purchace in both Cables are one way, which cannot be in a Capftern near fo conveniently done

But then thefe forts of Windleffes may be more properly term'd, or reduc'd to the Leaver, than the Wheel, fince the motion in thefe can be but continued for a fhort fpace, as may be anfwerable to that little diftance between the Fulciment and the Weight; but thofe Vertical Windleffes or Capfterns, may make continual Rotations without any Intermiffion or Difcontinuance

In this Figure, 1. 2 being the extream length of the Windlefs; 3. 4 the Checks of the Windlefs, in which the Windlefs turns; 5 a Stander to apply a Pall to ftop the Windlefs *A* the Windlefs, and *B* the Deck, *66* are the Hawse Holes of each fide, where the Cables come in; 7. are the Cables of each fide, 99 the Handfpokes or Leavers, and 8. the Holes for the Handfpokes.

The Handfpokes in this Pofition, feems to be Perpendicular from the Horizon, and fo they may be allow'd to be, the number is 6, the Proportion between the Semidiameter of the Windlefs, and the length of the Spoke is as 1 to 7 and on occafion, there may be two Men applied to every Spoke; nay, in *extra* forcing, there may be fome halling with Ropes faftened to the ends of the Spokes. But then you are to obferve, that when thefe Handfpokes make $\frac{1}{4}$ of a Revolution, and make a right Angle to their prefent Perpendicular Pofition, or becomes exactly Horizontal, then they are fhifted into the firft Pofition before they can purchafe any more. The Windlefs by this fhifting is ftop'd, the purchafe ceafes, and not only fo, but the gathering Motion is retarded, and there is at fome times a ftrain required, almoft equal to what it was at firft; but in the Vertical Windleffes, there is no fuch retarding Faculties happen, but the Motion is fteady and perpetual, according to the Power applied, which can be much greater than can poffibly be plac'd to any Horizontal Windlefs

For the clearer Explication of this Faculty, it will not be amifs to confider the Form of it, as it will appear, being more fully expofed to View in the Diagrams *I* and *K*.

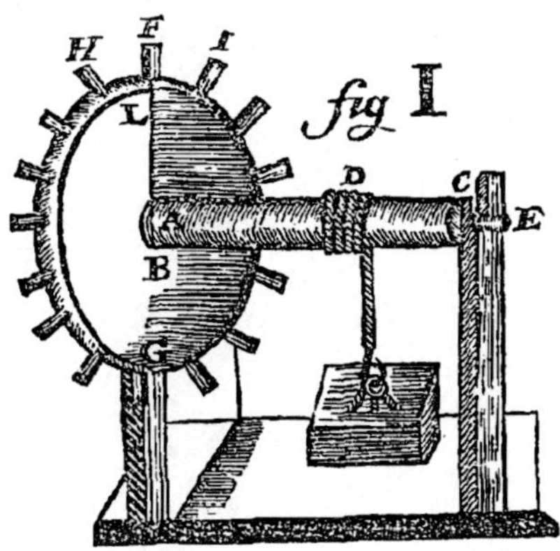

Firft in Figure I where *B C.* reprefents the Cylinder, or Spindle of the Capftern or Windlefs; which is fuppofed to move on a fmaller Axis. At E or Toe of the Capfterns, *T.* (which being all one in Comparifon to the feveral proportions, as if it were a meer Mathematical Line) *L. G.* is the Rundle or Wheel (or in a Capftern the Thrum Head) where the Spokes *H. F. I.* are put, imitating the Capftern Bars or Handfpokes in a Windlefs; *D.* the Place of the Cord, or the Whelps in the Capftern.

The

The Force of this Instrument consists in that Disproportion of Distance there is betwixt the Semidiameter of the Cylinder *A B*, and the Semidiameter of the Rundle, with the Spokes *F A* For let us conceive the Line *F. B* to be as a Leaver, wherein *A* is the Center or Fulciment, *B* the Place of the Weight, and *F* of the Power · Its therefore Evident, that by how much the distance *F A* is greater than *A. B.* by so much less need the Power be at *F* in respect of the Weight at *B* Suppose *A. B* to be as the tenth part of *A F.* then that Power or Strength, which is but as a Hundred Pound at *F.* will be equal to a Thousand Pound at *B*

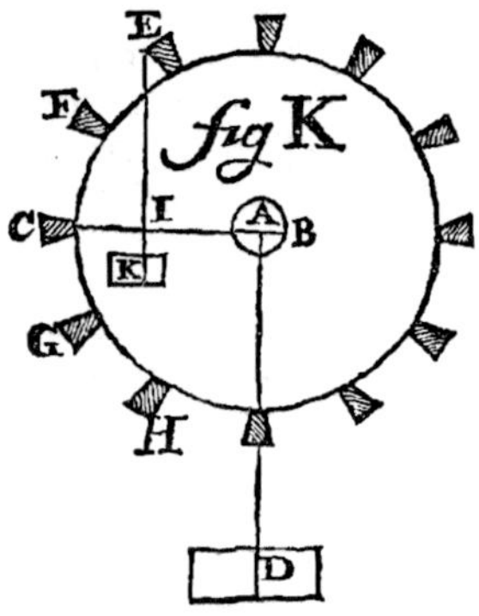

Figure K Suppose *A B* for the Semidiameter of the Axis or Cylinder,and *A C.* for the Semidiameter of the Rundle with the Spokes; then the Power at *C.* which will be able to support the weight; *D.* must bear the same Proportion unto it, as *A B.* doth to *A C.* so that by how much shorter the distance *A B* is in comparison to the distance *A C.* by so much less need the Power be at *C.* which may be able to support the weight, *D.* hanging at *B.*

And so likewise it is for the other Spokes or Handles *E, F, G, H,* at either of which, if we conceive any Power which shall move according to the same Circumference wherein these Handles are placed, then the strength of this Power will be all one, as if it were at *C.* But now supposing a dead weight hanging at any of them, (as at *E*) then the disproportion will vary, the Power being so much less than that at *C.* by how much the line *A. C.* is longer than *A I* the weight, *K* being of the same force at *E.* as if it were hung at *I.* in which Point the Perpendicular of its Gravity doth cut the Diameter.

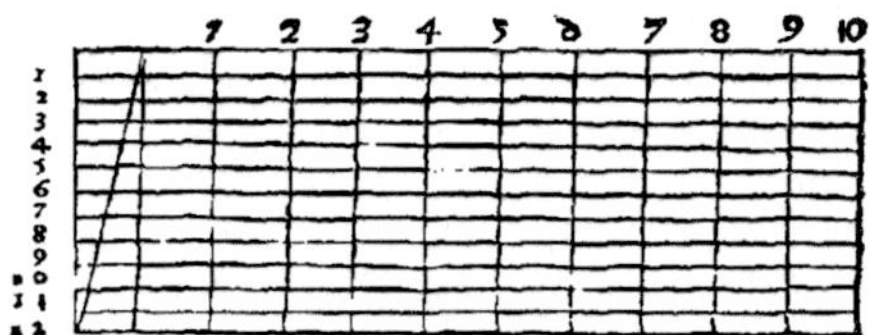

REASONS

REASONS

Publiſhed by Mr. *John Cocks*, late Chamber-keeper to His Majeſty's Moſt Honourable Privy-Council,

And Humbly offer'd for a BILL

To Breed Shipwrights, more experienced in the right and perfect Knowledge of the Uſe of their Tools, and in the practick Part of their Trade, and the due Obſervation of General Rules, for the more Firm and Well Newbuilding, Rebuilding, and Repairing of Ships and Veſſels; in Anſwer to the Maſter Shipwrights Propoſal, very well approved of in the Joynt Opinion and Reports, and in the Petition of the Fair-dealing Merchants within mentioned.

For the Caſe is clear and plain, where there is no General Rule Eſtabliſhed, no Fault or Tranſgreſſion will be own'd, nor diſcover'd, by ſome particular Clandeſtine Traders in Shipping, tho' it is common to find great Damages, and Loſſes, and the Errors and Deceits, and unskilful Workmanſhip in Ships and Veſſels, are manifeſt and plainly diſcover'd, and known, both at Sea and Aſhore.

IN the Year 1691, the Maſter-Builders and other experienced able Maſter-Shipwrights, in their humble Petition did ſet forth, That by many Years Experience, they did obſerve and find great Diſorders and Abuſe in the Practice and Government of the Shipwrights-Trade, and alſo many Difficulties and great Hardſhips that attended the fair dealing Maſter-Shipwrights, and Surveyors of Ships and Veſſels, for want of able Shipwrights well experienced in the right and perfect Knowledge of the Uſe of their Tools, and in the Practick Part of their Trade, to perform true and good Workmanſhip in their Undertakings; and alſo propoſed ſeveral particular regulating Clauſes, for the more Firm and Well-building, and better Survey of Ships and Veſſels, in Order to prevent the many evil Practices that are growing worſe, that appear in the Shipwrights-Trade, and other neceſſary regulating Clauſes, to amend and renew their Antient Charter, which ſaid Propoſal upon Reference, was deliberately conſidered and approved of, by the Joynt Opinion of the principal Officers and Commiſſioners of the Navy, and Corporation of *Trinity-Houſe*, that it would be for the Service of the Royal Navy, and the Advantage of the Shipwrights-Trade in particular, and for the Safety and Encouragement of Navigation in general, to have the Shipwrights-Charter renewed and confirmed, which ſaid Joynt Opinion is approved of by the late Lords Commiſſioners of the Admiralty, and by His late Majeſty King *William*, who approved of, and confirm'd the ſame in Council; and upon Reference, was alſo approved of by his Royal Highneſs the late Prince of *Denmark*, Lord High Admiral of *Great Britain*; and her late Majeſty Queen *Anne*, has been ſince likewiſe moſt graciouſly pleaſed to approve of and confirm the ſame in Council: That upon referring the ſaid Propoſal and Report to Council, learned in the Law, in Order to renew the ſaid Charter, their Opinion and Advice is the ſame as it has been before, on the like Reference, (*Viz.*) That there are ſome neceſſary and uſeful Clauſes in the Shipwrights antient Charter, (which is ſurrender'd in Order to be amended and renewed) and alſo in their ſaid Propoſals ſo well approved of and confirmed, as aforeſaid, that cannot be made Practicable, nor of Uſe to the Shipwrights-trade nor to the Royal Navy and the Merchants Service, without a Confirmation of the ſame by Act of Parliament to Ground the Shipwrights New Charter upon.

Shipwrights Propoſal for a General Rule to be obſerved and put in practice, was one main Reaſon that gained the Joynt Opinion of the Principal Officers and Commiſſioners of the Navy, & Corporation of Trinity House, and their Report is alſo well approved of and confirmed

[illegible] of Council [illegible] ed in the Law, [illegible] Opinion & Report

That in Purſuance of the Joynt-Opinion and Reports, on the aforeſaid Propoſal, an Eſſay by way of Specimen, is prepared for ſerviceable Proportions of the principal Materials of Wood and Iron, uſed in Ships and Veſſels, ſuitable and due to their Burthen, from 30 Tuns, to 1300 Tuns, in order to be further conſidered and affirmed by a Majority of the Maſter-Builders, and the experienced Maſter-Shipwrights, before they are enter'd fair in the Scheme and General Rule, annexed to the ſaid Specimen, in Order to be confirmed, eſtabliſhed and put into Practice, as a General Rule for the Scantlings, and the ſhifting of the Work, or the Scarph of the Work, That is the Well-placing of the principal Materials, by giving a ſuitable Diſtance of the Butt-ends of ſome particular Timbers, and Planks, and thick Stuff, from each other, whereby to have a good and ſerviceable Gravitation to each other, by Attraction of Parts, and for the Sizes of the Iron-work, and the Well-placing of it in ſome particular and moſt ſerviceable Parts and Places in each Ship or Veſſel, and alſo the number of Threads of Hair, and of White and Black Okeham, which ſaid Proportions are not to be leſs than a ſuitable Proportion due to the Burthen of every Ship or Veſſel, for the better Security and Safety of the Lives of His Majeſty's Subjects, and the common Freight of Merchants Goods, and may be greater at the Diſcretion of the Owners, or Maſters, or Chief Commander, or the Maſter-Builder, or either of them, when their Ships and Veſſels are deſigned to be Freighted with a dead-weight Lading, that Strains, Tries, and Proves the Scantlings and Gravitation, and the Truth of the Work, and of the Workmanſhip, alſo leaves it to their own Diſcretion, Skill and Judgment, as they or either of them think proper and fit for to New-build, or Re-build their reſpective Ships or Veſſels, for Burthen or for Sailing, as they pleaſe, and alſo to name and have any Shipwright or Shipwrights they pleaſe, to ſurvey them upon New-building, Re-building, or Repairing, always obſerving a proportionable main Breadth to her Length, and Height of Breadth, with a ſerviceable Breadth and Length of Floor, to give her a good Bearing above the Surface of the Water, and a clear Entrance afore, and clean Run aft, to make a free Paſſage, and ſtrong Currant of Water to the Rudder, whereby to Govern her on all Occaſions, with a ſuitable good Bow and Buttock to ſupport and give her Life to riſe in a Head-Sea; to wit, that Ships and Veſſels be well Weighed and Conditioned, and not over-charged with taunt ſtanding Maſts, and diſproportionable Yards, to create an ungovernable Force and Strain, more than her Capacity, or ſolid Content her Hull and Lading can balance, in diſturbed common Seas and Weather, and that the principal Materials of Wood and Iron uſed in Ships and Veſſels, as in the aforeſaid Specimen, and General Rule, are particularly named and inſerted, be ſo well gravitated to each other, and faſtned firm and ſecure, by good Workmanſhip, as to bear the great Power, and Strain of the Sails, and diſturbed Seas and hold out tight, and thereby prevent many Sea damages, extraordinary and total Loſſes in Voyages.

19 Char. II [illegible] for [illegible] Proportion of [illegible] for House, [illegible] conſidered and affirmed by [illegible] Maſters. The Neceſſity and Service is much greater for able Artificers, to conſider of [illegible] a General Rule of [illegible] Proportions, for the principal Materials uſed in Ships and Veſſels.

Note, On a [illegible] Gravitation, and the firm and well faying and faſtning of the principal Materials by good Workmanſhip The [illegible] and Service, and Safety of the Ship or Veſſel, [illegible] Lives [illegible] Mens Lives wholly depend.

And foraſmuch as many Credible and Eminent Merchant-Freighters, and the Owners of Ships and Veſſels, who obſerve and find, that they are the greateſt Sufferers by Sea damage Extraordinary, and by the Total Loſs of their Goods and Eſtates in Voyages, are of Opinion, one main Reaſon, and Cauſe of the ſaid great Loſs in Voyages, is the Diſorder and Abuſe in the Practice and Government of the Shipwrights Trade, and do agree with the Joynt-Opinion and Reports on the Shipwrights Propoſal, and the Opinion and Advice of Council learned in the Law aforeſaid; And therefore the ſaid Merchant Freighters and Owners (by their Petition) do humbly pray the Honourable Houſe of Commons for Leave to bring a Bill for Regulating Clauſes, to ground the Shipwrights new Charter upon, whereby to make it Practicable,

Petition of the Merchants and Owners of Ships, to the Honourable Houſe of Commons, and their Reaſons why they joyn in Opinion with the Maſter Shipwrights, and pray for their Propoſal of a General Rule to be [illegible] in Practice.

Practicable, as well for the Good of His Majesty's Royal Navy, and Merchants Service, as for the Encouragement and Good of Trade and Navigation in General.

A due Observation of a general Rule will prevent and save many poor Sea-men and their Families from so often begging Charity about the Countries, and in the Cities, Burroughs and Corporation Towns

A general Rule will be a more certain Proof of Marine works, and for the Interest of every Person concerned in Trade and Navigation

That notwithstanding the strange Notions and groundless Objections, that some particular Persons have had and made, with design to Amuse and Deceive others, on purpose to gain time to carry on and encourage the Evil Practice of Clandestine Owners of Ships, and Traders in Sea-Affairs, Ship-Jobbers, that New build and Repair by the Great or Lump, and Task-Masters, and Undertakers, and Insurers of Ships and Vessels, it is demonstrable and certain, That the Method in the Specimen and General Rule annexed to it, when Confirmed and Established, and put in Practice, according to the good Intent of the foresaid Proposal, will be a better Proof and more certain Way and Means, both to Incourage and Improve the Fair-dealing Traders by Sea, and Owners of Ships, and consequently Navigation in general, in His Majesty's Dominions, in regard it is a received General Opinion, That it will prove it self to be for the Interest and Good of every particular Fair-dealing Merchant-Freighter and Owner of Ships and Vessels, and Master-builder and Shipwright employed in the Shipwrights Trade, and every Mariner and Passenger, and for the Interest and Good of every particular Shop-keeper and Inland Traders, *&c* as well the Seller, as the Buyer, (by preventing their being often deceived in their Wholesale and Retail Trade, in Dry Goods and Wares, by Sea-damage extraordinary, which is generally Ship-damage, and comes through the Defects, and extraordinary Leaks, in Ships and Vessels) and also for the Interest and Good of all Persons concerned in Trade and Navigation to assist and help a general Good, where the Safety of their Lives, Goods and Estates, in a great Measure depends.

And on the contrary it is [illegible], against the Interest of every Person concerned in Trade and Navigation, to leave Clandestine Dealers and Insurers to themselves and without the use of a general Rule, whereby to prove the goodness of the Work and Workmanship in Ships and Vessels

That on the contrary, To leave every Insurer, and Clandestine Dealer and Trader in Ships and Vessels, to themselves, without the regular Method of a general Rule to prove the Truth of the Work, and of the Workmanship, or any other known fair Way in their Undertakings, and Performance of suitable Scantlings, and Gravitations of the Attractive Parts, and Goodness of the principal Materals of Wood and Iron, and the well placing of them in some principal and most serviceable Parts in Ships and Vessels, and more particularly by the greater Lump, where it is common to have no Inspection or Survey whatever, before they are finished for Sale, by the way of Trade, and ready to enter and receive Mariners and Passengers and Merchants Goods on Board, who are very near concerned, and often much dissatisfied, that they have no fair, nor true Account of the firm and well New-building, and Goodness of the Ship or Vessel, nor of her sufficient Repairs, where they Adventure their Lives, Goods and Estates.

Also it is very severe and hard for Seamen to Pump a defective leaky Ship a long Voyage, to save the Ship and Goods, and when they are paid to have Money stopped and taken out of their Wages for Sea damage extraordinary

That it is well known when Ships and Vessels prove so extraordinary Leaky, by Defects, or by their Insufficiency and Deceits, that they founder, and the Seamen lose their Lives; And when it so happens, that any of them save their Lives, all their Wages is kept from them, and lost for the outward, or for the home Voyage, when the Founder happens, notwithstanding the said Seamen have had extraordinary Work and Labour, by their excessive Pumping, during the time of a long Voyage, to save the Ship and Merchants Goods, yet the aforesaid Clandestine Owners and Insurers, neither in a Body by Partnership, nor single of themselves, seldom or never have any regard to relieve or help the poor distressed Seamen, that save their Lives and have lost their Wages, nor their helpless Families, the Wives and Children of them that lost their Lives by foundring as aforesaid; and it is too often known,

that

that in their diftreffed Conditions they are forced to beg the Charity of well-difpofed People in and about the Country, and in the Cities, Burroughs, and Corporated-Towns of *Great Britain*, or otherwife are obliged to return and beg their Way to the particular Parifhes where they were Born, or were Inhabitants laft, and are by their Neceffities forced to depend on their Charity, to fubfift and keep them from ftarving. Therefore, and for the Reafons aforefaid, it is with humble Submiffion conceived, That fuch known Evil Practices do in a great meafure tend not only to deftroy Seamen and impoverifh their Families, but alfo to deftroy the Trade and Navigation of *Great Britain*, and is equal to that of leaving open the Gates, and many great Breaches, in the Walls of a fortified City, or Town, to let in a known common Enemy by Confent.

And alfo it is apparent, that His Majefty and the Merchant Freighters, that adventure their Goods and Eftates in Ships and Veffels, have no fair Account nor near Eftimate of the great Lofs by Sea-damage to Merchants Goods in one Year, nor of the number of Ships and Veffels, and of Seamen and Paffengers that have loft their Lives in any one Year, by extraordinary Leaks, thro' known Slights and Defects in the Hulls of Ships and Veffels, that plainly appear in the Voyage in fair Weather, and common difturbed Seas and Weather, and the faid Defects and extraordinary Leaks in Ships and Veffels, are too often neglected, or wilfully flighted in Repairs, and continued from Voyage to Voyage.

No Man lofes his Life Afhore, by an unnatural Death, but the Caufe of it is enquired into by a Jury, but when a Hundred or more Men lofe their Lives in an infufficient and deceitful Ship, there is no Inquiry for a true Account of that Lofs, nor any known [illegible] nor general Knowledge [illegible] the [illegible] great Lofs.

And it is to be obferbed, which is very abfurd, that fome particular Owners of Ships and Veffels, and Merchant Freighters, and other Sea-faring Traders, are fuch great Strangers to their own Intereft in the breeding of able Shipwrights, to the practick part of the Shipwrights Trade, (which cannot be well learned afhoar, and at Sea, in lefs than Seven Years time, with great Induftry and Diligence, Care and Pains) So they neglect and wholly obftruct the only fair Way and Method in a great Undertaking of folid Work, that is very ferviceable to them, as well in the Improvement of their Eftates, as in preventing the lofs of their Eftates. For that it is known, there are many vagrant Apprentices and Journey-men Shipwrights, that fhelter themfelves from place to place in Seaport-Towns, and from Ship to Ship where they are not known, that practice the Shipwrights Trade afhoar, and take upon them the Charge and Care of Ships and Veffels at Sea. Alfo it manifeftly appears, at the Arrival and unloading of Ships and Veffels, there are many great Damages by Salt-Water, commonly difcovered and found in Merchants dry Goods and Wares, and the Lives, Goods and Eftate of his Majefty's Subjects that adventure and trade by Sea, are very much concern'd, and too often totally loft by Deceits and Errors in the principal Materials, and the unskilful and infufficient Workmanfhip in Ships and Veffels. Therefore, and for the Reafons aforefaid, why fome particular Owners and Merchant Freighters of Ships and Veffels, do not forward and encourage the Mafter Shipwrights, to anfwer and make good their Propofal in 1691, that they may Effectually perform their Undertakings, and their Workmen and Apprentices earn and deferve their Wages. Being duly confider'd, and well weighed, is very ftrange, and ftill admirable. In regard it will prove to be grounded on good Reafon, and fair in it felf (and at this time much wanted to be put in practice) whereby in a great meafure to prevent and fave every Year many confiderable Damages to Merchants Goods of great Value, and total Loffes in Voyages as aforefaid, and alfo to relieve and maintain the poor, aged, and difabled Cripples of the Shipwrights Trade, of which, Numbers both in their Youth, and in Old Age, by Falls and Bruifes, and Accidents that often happen, (fince the Increafe of Ships of great Burthen)

Vagrant Shipwrights Apprentices, and Journey-men are a great difappointment in Undertakings, and of evil Confequence to fair dealing Owners, and Merchant Freighters of Ships and Veffels.

And to keep a Shipwrights Apprentice the greateft part of all his Seven Years time of his Apprenticefhip at Sea, does not only deprive him of his Trade for his Life time, but alfo [illegible] the breeding of [illegible] Apprentices that [illegible] had fome Experience of the [illegible] ashore And it would be good Service [illegible] to know the Ufe of a Ship, or to learn Trade at Sea, which is [illegible] a great Difappointment in Undertakings and of [illegible] Confequence to [illegible] ing Owners and Merchant Freighters, and to Trade and Navigation in general.

as

as well in the Royal Navy Service, for the Defence and Security of this His Majesty's Kingdom and Dominions of *Great Britain*, as in Merchants Service, where they are Objects of great Pity, having no Relief, save only Parochial Charity.

A true Observation in the Voyage in a publick Journal, to shew the length of time that Ships are Pumped, and the Weather, &c always to remain and be kept on Board of every Ship and Vessel after they are unladen and laid up, will be of good Service to prove the Truth of this Clause whereby to discover the main Reason and Cause of so much Sea Damage extraordinary in the Voyage In order to prevent and save the like great Damage the next Voyage, for that it is well known, Journals commonly taken by some particular Officers in Ships and Vessels, relating to Navigation, are always carried away by the said Officers when every Ship is discharged and laid up, and therefore private Journals are of no Use nor Service to the Ship for the next Voyage Also it is to be observed, that Navigable private Journals, very seldom, and many of them do never set down the true length of the time that Seamen pump a Leaky Ship or Vessel extraordinary in fair Weather, and in common Seas, and Weather apart and distinct from their pumping in Disturbed Violent Seas, and Stress of Weather.

And so it is, *may it please your Honours*, the Case is clear and plain, where there is no general Rule Established, no Fault or Transgression will be own'd, nor discover'd by some particular Owners and Merchant Freighters and Traders in Shipping, tho' the Deceits and Errors in the principal Materials, and in the unskilful and insufficient Workmanship in Ships and Vessels, are plain and manifestly known at Sea, by the great Damages and Losses when extraordinary Leaks appear, which are discovered there by the length of the time the Ships and Vessels are pumped in fair Weather, and in ordinary common Seas and Weather. And the Shipwrights is a serviceable and solid Trade, wherein there is a great variety of Workmanship, which cannot be well perform'd without long Experience and great Industry, Diligence, Care, and Pains. And the Lives, Goods, and Estates of many of His Majesty's Seafaring and Trading Subjects are very near and much concern'd. And notwithstanding the joynt Opinion and Reports, and the Petition of the fair dealing Merchant Freighters and Owners of Ships, that very well approve of an Established general Rule in the Shipwrights Trade as above mention'd; yet the fair Method of an establish'd general Rule to prevent extraordinary Leaks and Pumping, and to save great Damages and Losses every Year, is wilfully neglected, and wholly obstructed by some particular Clandestine Traders in Shipping, namely some particular Owners and Merchants, and Ship-Jobbers, and Task-Masters and Undertakers from one to another, and Insurers, that have no manner of Regard nor Concern for the Loss by Sea Damage extraordinary, nor for the great Loss of other Mens Lives, Goods, and Estates in Shipping.

All which as is humbly conceived, will be thought sufficient Grounds to bring in a Bill for Limiting the Master Builders and other able Master Shipwrights to a certain . . . . time for to consider of, and affirm the suitable Proportions particularly nam'd and ascertain'd in the Specimen, and general Rules, according to the well meaning of their Proposal aforesaid, without any Loss of more time And is humbly submitted to the Knights, Citizens, and Burgesses of the Honourable House of Commons of Great Britain *in Parliament Assembled.*

The

The Contracting Part IN SHIP-BUILDING Full and Methodical.

The Manner of the Law-part in Ship-Building, or the Nature of Contracting by Indenture, for Building any New Ship or other Veſſel: Alſo what other Conſiderations ought to be in Refitting or Hireing Ships.

And firſt to the Indenture for New-Building

THIS Indenture made the day of in the Year of our Lord Between *A. B.* of ſuch a certain Place and County of the one Part, and *C. D* of the ſame, or ſome other Place, of the other Part, *Witneſſeth*, That the ſaid *C D* for the Conſiderations hereafter expreſs'd, doth Covenant, Promiſe and Grant, to and with the ſaid *A. B* that the ſaid *C D.* his Executors, Adminiſtrators and Aſſigns, ſhall and will at his or their own proper coſt and charges, well and in workman-like manner, Erect, build, and Launch (off from ſome certain Place, pitch'd on for that Purpoſe, without Prejudice, and deliver her Water-born, or Floating) one good and Subſtantial Ship or Frigat, of good, ſound, and ſerviceable, well ſeaſon'd New Timber, and Plank of *Engliſh* Oak, excepting three or four Strakes of well ſeaſon'd ſound Elm Plank, from the Garboard Strakes upwards, or otherwiſe white Crown'd Eaſt Country Plank for the Outſide of the Ship under Water; and that the ſaid Ship or Frigat ſhall contain in length upon the lower Gun-deck, from the Rabbit of the Stem, to the Rab- *Length* bit of the Stern poſt, meaſur'd on the a direct ſtreight line in the Midſhips Foot; breadth from the Outſide of one Plank to the Outſide of *Breadth* the other, at the extream or largeſt part in the Midſhips, meaſur'd directly thwart the Ship, by Horizontal and Perpendicular Parallels Feet Inches Depth in Hold from the Cieling or Foot-waleing in the Hold, to the upper *Depth* part of the Gun-deck Beam meaſur'd at the Foreſide of the Mainhatch way by a Perpendicular line, drawn from hanging the Line of the ſaid Deck Feet Inches; breadth at the Tranſum that lays under the Gun-ports of the low- *Transum* er Deck meaſur'd by a direct ſtraight Line, from the after upper Corners Feet *Breadth* Inches · Rake aft from the lower part of the Keel, to the upper part of *Rake of Post* the ſaid Wing Tranſum meaſur'd by a Perpendicular drawn from the Keel Feet Inches, which may properly be term'd the Rake of the Stern Poſt The *Keel* Keel to be of Elm, not in more pieces than to be inches ſquare in the Midſhips, and continue that Subſtance forward, but taper'd aft to Inches in due Proportion, to be ſheath'd with a falſe Keel Inches, and to be ſcarph'd *False Keel* one piece over another ſideways Feet, and thoſe Scarphs to have each Bolts of Inch Diameter, Sarcer headed, Clinch'd or Riveted, and laid with Tar and Hair. Stem to be very Sound and Subſtantial, and not in more pieces *Stem*

 than

than Bignefs Fore and Aft Inches, and thwartfhips Inches, the Scarph of the Stem to the Scarph of the Keel to be as 8 to 9, and to be Bolted, Hooked and Tabled, in Proportion to the Scarphs of the Keel, and alfo laid with Tar and Hair, to have a falfe Stem or Apron of the infide on the main Stem, half the thicknefs of the main Stem, and twice the breadth, and the Scarphs one Foot long. The Stern Poft Sound and not Knotty, neither too frow or tender grain'd, to be Inches thwartfhips at the Head, and Inches Fore and Aft, and Inches Fore and Aft below on the Keel, and as big as the Keel thwartfhips, to have a falfe Poft within fide well joined to the main Poft Inches Fore and Aft, and fufficient to fupport the Hoodings-ends, or after Butts of the Planks; to allow of another Falfe Poft without fide, which fhall be as 1 to 3 to the breadth of the main Poft below, even with the upper Edge of the Keel, every one of the Pofts to be tenon'd into the Keel ⅓ of the Keels depth, and the main and aftermoft falfe Poft to be connex'd to the Keel with one Subftantial Dovetail of Iron, on each fide, to each of them, and the Dovetails or Iron plates to be Inches broad, and part of an Inch thick, bolted through each Dovetail, and the Bolts to be clinch'd The Rifing or Dead wood aft to be Feet long, and of fufficient breadth thwartfhips, that the Garboard Strake may join, or fay, to keep the Water out in cafe the after part of the Keel is bent of, the Dead wood to be tenon'd into the Poft, and to have a Knee, whofe Arm upon the Poft fhall be Feet long, and the Arm on the Dead wood Feet long, to be Sound and Subftantial in Proportion to the length, or otherwife thwartfhips Inches, and in the Throat or Bending Inches without a Chock, and at the ends Inches, which Knee and Dead wood fhall have one Bolt, in every Inches of Diameter, Sarcer headed, and if fuch Bolts are drove through the Keel, they fhall be there Clinch'd · The Rifing or Dead wood forward to be Feet long, and Inches broad, at the foremoft end, fitted to the Apron of the Stem, to be Inches deep at the after end, and Inches broad The Floor-timbers to be Feet length, bignefs Fore and Aft Inches, up and down on the Keel Inches without the Chock, and Inches in and Out at the Floor Timber head; the fpace between the Floor Timbers to be Inches; to cut Limber Holes of each fide the middle Line Inches of Inches fquare; and every other Floor Timber to be bolted through the main Keel with a Bolt of Inches diameter, and clench'd there · The lower, or firft tire of Foot-hooks to be Foot long, and Inches fore and aft below, and as big as the Floor Timber in and out, and to taper in due Proportion each way, according to a diminifhing Line, drawn from the bignefs of the top Timber at the head; fo that the bignefs of this Foot-hook at the head fhall be Inches fore and aft, and Inches in and out; the Scarph or over-launching of the Floor Timber, and this tire of Foot-hooks, fhall be at leaft Feet; fecond Foot-hook foot long, inches fore and aft below, and inches thwart-fhips, inches fore and aft aloft, and inches thwart-fhips; third Foot-hook foot long, inches fore and aft below, and inches thwart-fhips, and inches fore and aft aloft, and inches thwart-fhips; fourth Foot-hook foot long, inches fore and aft below, and inches thwart-fhips, and inches fore and aft aloft, and inches thwart-fhips: Top-timber foot long, inches fore and aft below, and inches thwart-fhips, and inches fore and aft aloft, and inches thwart-fhips: Obferving, that neither of thefe Timbers fhall have any Chock to help the Compaffing of the Piece, that fhall exceed at either end of the Timber above ¼ of the length of the Timber, nor more than ⅓ of any Timber's refpective thicknefs; and that the Timber fhall have his full Subftance in the middle, without any Defect to weaken the middle part, but that the faid Proportion of Chocking fhall diminifh to a point, or Wedge fafhion, towards the middle of the Timber. The Kelfon not to be of more pieces than and that the Scarph being foot long, hook'd and butted, and as near as poffible to be placed between the Scarphs of the Keel, and to be inches up and down, and inches thwart fhips in the Midfhips, and taper'd aft in due Proportion, fcored upon the Floor Timbers inches, and to be bolted through every other Floor Timber, and

the

Falfe Stem · *Stern Poft* · *Falfe Poft within* · *Falfe Poft without* · *Dead wood* · *Knee on the Dead Wood* · *Dead Wood forward* · *Floor Timbers.* · *Lower Foot-hooks* · *Second Foot hook* · *Third Foot-hook* · *Fourth Foot-hook* · *Top-timber* · *Kelfon.*

the Keel where they ſhall be clench'd, and the Bolt to be Inch diameter Obſerving, that the Kelſon ought to be placed as far forward and aftward as it poſſibly can be placed In Hold to put in one Strake of inch Plank at the feet of the lower Foot-hooks, and Strakes or Sleepers, or thick Strakes of each ſide the Floor Timber-head, the thickeſt that is placed on the Floor Heads and ſecond Foot-hook Heels, ſhall be inches thick, and inches broad, the reſt to be inches thick, and inches broad, and to taper forward and aftward in due Proportion according to the tapering of the Ship. To have two Srakes of Orlop Clamps on each ſide, of inches thick, and inches broad, and alſo two Strakes of each ſide of Gun-deck Clamps of inches broad, and inches thick. All which Clamps to be ſcarph'd, with what is term'd *Flemiſh Scarph*, hooked and butted, and to be twice as long as the Clamps are broad, and half the breadth added unto it, which may be a ſuitable Proportion for the length of all Scarphs, and all the reſt of the Foot-waleing to be inches thick, and inches broad, and taper'd in due Proportion, as aforeſaid: To put in Beams for the Orlop inches fore and aft, and inches up and down, of them to be placed before the Maſt, and of them abaft the Main Maſt. To have bends of Riders, that is, Floor Riders, and Foothook Riders, the Floor Riders length feet, to be inches fore and aft, and inches upon the Kelſon, and inches deep at the Floor Timber head, the Foothook Riders length feet, to be inches fore and aft, and inches deep; the Floor to be bolted in every inches ſpace, with Bolts of diameter, the Foot-hook Riders to be bolted in every inches ſpace, with Bolts of diameter; the Floor Rider Bolts to be clench'd without board, and Caps of Lead nail'd over the Clench; the Foothook Rider Bolts to be clench'd within board. Obſerving, that all Bolts under Water are made of very good ſound Iron, wrought very true, and be drove very ſtiff. To lay an Orlop, or Platform, in the Hold, proper and convenient, according to the Uſe the Ship is deſign'd for, with a ſufficient number of ſizable Beams, knee'd at each end with Knees of inches ſided, and inches in the throat beſides Chock; to lay your Carlings feet aſunder, and to be inches thwart ſhips, and inches up and down, and be ſcored into the Beams inches; to lay the Ledges inches aſunder, and to be inches up and down, and inches fore and aft; to lay the Flat with Deal, or Oak, according to the Uſe. Which being a Matter ſo very various, it will be to little purpoſe to mention the Store Rooms, or other Contrivance in the Hold, until the Uſes are reſolved on. Top Riders to be feet long, and inches fore and aft below, and inches thwart-ſhips, and inches fore and aft aloft. and inches thwart-ſhips to be bolted in every inches, with a Bolt of inch Diameter, and alſo to have two Bolts through the Rider and the Beam by which he is placed, with Bolts of Diameter, and well clinch'd, to have a Step for the main Maſt, of a ſound clung Piece, being inches fore and aft, and inches upon the Kelſon, and foot long, to have a Pillar under every Beam in the Hold, both Gundeck and Orlop, of inches ſquare. The lower Gundeck Beams to be inches up and down, and inches fore and aft, either ſcarph'd in two Pieces, or in one intire Piece, obſerving if they are ſcarph'd, that the Scarph ſhall be ⅓ of the Length, and to be tabled with hook and butt, and bolted in every inches, with Bolts of inch Diameter To lay the Beams with regard to the Hatchways, Maſts and Ports, according to the Uſe of the Ship, that there may lay one Beam under every Port, and one between, or otherwiſe to have a certain Number between Stem and Stern, the main Hatchway to be feet between beam and beam, and feet thwartſhips, fore Hatchway, feet fore and aft, and feet thwartſhips, after Hatchway, feet fore and aft, and feet thwartſhips, the beams to be kneed at each end, with two Knees, one hanging, and one lodging Knee, the up and down arm of the hanging Knee to be feet, and the other arm to be feet, and to be in-ches

Foot W[illegible]s

Orlop Clamps, or Middle-band, and Gundeck Clamps.

Orlop Beams

Riders

Platform.

Top Riders

Main Step

Pillars

Lower Gundeck Beams.

Knees Hanging

ches fided, and inches in the Throat To have no Chock, and to be bolted in every inches, with Bolts of inch Diameter To have a Ring, and a Forelock, or Iron Key, to every Bolt in and out. And every end Bolt fore and aft, the Arm of the lodging Knee fore and aft, not lefs than feet long, and the other Arm not lefs than feet, to be hooked in the Beam, and fided inches, and inches in the Throat, befides the Chock. To be bolted in every inches, with Bolts of inch Diameter To have a *Carlings* Ring and Forelock on every Bolt. To have Tire of Carlings, on each fide the middle Line, the Tire on each fide the middle Line, to lay in due range, to make the fides of the Hatchways, the other Tires to be equally divided, between them and the lodging Knees; and to lay in due range according to the Tapering of the Ship, on each refpective Plan: And to be inches broad, and inches up and down, fcored into the Beam inch. To be mention'd, either Oak or Fir, according to the Ufe of the Ship, *Ledges* but in the lower Decks they are generally Oak, the Ledges to lay inches afunder; and to be inches fore and aft, and inches up and down. Scored into the Carlings inches, and to be of the fame Timber that the *Waterways* Carlings are of. The Waterways to be inches thick, chin'd away to the Thicknefs of the Flat of the Deck, and the Spirkitrifing, always Oak, very found, and free from Defects: To be at leaft 12 inches befides the Chine. All *Flat of the Deck* the reft of the Deck to be of well feafon'd Oak-plank, either Englifh, or white-crown'd Eaft-Country. Length of each Plank at leaft feet, breadth in the Midfhips each inches, and Thicknefs inches. Diminifhing the breadth aft and forward, in due Proportion, according to the Tapering of the Plan; all the Flat of the Deck to be nail'd at every Beam, in every Plank, with two Nails, that every Hundred fhall weigh Pounds. And alfo to be treneld in every Ledge, and Carling, with one or two Trenels, according to the breadth and thicknefs of the Strakes approved on, with Trenels of inch Diame- *Lead Scuppers* ter To put out lead Scuppers, on each fide, of Lead, that every foot fhall weigh Pound, to make as many Hatches as fhall be thought pro- *Main Hatches* per (mentioning the fame) which fhall be made of Oak Ledges inches up and down, and inches fore and aft, and cover'd with 2 inch Plank; the Comings to be of inch Plank, laid with Tar and Hair, and nail'd with Nails of inches length; and every hundred Weight fhall weigh Pounds. *Other Hatches* All the other Hatches. The Ledges fhall be to the main Hatch Ledges, as 4 to 5, and Plank, as 3 to 4 Comings, the fame as the Comings of the main Hatch, for height and breadth, as 4 to 5; with convenient Scuttles in fome of the Hatches, according to the Ufe of the Ship, and mention'd to have *Well* a Well under the Deck, about the main Maft, of feet fquare: And that to be made firft, with Stanfhons or Pillars, and cover'd with inch Oak Plank, as high as the Orlop; the Pillars to be inches fquare, and the Plank to be nail'd with two Nails in every Pillar, of inches long, and every Hundred of them to weigh Pounds All the Well above the Orlop may be ordinary Deals, nail'd to the Pillars (which fhall not ftand more than feet afunder, having one in each Corner) with twenty four penny Nails. To have *Manger* a Manger on the lower Deck (if the Ship carries her Hawfe-holes there) built with inch Plank foot high from the lower Deck, which fhall be brought aft from the Stem, on the direct middle Line of the Ship feet, the Plank to be well rabbited one into another, with Channels of half the Thicknefs of the Plank, and joyn'd to endure Calking To be nail'd at the fide, with Nails of inches long, one Hundred of them weighing Pounds To be groved into two fubftantial Pillars, in the middle of the Ship, which fhall be bolted in to the Beams, with Bolts of inches Diameter The Pillars to be inches thick, and inches broad; fecured in every refpect: Sufficient to make a Step for the Bowfprit: To have 4 Scuppers of inches Diameter in the Manger, of the like Lead that makes them Scuppers in the other *Hawfe Piece* Part of the Deck. The Hawfe fhall not be lefs than feet broad, and equal in Thicknefs to the Ships Timber at that Place, and the Plank both within board

board, and without board, having in each Hawse-piece, a hole cut near the middle of the piece of Inches diameter, to place pair of Bit pins for to belay the Cables to, one pair of which shall stand Feet from the Stem, measur'd direct on a middle Line, and to be Inches square, the Cross-pieces to be Inches fore and aft, and Inches up and down, the other pair of Pins to stand Feet from the Stem measured as aforesaid, and to be Inches square, the Cross-pieces to be Inches up and down, and Inches fore and aft, and each Cross-piece and Bit-pins to be of a suitable length, sufficient to take two turns with the Cable sizable for such a Ship, and the Cross-pieces to be fastened with two pair of substantial Hooks and Eyes, to the Bit-pins, for the conveniency of taking them off to calk under, to have a substantial Spur or Knee against each Pin, whose Arms shall be, that on the Deck Foot long, and the other Foot long, to be sided Inches, and bolted in every Inches space with a Bolt of Inch diameter; also the Pins shall each of them have two Bolts through the beam they stand against (they being let into the beams one Inch and half) the Bolts to be Inch diameter, and the Pins to continue the substance of the Head two Foot under the lower edge of the Gun deck beam, and from thence to the lower end they may be taper'd by a straight Line, to make the lower end $\frac{2}{3}$ of the substance of the top To have breast Hooks in the Hold, between the lower Deck breast Hook, and the fore Step, which shall be equally spaced, also to have one Hook under each Deck, and one under the Hawse holes, which breast Hooks shall be Foot long, and the lower Deck breast Hook shall be Inches sided, and Inches within a Foot of the ends, and Inches in the middle besides the Chock, them below that lower Deck shall be Inches sided, and Inches within one Foot of the end, and Inches in the middle besides the Chock, them above the lower Deck to be Inches sided, and Inches within one Foot of the end, and Inches in the middle besides the Chock, they shall have one Bolt through each and through the Stem, and all the other Bolts shall have not above Inches between Bolt and Bolt, and to be Inches diameter, and belayed with one Ring and a Forelock to each Bolt To have a Step for the fore Mast Inches broad, and Foot long, to have Inches depth above the Kelson, without a Chock, and to be cross bolted, if it be possible, through two Floor Timbers, that the Bolts being two tire shall not be above Inches asunder, and Inches diameter, well clench'd To have two strakes of Spirkit-rising of Foot long each Plank, except the foremost and aftermost to help the shifting the Butts, to be Inches thick, and Inches broad, hooked and tabled one into another two Inches, two have Port-holes of Inches fore and aft, and Inches up and down, and to be Inches from the lower Deck to the Cell, to put in Cells for the same below and aloft; that below to be Inches up and down, and that aloft to be Inches up and down, and both of them to answer the thickness of the Timber the other way, also to make two Port-holes in the Counter, of the same Dimensions in every particular. To place Partners for the Main Mast of long, Inches broad, and Inches thick, to score the Beams and Carlings into them one Inch, to make them in two pieces of Inches breadth of each side, and the middle piece in the Wake of the Mast to be Inches broad, rabbited one into another half the thickness of the Partners, and to be bolted at each end in every Inches, with Bolts of Inch diameter, and to be trenel'd in the Carlings with Trenels of Inch diameter To place Partners for the Fore-Mast of Foot long, Inches broad, and Inches thick, the two outside pieces to be Inches broad, and to be bolted with Bolts of Inches diameter space between, and the other Work to be according to the Method mention'd of the main Partners To fix a piece for to step the Jeer Capstern in from the main Hatch to the fore Hatch, to be Inches broad, and Inches thick, in the Wake of the Sweep of the Whelps of the said Capstern, and to raise the other part thwart-ships with Chocks; to score the said Step upon the

Bit-pins. *Cross-pieces.* *Breast-hook.* *Fore Step.* *Spirket-rising lower Deck.* *Port-hole.* *Main Partners.* *Fore Partners.* *Step of the Jeer Capstern.*

Beams and Ledges one Inch, and to faſten it with Nails in every Beam, proportionable to the faſtening of the Plank on the flat of the Deck. Main Capſtern Partners to reach from the after Hatch, to the Fiſh-room Hatch, to be Inches broad and Inches thick, ſcored over the Beams and Ledges one Inch, and to be faſten'd in every Beam with Nails of Inches long, to be no more aſunder than they are in the flat of the Deck, alſo trenel'd in the ſame proportion according as they are nail'd: To have two Pillars ſhoulder'd, in the Hold the Pillars equal in bigneſs to the Pillars of the other Beams, but the ſhoulders to project of three ſides Inches, to have a Step from thoſe two Pillars for the Step of the main Capſtern, which ſhall be Inches up and down, and Inches thwart-ſhips, and to hold the Subſtance from end to end. To have a Step for the Mizon Maſt in Hold of Foot long, and Inches ſided, to be Inches up and down within a Foot of the end, and Inches in the middle without a Chock, and to be bolted in every Inches, with a Bolt of Inch diameter. The Partners of the Mizon Maſt to be Feet long, Inches broad, and Inches thick, to be ſcored over the Beams and Ledges one Inch, and faſten'd in proportion to the faſtening of the main Capſtern Partners, all the reſt of the flat of the Deck to be cover'd with Inch Plank faſten'd as afore-mention'd: To raiſe the Hatches from the Deck Inches: To have a turn'd Pillar under every Beam of the upper Deck Inches ſquare at the lower end, and Inches ſquare at the upper end, tenon'd below and aloft into Beam and Deck one Inch and half, to have a ſufficient number of Ladders, or Stair-caſes, (according to the Accommodation requiſite) to go from one Deck to another, and alſo into the fore and after Cockpits, mentioning the number and places where they ſhall ſtand, the ſides of the Ladders to be Oak of Inches broad, and Inches thick, ſtanding at an Angle of with the Deck; the Steps to be Oak or Firr of Inches thick, and to ſtand Inches aſunder, each Step rounding outward in due proportion, to beget a more eaſy going up and down, and to be let into the ſides half an Inch, to be nail'd with three Nails at the end of every Step with 20 *d* Nails; to have two Braces at every Ladders back, dovetail'd into the ſides Inches, and nail'd with Nails. To particularize the nature of the winding and flying Stairs would almoſt take up a Contract, which being ſo ſeldom uſed in the Contracting Yards, I ſhall not be ſo tedious to mention here. To have Tranſums, the Wing Tranſum to round Inches, and to be Foot long, Inches up and down, and Inches in and out at the Stern poſt, beſides what is ſcor'd over the Poſt, to be Inches in and out at the ends, to be an entire piece by reaſon of its being rabbited at the upper and lower Edge upon the outſide for the Plank, and to be hook'd within ſide for the Tranſum Knees. The lower Deck Tranſum to be Inches ſided, and all the other below the Deck to be Inches ſided, and each to be Inches in the middle, beſides the Chocks, and ſhaped at the ends according to the Faſhion-pieces which ſhall be ſided Inches. All the Tranſums to be ſcored into the falſe Poſt Inches, and home to the foreſide of the Rabbit of the Poſt; the Faſhion-pieces to be trenel'd to the Tranſums with a Trenel of Inch diameter, and the Tranſums bolted to the Poſt with one Bolt drove into every Tranſum through the Stern-poſt, the ſpace between the main Tranſums to be Inches, and to have a falſe Tranſum between the main Tranſums of Inches thick, and Inches in and out, to have a Tranſum at the upper end of the Poſt under the Helm port, which ſhall be Inches thick, and Inches in and out, prick'd home to the Counter-plank, to have a Tranſum under the upper Deck, of Inches up and down, and Inches in and out; every one of thoſe Tranſums to have a Knee at each end, the Wing Tranſum Knees Arm fore and aft to be Feet long, and the other Arm to be Feet long, and to be Inches thick up and down, and Inches in and out within a Foot of the ends, and Inches in the throat, the ſame way beſides the Chock, to be bolted in every Inches with Bolts of Inch

diameter,

diameter, and well clench'd The Deck Transum Knees fore and aft Arms to be Feet, and the other Arm Feet, to be sided Inches, and well grown, being Inches in the throat besides the Chock, and to be bolted in every Inches with a Bolt of Inch diameter, and every other Transum Knees Arm fore and aft under the lower Deck to be Feet, and the other Arm to be Feet long, and Inches sided, to be well grown, and to be Inches in the throat besides the Chock, and to be bolted in every Inches space with a Bolt of Inch diameter, and all well clench'd, or forelock'd. The Helm port Transum Knees fore and aft Arm to be Foot long, and the other Arm Foot long, to be sided Inches, and Inches in and out at the ends, and Inches in the throat besides the Chock, and to be bolted in every Inches with a Bolt of Inches diameter, and well clench'd. The upper Deck Transum Knee to be equal in bigness to the upper Deck Lodging Knees, both in bigness and fastening
The upper Deck Clamps to be foot long each, and scarphed with *Flemish* *Upper Deck Clamps*
Scarph Hook and Butt, Scarph Foot long, as was aforesaid; the breadth to be from the upper part of the Ports of the lower Deck to the Deck Line, only the thickness of the upper Deck Knee taken out, to shut up between the Clamps and Spirketing with plank of Inches thick, upper Deck Beams to *Upper Deck Beams*
be intire, to round upwards Inches, and to be Inches fore and aft, and Inches up and down, to be let into the Clamps at each end Inches, and to lay directly over the Beams of the other Deck for the conveniency of Pillaring. The perpendicular height between the upper edge of the lower *Deck Height.*
Deck Beam at the side to the upper edge of the upper Beam shall be Feet, the Beams to be knee'd at each end with two Knees, one lodging and one hanging; the up and down Arm of the hanging Knee to be Foot long, and the other Arm Foot long, to be Inches in and out at the ends, and Inches in the Throat, having no Chock, and bolted at every Inches with a Bolt of Inches diameter, and well clench'd The lodging Knees fore and aft *Upper Deck Knees*
Arm to be Feet, and the other Feet, to be well grown, and Inches in the Throat besides the Chock, and bolted in every Inch space with Bolts equal to the hanging Knees, but to be forelock'd To have Tire of Carlings, or long coming Carlings to make the Hatch-ways, according *Carlings*
to the Use of the Ship, the Tire of Carlings next the middle Line to make the Hatch-ways, and the other Tires to be equally divided between the Hatch ways and lodging Knees, and to lay in due range according to the tapering of the Ship, to be Inches up and down, and Inches thwart-ships, but the coming Carlings, if any to be, Inches up and down, and Inches thwart- *Coming Carlings*
ships, and all the Carlings to be scor'd into the Beams one Inch and half; the Ledges to lay Inches asunder, and to be Inches up and down, and *Ledges*
Inches fore and aft, to be scored into the Carlings. All which Carlings and Ledges may be Firr, except in the Wake of the Fire-places. Flat of the Deck, the Water-ways to be Inches broad, and Inches thick, and *Flat of the Deck*
chin'd to make the thickness of the Deck Plank and Spirket-rising, to lay three or four Strakes of *English* Oak Plank of Inches thick next to the Water-ways, and all the rest of the Flat of the Deck from the Bulkhead of the Fore-castle quite aft, may be well season'd *Prussia* Deal or Inches thick, and Feet long, equal to the length of the Plank or longer, and to be nail'd in every Beam with Nails of Inches long, every Hundred to weigh Pounds, and not to be above Inches asunder thwart ships, to have Nails in every Ledge at the same distance asunder, of Nails Inches long, and every Hundred to weigh Pounds To have Port holes of each side *Upper Tier*
on the upper Deck, exactly between those below, the length fore and aft Inches, depth up and down Inches, and height from the Deck Plank Inches To have two Cells, one below of Inches up and down, that aloft Inches up and down, and to be answerable with the Timber the other way, to have a String or pieces of well-season'd Oak, the upper edge to make *String and*
the lower Cell of the Port, to be Foot long each piece, and Inches *the Port*
broad,

broad, and Inches thick, to be ſcored into every Timber one Inch, and to be put or join'd home to the outſide Plank, being placed perpendicular from the ſtanding of the Timber, and bolted through every Timber with a Bolt of *Spirketing.* Inch diameter well clench'd, the Plank between that and the Water-way to be Inch thick, and Feet long, and fitting the diſtance between with one *String above the Ports* breadth; to have a String above the Ports of Fir Inches thick, and Feet long, and broad enough to reach from the Plansheer to the upper part of the Port in the Waſte, and under this String to have filling ſufficient, that the *Gratings or Hatches.* Work about the Timber heads may be calk'd. To have Hatches or Gratings ſufficient according to the Uſe of the Ship; and ſuch Hatches or Gratings raiſed with Comings and Head-ledges, to keep the Water from between Decks, but ſpecified what ſort and quantity of Hatches, or Gratings, you require, as was *Topſail Sheet Bits and Gallows.* done by the lower Hatches. To fit Topſail Sheet-bits, or Gallows, Inches ſquare, and to be Foot long, ſtep'd through the main Partners; to have one ſhiver in each piece of Inch thick, and one of Inch thick, each to be of the diameter of the pieces at the upper Deck; to have a croſs piece of Inches deep, and Foot long, and of the thickneſs that the ſide pieces are ſquare; the ſide pieces to be tenon'd into the croſs pieces half the depth of the croſs piece, with a Tenon of Inches broad, and a quarter of the ſquare for thickneſs, pin'd with wooden Pins; to have a Fidd, or piece of well ſeaſon'd *Engliſh* Oak, of Inches long, Inches deep, and Inches thick, let through the ſide pieces thwart-ſhips, Foot from the Deck, to be-*Jeer Bits* lay the Topſail Sheets to. To have a pair of main Jeer-bits Inches ſquare at the head, and as low as the lower edge of the upper Deck beam, and then to taper downwards to ⅞ of what they are aloſt, and to ſtep in the main Partners, where they and the Topſail Sheet bits ſhall have one Bolt through the Partners of Inch diameter; alſo each of the four to have two Bolts in them, drove through the upper Deck beam of Inches diameter, and well clench'd, the ſhivers equal in bigneſs to the ſhivers in the Topſail Sheets, according to the ſquare of the pieces, and of equal number; to have a croſs piece for the Jeers to be belay'd to the upper edge, of which to lay Inches from the Deck, and to be Inches ſquare, and Feet long, and the head of the Bits to be Feet above the Deck, to have Partners for the Jeer *Jeer Capſtand Partners* Capſtand of Feet long, Inches thick, and Inches broad, to have them in two pieces of equal breadth, and to have half an Iron Hoop of Inches broad, and half an Inch thick, fix'd in each, and the pieces to *Jeer Capſtand* be bolted at each end, to take up and down. To have a Jeer Capſtand Inches diameter in the barrel, and to be made in a true Proportion according to ſuch a diameter, to have a Thrum head with Bar-holes, and ſuch a number of Bars fitted Foot long each, of Aſh. To have two Engine Iron Falls of Inches ſquare, fix'd according to Cuſtom: To have a main *Main Capſtand* Capſtand of Inches in the barrel, with a Thrum-head, and Bar-holes, and ſuch a number of Bars of Aſh of Foot long, with two Engine Iron Falls of Inches ſquare, and fitted in every reſpect in a due Proportion, according to the dimenſion of the barrel, and Cuſtom of the Work. To put *Scuppers.* out Lead Scuppers on each ſide the Ship, of inch diameter, and of ſuch *Forecaſtle and Quarter-deck* Lead that ſhall weigh every foot ſquare pound. The Beams of the Forecaſtle and Quarter-deck to be inches up and down, and inches fore and aft, the Quarter deck beams to be intire, and lye foot aſunder, the Forecaſtle beams to *Clamps* lye foot aſunder. The Clamps of the Forecaſtle to be of one Piece inches broad, and inches thick; That of the quarter Deck, to reach from the Drift, at the main Maſt, to the great Cabbin, and ſhall be inches thick and inches broad, and in the Wake of the great Cabbin, there *Elm-String.* ſhall be a String of Elm, into which the Beams ſhall be dove tail'd, and bolted with Bolts of inches Diameter. Alſo the String ſhall be bolted through the Side, with a Bolt at every inches Diſtance, and of inches Diameter, well clench'd, and ſhall be inches up and down, and inches in and out, and cut as the Figure A: And all the other Plank, or Deals, that

that shuts in between the Clamps Strings, and Spirkitting, shall be inches thick, shifting the Butts clear one of another, at least feet Every other Beam in the Forecastle, and Steeridge, to be knee'd with a hanging Knee, whose up and down Arm shall be feet, and the other Arm feet, to be sided inches, in and out at the Ends inches, and in the Throat inches, to be bolted in every inches, with a Bolt of inches Diameter, and well clench'd To have round projecting Bulkheads, to the Steeridge and Forecastle, as usual, with Stanshons, convenient for a Door of each Side, of foot in the Clear, the Door to go into Leaves, and a Porthole of inches square, cut in him; and to lay inches from the Deck, and hung to the Doors with hinges, of the fashion inches broad, and the Part of an Inch thick, to be nail'd with Nails in each of penny Nails. The Doors to be hung to Stanshons, of inches square, and to be rabbeted the Thickness of the Doors; the Hinges to be of the fashion, nail'd with Nails of penny Nails, putting Lead under the Head of all Nails that goes against Iron. To put up Stantions between the Door, equal in Bigness, and convenient to make Lights, of inches, up and down, and inches thwart, which is for the Steeridge Bulkheads, but in the Forecastle Bulkhead, there is Stantions put up between the Doors, convenient to hang a Bell to, and be rather bigger than the Door Stantions, to the Side of the Ship: Of each Bulkhead, there is Stantions put up, to make Doorways for Cabbins, to make them clear of the Guns; and hang them Doors equally as well as the Doors of the Steeridge and Forecastle: To cover all the Stantions with well season'd *Prussia* Deal, of inches thick, and lin'd within Side, between the Stantions, with Deal of thick; and to nail it with Nails no more than inches asunder: To have Basis to step the Stantions on, of inches thick, and inches fore and aft: To lay under it Tar, Hair, and Hair Size in the Seams, being first well calk'd; and to nail the Basis with Nails, that every Hundred of them shall weigh Pounds, and not to be but inches asunder. To have Rails and Brackets for Ornaments, as usual, the Beams in the Wake of those Bulkheads, to be double knee'd, and to have a Standard at each End of the Basis; the up and down Arm to be foot, and thawartships inches, to be sided inches, well grown; and to be inches in the Throat, bolted with Bolts of inch Diameter, and to be no more than inches asunder To have Ports on the quarter Deck inches, fore and aft, and inches up and down, and to lay inches from the Plank of the Deck, which Plank of the quarter Deck, and Forecastle, shall be, First, The Waterways shall be *English* Oak, of inches thick, and inches broad, to be chin'd away to the Thickness of the Spirkitting, and flat of the Deck, which Plank in the Flat, shall be inches thick, laying out as far as the Guns, and all the rest of the Flat to be well season'd *Prussia* Deal, of the same Thickness, and nail'd in every Beam, with Nails of inches long, that every Hundred shall weigh Pounds, laying inches asunder, and to wind Oakam about the Heads of each Nail, to preserve the Head, and to hinder Leakage. The Spirkitrising of the quarter Deck, to be Plank of inches thick, and broad enough to cover the lower Cell of the Port; and all the other Part, up to the Timber Head, shall be Deal of inches thick; except the Clamps of the Coach and Roundhouse, which shall be according to the different Lengths of such Parts, which always will be various, according to the Height of the Ship To space the Timbers in the Stern, so as to have Lights in the great Cabbin, such Timbers to be step't in the Wingtransum inches, and bolted with a Bolt of inch Diameter To order them to make a Counter, to project (and lay Parallel to the Sternpost) feet To round the Stern outwards inches, the Timbers to be inches square at the Wingtransum, and truly diminish'd upwards to inches, they may be in two Pieces, and scarph'd just above the Knuckle. To have a Transum under the Lights of the great Cabbin

Arm | *Bulkheads of the Steeridge and Forecastle* | *Quarter Deck Ports* | *Waterways.* | *Flat of the Deck* | *Spirkitting.* | *Clamps of the Coach* | *Stern.*

bin inches, up and down, and inches in and out, which shall be Knee'd at each End, with a Knee sided inches; the fore and aft Arm shall be feet, and the other Arm to be feet: To be inches in and out at the Ends, and inches at the Throat, without a Chock, and be bolted in every inches, with Bolts of inch Diameter, well clench'd: To have a Deck transum, under every Deck, and all the other Lights which shall be knee'd, and bolted, and in every respect proportionable, as the Timbers of the Stern are at the Place where the Transums are fix'd. To have a Gunel at the Top of the Tafferal, from one side of the Ship to the other inches up and down, and inches fore and aft, and to project in the Midships, for the Conveniency of Leting the half Part of the Ensign Staff into it: To have Rails without side, against every Transum, embossed in Form, and to be bolted through every Timber and Transum, with a Bolt of inch Diameter, and well clench'd; the Rails under the Lights to be channell'd, to keep the Water out, and all the other Part of the Stern to be cover'd with well season'd Deal, of inches thick, nail'd with Nails inches asunder, in every Timber: To have Ports made in the Stern, ranging with the Ports of the Deck: To have a carved Tafferal with such a Figure as shall be order'd, and all other convenient carved or painted Works for Ornaments, being particularly specify'd. To have Gratings on the quarter Deck feet long, and feet broad; to be made with Ledges to round inches, and to be inches square, the Battons to be Oak of inch broad, and inch thick, nail'd with two Nails, at every Intersection of perny Nails. To have a Grating on the Forecastle foot long, and feet broad, and be made after the said fashion: To raise each on the Deck, with a Coming of inches broad, and inches thick, and Head Ledges answerable to the Round of the Ledges, to lay them with Tar and Hair, and nail them in every inch Distance, with Nails of pence one Hundred. To have Foretopsail Sheetbits, and Jeerbits step'd, in the upper Deck's Forepartners, and to be inches square at the Head, and feet long above the Forecastle Deck, to continue the Substance down to the lower Edge of the Beam; and then to taper, and be at the lower End, ⅔ of what they are aloft, except it is required to make a Shiverhole in the Forecastle for the Jeers, and then to continue that Substance quite down, and to be bolted in the Partners, with a Bolt of inch Diameter, and to have two Bolts in the Beams through each Piece, of Bolts of inch Diameter, well clench'd. To have two Shiverholes, one of inch thwartships, and the other of inch; to have a cross Piece of foot long, and as square as the Bitts To have Forepartners on the upper Deck, of foot long, inches broad, and inches thick; to be scored over the Beams and Carlings one inch, and be bolted at the Ends, with Bolts of inch Diameter, two at each End of a Piece To have Mizonpartners of feet long, inch broad, and inches thick, to be either bolted or spiked in every Beam, with a Bolt or Nail, which shall weigh Pound; and to be placed inches asunder thwartships. To have Catheads on the Forecastle, to steave in every foot without the Forecastle inches, and to be inches square, or inch deeper, to continue the Substance one foot within the Side, and to lay a-thwart the Ship directly with the Beakhead, and bolted in every inches, through the Forecastle Beam, with Bolts of inch Diameter, and to have a Piece in the middle, between the two Cat-tails, answerable to the Substance of the Tail, at feet within the Side; and to be hook'd, and tabled down to the Tails, and bolted after, and in the same Manner, all a thwart under such Parts, being first laid with Tar, Hair, and Hair Size in the Seams, and the Bolts to be well clench'd: To have Shivers cut in each Cathead, of inches, and a Snatchblock fix'd on the Gunel, suitable to the Cathead To have a Supporter under each Cathead, to reach out within inch of the Shiverholes; and to be bolted through the Side, with a Bolt at every inches, of inch Diameter; to range

Grating on the Quarter Deck · *Grating on the Forecastle* · *Foretopsail Sheetbits and Jeerbits* · *Forepartners* · *Mizonpartners* · *Catheads* · *Supporter.*

truly

truly Circular, with either the lower or middle Rail of the Head, the Cathead to have an Iron Hoop, exactly fitted, just without the Shiverholes, and nail'd with four Nails, to be inches broad, and inch thick The Knee of the Head to be shap'd, according to the Figure in a Draught, drawn for the Purpose; to be in no more Pieces than and the main Piece to be foot long, and inches in the Throat, besides the Chock, and to fay to the Stem feet, to be as thick as the Stem, and diminish outward from the Stem inch in one foot; to be at the upper End inches thwart; to lay the upper Part at the Stem, direct with the lower Gundeck: To have one Bolt at the Throat, through the main Piece, and into the Ship of inch Diameter; the rest of the Bolts to be within inches one of another, and to be in Proportion to the Throat Bolt, according to the Length, and all to be well ring'd, and forlock'd, with in side; and all the rest of the Pieces, that makes the fashion of the Knee, may be fasten'd to the main Piece with Bolts in every inch of inch Diameter. To have a Gripe, of the Thickness of the Stem, to be fix'd from the end or foresoot of the Keel (into which he shall be tenon'd half the Thickness of the Keel; and the Tenon to be inch square, with a Dovetail on each Side inches thick, inches broad, inches long, with two Bolts) to run upwards foot above the lower Part of the Knee, and to be bolted through, and belay'd within side with a Ring and Forlock: To be inches asunder, and inches Diameter To have two Cheeks of each Side, which shall be inches sided in the Throat, and inches in and out, and inches at the after End up and down, and inches in and out, and inches at the foremost End, up and down, and inches in and out: The upper Cheek may be $\frac{1}{7}$ less than the lower, and both to answer the Sheer of the Wale, and cutting down of the Knee; to be well grown, the lower one to lay with the cutting down of the Knee, and the other to lay inches above it, from one upper Edge to the other, and be bolted in every inch space, with a Bolt of inch Diameter The after Arm of each to be feet long, and the other to be feet long. To have a Lyon, or other Figure upon the Knee feet long from the Crown, to the hinder or lower Claws, to be inches fore and aft at the Breast, and inches thwart after it's carved, and to be cut or carved, according to a due Proportion from that Bigness, and shap'd and smoothly carved, according to the Use and Custom of Carving The upper Rail to be shaped truly Circular, and to be inches in and out, at the after End, and inches fore and aft, to be inches fore and aft at the Foremast End, and inches thwart, and to taper by a diminishing Line, to be fasten'd at the after End, with two Bolts of inch Diameter, and nail'd at the foremost End. The middle Rail to be inches in and out, at the after End, and inches up and down The lower Rail to be inches square, at the after End, and both to diminish forward one inch in a foot To place Timbers, one at the Stem inches sided, and the other to diminish forward half an inch in each, and to lay inches asunder. To have a Trailboard from the Stem, to the Claws of the Lyon, groved in every way, and to be inches thick, and inches up and down. To have a Lace upon that, tenon'd into the Stem, $\frac{1}{4}$ of the square of the Lace, which shall be inches To have a Kelson, on the Timbers of foot long, and inches square, at the after End, and inches square at the foremost End. To have a Stander on that, bolted to the Stem, and through the Kelson, Lace and Trail inches into the Knee, the Bolts to be inches asunder, and of inch Diameter, the Stander to be inch thwart, and inch in the Throat, well grown. The Beams, or thwart Pieces, one to be placed close to the Stem, and to be dovetail'd into the upper Rails, to be inches up and down, and inches fore and aft, to be bolted into the Stem, with two Bolts, of inch Diameter; and to have two Knees at each End inches sided, and inches in the Throat, to be bolted in every inches, with one Bolt of inches Diameter To have another Beam feet above that of

inches

Head. Gripe. Cheek. Lyon. Upper Rail. Middle Rail. Lower Rail. Timbers. Trail. Lace. Kelson. Stander. Beams.

inches up and down, and inches fore and aft, and to have one Knee at each End inches sided, and inches in the Throat, and to be bolted in every inches space, with a Bolt of inches Diameter To have thick Pieces for the Foretack, fix'd between two Timbers, of inches thick, and bolted at each End, through the Timbers, with two Bolts, of inch Diameter. To have a Quafe (or a Piece made Saddle fashion) on the Locks of the Lyon, from Rail to Rail. To have Gratings in the Head, as many as can be well placed, from the Bow of the Ship, to the foremost cross Piece, only in the Midships lay Carlings between the Beams inches up and down and inches thwart, to lay feet asunder, to have Houses of Easement in the Head, to have three Eyebolts for the Horses, of inch Diameter, to cut Holes in the Knee, for the Gammonings and

Beak Bobstay To have a beak Bulkhead feet abaft the forepart of the Stem; the Stantions to be inches square, and to stand so as to make Doorways, answering the Forecastle Bulkhead Doors, and to be inches broad; the Stantions to be rabbitted half the Thickness of the Door one way, and the whole Thickness the other, to make Ports equal in Height to the Ports of the Side, at which Height a Collar Beam shall be placed, from Side to Side, to be inches up and down, and inches fore and aft, to be knee'd at each End, with one Knee inches sided, inches at the Ends, and inches in the Throat, to be bolted in every inch, with Bolts of inch Diameter, the Beam to be rabbitted for inch Plank, to lay the Beakhead, and nail it at each End, with Nails inches asunder, every Hundred of them to weigh Pounds. To cover the forepart of the Stantions with *Prussia* Deal inch thick, and to nail it with Nails in every inch space To step the Stantions into the Collar Beam inches, and bolt them, or nail them at the upper Part with Nails, that every hundred Weight shall weigh Pounds, and be inches long. To make Doors and Ports of ordinary Dealboard, lin'd with Elmboard, and nail'd in every inch, with penny Nails To garnish this and all the Bulkheads, with Rails and Brackets as customary, to have a House or two Houses of Easement, project semicircle fashion by inches radius close to the side, wrought with Stantions and Deal, by the same dimensions as the other part of

Gallerys the Bulk-head To have a Gallery on each side Foot long on the side, measured from the upright of the Stem on the sheer of the Ship, and to project Feet, the lower Stool to be Foot long, Inches broad, and Inches thick, and to lye ranging with the sheer of the Wales, level from the Ship side, and as high in the middle as the Plank of the upper Deck;

Stools to have another Stool of Foot long, Inches broad, and Inches thick, and to lay after the same manner with the next Deck upwards, and so to lay a Stool successively at every Deck, and such Stools to be bolted through each Deck, at every inches distance, with a Bolt of inch diame-

[illegible] ter. To have Rails feet high from the Stools, to make the lower Part of the Lights, to bring on *Prussia* Deal inches up and down, from Stool to Stool, and nail it at the Stools, with penny Nails, at every inches distance, to finish the Gallery in every respect, according to the Figure, laying Lead over the upper Stools, to keep the Water out, it being first calked with parceling of Canvas: To have Lights on each Side inches up

[illegible] and down, and inches thwartships. To have quarter Pieces carved inches sided, and to answer the Shape prescribed in the Mode of the Stern, and to be bolted at every foot distance, with a Bolt of inch diameter.

Rudder To hang on a substantial Rudder feet long, inches in and out at the Head, and inches thwart, the main Piece to be inches broad at the lower end, and as thick as the Post, as high as the Waterline, or feet, and from thence to diminish bigger upwards, to the Scantling prescribed, to continue inches thwart foot down from the great end, and inches fore and aft, to have Fir brought on of the aft side, to make the Rudder inches broad at the lower end, and inches foot high, but

if

If there wants any Subſtance next the Poſt, to be made out with Oak, to bard him each way for traverſing, according to the Angle the Tillar will make; to have Braces inch thick at the Hole of the Pintel, and inches thick at the Shoulders, fairly diminiſhing to inch at the End; and to be inches up and down. To have the Seams well calked under them, and to be parcell'd in the Wake. To be nail'd with Nails of inches long, and every Hundred to weigh Pounds; and be ſet inches aſunder To have Gudgeons to be drove through, and be well forlock'd within ſide, and to be inch diameter To have Pintels as broad as the Braces, and inches long; the Shoulders to be of the ſame Subſtance with the Braces and nail'd in every reſpect as well. To lead the Forepart of the Rudder, and alſo the Poſt turning the Lead, and nailing of it with Lead Nails, on the Side of the Rudder; to bolt the Pieces that makes the Rudder, together with Bolts, of inch diameter, in inches diſtance, to have two Rings at the Back of the Iron to make faſt a Rope or Tackle. To have a Tillar fitted to the Rudder foot long, and inches up and down, at the Forepart of the Rudder Head; and inches thwart, to taper to inches up and down, at the Aftpart of the Rudder, and inches thwart, and to plate the Head of the Rudder with Plates, to help the Strain of the Tillar; and to drive on Hoops, to ſtop the Tillar in the Rudder Head, by a Bolt drove through the Tillar, at the Aftpart of the Rudder Head of inch diameter; the Tillar to be at the Foremoſt End, inches ſquare, and there to have an Iron Gooſeneck fitted on, to put the Whip ſtaff on; which Neck ſhall be let on upon the Tillar, and have a Strap of each Side, of foot long, inches broad, and nail'd with ſingle Port Nails, the Hoop of the Neck to be inches broad, and inch thick; the Part of the Neck that extends from the Tillar, to be inches long, and inches ſquare, the other Part of the Neck to be inches long, and inch diameter, made round, only to have Shoulders left anſwerable with the other Part, inches from the bend. To have a Forlock Hole at the End, to ſtop on the Whipſtaff, which ſhall be a Piece of Aſh foot long, made round, inch diameter at one End, and inch diameter at the other; to have an Iron Hoop at the great End of inches broad, and inch thick, and to have a ragged Bolt, with an Eye made big enough for the Gooſeneck to go into To have a Plank fitted up to the upper Deck Beams, truly circular from Side to Side; which Sweep (as it's term'd) ought to be an Arch of a Circle, made by the Tillar, making the Rudder Head the center. To have an Iron Cleat fitted to the Tillar, of inches long, inches broad, and inches thick; to be bolted to the Tillar, with two Bolts, of inches diameter, ſarcer-headed, and forlock'd, which Cleat to be fitted after ſuch a manner, that it may ſlide on the Sweep, and hang the Tillar up to it To have a Plate of Iron let in artificially into the Sweep, for the Cleat to ſlide on; the Sweep to be inch Plank, inches broad, and to have Cleats at each End, of Wood, to ſtop the Tillar's going too far To have a Wheel or Reel fitted on the Quarter Deck, with Blocks in the Gun Room, and Bolts drove for traverſing the Tillar, without the help of a Whipſtaff, the Wheel to be foot diameter, made with Elm, Quarter of inches ſquare, the Reel or Cylinder to be inches diameter, and inches long, having Iron Axis fitted at each End, with Iron Plates round the Axis: To have Iron Stantions, or Supporters, to lay the Axis in; inches high from the Deck, and ſupported with Braces on each Side. To have Blocks in the Gun Room, well faſtned to the Beams; and Shiver Holes in them, big enough for a inch Rope to reeve in: To have an Eye Bolt on each Side, to laſh a Block for the ſaid Rope, the Eye Bolt to be inch diameter, and faſtned without ſide. To have Standers on the lower Gun Deck Pair; one pair againſt the Foremaſt, one pair againſt the Bitts, one pair againſt the Cheſtree, one pair againſt the Mainmaſt, one pair againſt the Maincapſtern, one pair againſt the Mizonmaſt; to be inches ſided, and inches in the Throat, without

Tillar. Gooſeneck. Whipſtaff. Sweep. Cleat. Wheel and Reel. Standers on the Lower Deck.

without any Chock, and inches at the Ends, to ftand upon the Deck, and that Arm to be feet long, the up and down Arm to be feet long; to be bolted in every inches, with Bolts of inch diameter, the Seams on the Deck to be well calked and fiz'd, laying Tar and Hair under; and all the Bolts to be well clench'd.

Upper Deck Standers. To have Pair of Standers on the upper Deck, a pair at each Bulkhead, a pair againft the Shank-painter Chain of the Anchors, a pair at the Cheftree, a pair at the Mainmaft, a pair at the Mizonmaft; to be fided inches, and inches in the Throat, and inches at the Ends, to be bolted at every inches, with Bolts of inch diameter, the Bolts to be belay'd as aforefaid, and the Seams and Deck ferved alfo as aforefaid

Quarter Deck Standers To have Pair of Standers on the Quarter Deck, one pair at the Bulkhead, and one pair againft the Mizonmaft; to be fided inches, and inches in the Throat, and inches at the Ends, to be bolted in every inches, with Bolts of inches, the Seams fized under.

Plank without Board. To Plank without Board from the Rabbits of the Keel, Stem and Stern Poft, Strakes of Elm Plank, of inches thick, inches broad, and every Plank, except fome afore and abaft for fhifting the Butts, to be from foot long, to foot long, to make good Calking Seams and Butts To have two Trenels in every Timber, which fhall go through the Outboard Plank Timber, and Inboard Plank; excepting one

Trenels Trenel left crofs in every 3d or 4th Timber, which fhall not be drove out again, when you come to bring on the foot Walcing, but remain to keep to the Outboard Plank; the Trenel to be inch diameter, of well feafon'd Timber; and to continue that bignefs of Trenel to the Floor Timber, and then the bignefs of the Trenel upwards, to be according as the Cube of the breadth of the Timbers, are one to another; fo that at the Toptimber Head, the Trenel

Oak Plank. fhall be inch diameter To have Strakes of Oak Plank, from the Elm, upwards of inches thick, inches broad, and feet long;

Thick Strakes and from thence to the Wale, to fwell bigger gradually: That the upper Strake fhall be inches thick, and inches broad, the next to him, inches thick, and inches broad; the next to that, or third, inches thick, and inches broad, the fourth, inches thick, and inches broad; and ftill if you have Timber by you, that will fuit to continue equal Lengths as

Sceling Strakes aforefaid To have every Strake extend to the Rabbit of the Stem ex-

Lower Wale cepting and they to be fhort of the Stem, but feet: The lower Wale to be inches up and down, and inches in and out, not in more

[illegible] Pieces than the Hafpin to be feet long, and following Piece for-

Strakes between ward feet long, after Piece feet long, to be The Strakes between

Upper Wale the Wale inches broad, and inches thick, the upper Wale to be inches deep, and inches in and out, and not in more Pieces than the Harping to be feet, following Piece feet; to be fcarph'd with *Flemifh* Scarph, inches long. To trenel all the Wales, and thick Strakes about the Wales, with Trenels of inch diameter; the Strake upon the Upper Wale to be inches thick, inch broad, and to fcarph the Butts of the Wales, fo that every Strake fhall over launch one another feet; and to have whole Planks between two Butts: The fecond Strake above the upper Wale to be inches thick, inches broad, and to butt at the Hawfe Pieces; but that below him, to be wrought his whole breadth to the Stem: To taper the Strakes up to the Channel Wale, to inches thick; and to work them of equal breadth, from the two Strakes above the Wale, to the

Channel Wale Channel Wale, to drive Trenels in every Timber, of inch diameter; the lower Channel Wale to be inches thick, and inches broad, on the Flat of the Side; the Strake between the Channel Wale, to be inches thick and inches broad, the upper Channel Wale to be inches thick, inches broad on the Flat, and both to be wrought according to Cuftom, the upper Edges fquare from the Timbers, to the thicknefs of the Plank, and then level out to the Edge; to have fuitable Lengths, that the Butts may give Scarf to the Ports; and no Butt to be under the Channels, nor in the Wake of the Chain Bolts; to be butted with plain Butts, and not fcarfed The Strake upon

upon the Channel Wale to be Oak, inches thick, and inches broad, and all the reſt of the Planks to be made of well ſeaſon'd *Pruſſia* Deal, of equal breadth quite up, not exceeding inches broad; and to be gradually taper'd to inches thick, and to be trenel'd with one Trenel (and one Nail of inches long; and every Hundred of them to weigh Pounds) in every Timber. To have a Planſheer from the Midſhip Drift, to the Forecaſtle Drift, of inches thick; to be nail'd in every inches, with a Nail of inches long, and every Hundred of them to weigh Pounds. To have a Rail ranging with the Height of every Drift, of inches up and down, and inches in and out, to gauge and ſet him truly circular, according to the Sheering of the Wales, and nailing him in every inches, with a Nail of inches long, and every Hundred of them to weigh Pounds To have a Rail of inches up and down, and inch s in and out, to lay at equal diſtance from the Channel Wale; which diſtance ſhall be inches to the lower Edge of the Rail, to be nail'd in every inches diſtance, with a Nail of inches long, and every Hundred of them to weigh Pounds. All ſuch Rails to be emboſs'd, according to Cuſtom; the upper and lower Edges of them to be Horizontal, making a Rhombus as the Figure A. To have Planſheers on all the Drift Rails, from the Mainmaſt aft, of inches thick; and to be nail'd in every inches Diamond faſhion, with a Nail of inches long, with Sheething Nail Head, to taper the Timbers upwards, letting them through the Planſheer, from the Mainmaſt aft; the Timbers to be inches aſunder. To have a Fife Rail fixed on the Timber Heads, inches broad, and inches thick, to lay equally diſtant from the Planſheer; and that diſtance to be inches, to the upper Edge of the Fife Rail; and to be nail'd at every Timber, with a Nail of inches long, the Waterway on the Forecaſtle to be ſcored about the Timber Heads, even with the Outſide of the outboard Plank; alſo to have a Gunel of inches thick, and inches broad, wrought after the Faſhion of the Waterway, and to be nail'd in every Timber, with a Nail of inches long; and every Hundred of them to weigh Pounds. To have an Oak Rail, upon the Outſide of this Gunel, emboſs'd, to be inches up and down, and inches thick, to leave the Timber Heads inches above the ſaid Gunel; and to be inches fore and aft, and inches in and out To have four Timber Heads inches long, above the Gunel, for to make Kevels, for the main and Foretack, and to be inches in and out, and inches fore and aft. To have main Channels for the Shrowds, foot long, inches broad, at the After End, and inches broad at the Foremoſt End, to be inches thick at the Side, and inches out; and then to be work'd away to inches thick, at the Outſide. To have the main Piece next the Side, inches broad; and to have Tenons let into each Piece, of inches thick, inches broad, and inches long in each. To fix this Channel's Foremoſt End, with the Forepart of the Mainmaſt; and to lay him ¾ of an inch below the upper Edge of the upper Channel Wale, to nail him at each End with Nails inches long, that every Hundred of them ſhall weigh Pounds. To bolt him at every inches, through the Ship Side, with Bolts of inch diameter. To have Chain Plates, which ſhall fit exactly from the upper Part of the Channel's outer Edge, to the middle of the lower Channel Wale, to be made as cuſtomary; inches thick, and inches broad; to be inches diameter at the bend of the Neck, and inches broad at the Foot, that goes on the Channel Wale: To have Dead Eyes, of inches diameter, bound with a round Iron of inch diameter, put to every Chain Plate To have a Chain Bolt drove through the middle of the lower Channel Wale, of inch diameter; and well-ring'd, and forlock'd, within ſide of the Ship To have Backſtay Plates in this Channel, of inch thick; and otherwiſe made and faſtned in every particular, as the Chain Plates. To have Ring Plates, to belay the Runners and Tackles to, of inches thick, wrought in Proportion to the other, and faſtned to the Channel

Pruſſia Deal

Planſheer

Rail ranging

Sheer Rails

A

Drift Planſheer

Fife Rail

Forecaſtle Waterway, Gunel.

Rail

Main and Foretack Kevels

Main Channel

Chain Plates

Backſtay Plates

Ring Plates

Channel Wale, as aforesaid. To have wooden Knees placed in the Channels, one Arm next the Side, to be inches long; the other to be as the breadth of the Channel, to be sided inches, and inches in the Throat; to be bolted in every inch distance, with a Bolt of inch diameter; the Knees to be placed feet asunder, having one at each End, as near as possible. To have a Stool for a Backstay, something abaft the Channel, of inches long, inches broad, and inches thick, to be fastned with one Bolt, of inch diameter, and a Nail at each End, the Chain Plate, Dead Eye, and Bolt, of the same Dimensions of the other Backstay Plates; and also fastned. To have a fore Channel on each Side, of foot long, inches broad at the Foremost End, and inches broad at the After End, to be inches thick at the Side, continuing that thickness inches; and then tapering of him to inches without side: To lay him with the Mast, and under the Edge of the upper Channel Wale, as was aforesaid; to nail him at each End, with two Nails of inches long, every Hundred to weigh Pounds: To bolt him at every inches distance, through the Side, with a Bolt of inches diameter. To have Chain Plates of inches thick, and other scantling Proportional, and placing of them, as was aforesaid of the Main; the Bolts also to be proportion'd to the Plates To have Backstay Plates; of inches thick, and other Proportions to the Main, and also placing in of them. To have Ring Plates, of inch thick, and other Proportions as aforesaid; the Bolts and fastning of them as usual. To have Knees in them; the up and down Arm to be inches long, the other to be as the Channel's breadth; to be inches sided, and inches in the Throat, well grown; to bolt them in every inch, with a Bolt of inch diameter. To have a Rail on each Channel's Back, inches square, imboss'd; to be nail'd in every inches distance, with a Nail of inches long, and every Hundred of them to weigh Pounds. To have Backstay Plates; inches thick, with a Stool, inches long, inches broad, and inches thick, to be fitted and fastned with the Plate and Bolt, in every Particular, as was aforesaid To have a Mizon Channel on each side, feet long, inches broad, and inches thick, bolted with Bolts equally spaced between the Ends, of inch diameter To have Chain Plates every way as big as the main Backstay Plates; and the Bolts to be answerable in every particular, and fastned. To have Spurs, made in Form as custom inches sided, and inches fore and aft. To have a Rail on the Back, inches square, and to be nail'd at every inch distance, with a penny Nail; all the Channels to be work'd off at each End, as customary; and the Mizon Channel to be plac'd feet under, and parallel to the Fife Rail To have Ports to every Port Hole; the lower Deck Ports to be inch Plank, lined with Elm or Oak, cut compassing, according to the Ship Side; to work the Lining inches thick, and the Outside Plank ranging with the Seams in the Sides, to nail the Port Diamond Fashion, in every distance, with penny Sheathing Nails. To have a Stop, of inches all round, to hang them Ports with two Hinges, of inches broad, and inches thick, at the biggest End; and inch big at the thinnest End; to be inch thick at the Edge; and the Eye to be inch big for the Hook. To place the Hinges, inches from the Ends of the Ports; and to be exactly as long as the Port Hole is up and down. To have a Bolt in the Hinge through the Port, inches from the Top, of inch diameter, and forlock'd within Side. To have an Iron Shackle, or small Ring Bolt drove through each Hinge outwards, and forlock'd; the Ring to be big enough to reeve turns of a inch Rope, to lash the Port in; the Bolt of the Shackle to be inch diameter: To have another Shackle drove inward, and forlock'd, to make fast the Port Rope to, and all the Shackles to be placed inches from the lower Part of the Port. To have a Ring Bolt, and an Eye Bolt, drove outward, on each Side of the Port; the Eye of the Eye Bolt, to be inches; and the Ring of the Ring Bolt to be inches diameter; and all the Bolts

to

Margin notes: *Stools for Backstays*; *Fore Channel*; *Chain Plates*; *Backstay Plates*; *Ring Plates*; *Knees*; *Rails*; *Stool of the Backstay*; *Mizon Channel*; *Chain Plates*; *Spurs*; *Rail*; *Ports Lower Deck*; *Stop Hinge*; *Shackle*; *Ring Bolts & Eye Bolts*.

to be, both Ring and Eye bolt, Inch diameter To have an Eye bolt drove over the Port, to lash up the Muzzle of the Gun, the Eye of the Bolt to be Inch diameter, and the Bolt to be Inch diameter, and all the said Bolts to be well forlock'd, to nail the Port-hinges with Nails of *Nails.* Inches long, broad headed, and every Hundred to weigh pounds, and to be Inches asunder: The upper Deck Ports to be made of *Upper Ports* of Inch thick, lined with Elm, cut answerable to the Compass of the Ship side, to nail them with penny sheathing Nails Inches asunder, the Stop to be inch, to have Hinges length, as aforesaid, *Stop* and bigness proportionable to the length, to be nail'd with such Nails as aforesaid, that every Hundred shall weigh pounds, and to be inches asunder, to have a Ring and Start, drove in inches from the lower part in *Ring & Start* the middle for the Port Rope the Port Hooks to be in all the Ports drove *Port-hooks.* through, and clench'd in the lower Ports, whose diameter shall be inches, and in the upper Ports of inches diameter, the turn of the Hook to be always as long as the Hinge is broad. If there shall happen to be any Ports requir'd to be made in two leaves or parts, then they shall be made in lieu of the *Half Leaves* Charge allowed for an intire Port in every respect To have one Ring-bolt and one Eye bolt of each side every Port to lash the Guns, of inch diameter, and to be forelock'd. To have a Chestree on each for the main Tack to *Chestree* be inches fore and aft at the Gunnel, and inches fore and aft at the upper main Wale, to be fix'd close to the Ship's sides, and bolted in every inches with a Bolt of inches diameter as far down as the lower Channel Wale, where he shall be inches in and out, and as thick as the Wale below, having a Hole cut through for the main Tack between the Channel Wale of inch diameter, and as far out as the Channel Wale, to have an Eye-bolt of inch diameter drove inches below the hole, to have a Bolster fitted at the upper end of the Chestree of foot long, and inches deep, nail'd with Nails of inches long, sizable, the Chestree to be placed feet before the Main Mast To have Shivers fix'd in blocks for the fore *Fore & Sprit-sail Sheet Block* and Spritsail Sheet feet before the Main Mast; the Shiver for the fore Sheet to be inches thick, and the spritsail Sheets inches thick, the Blocks to be bolted into the side with two Bolts at each end of inch diameter, well clench'd, to have a Shiver for the main Sheet fix'd in a block let through *Main Sheets* the sides, and bolted as the fore Sheets, and to be placed feet abaft the Main Mast above the Quarter Deck. To have Eye-bolts drove for the standing *Eye Bolts* part of the fore Sheets and main Sheets of inches diameter clench'd. To have a Block of each side with a Shiver of inch diameter for the main *Lift Blocks.* Lifts, which Block shall be inches long, inches in and out, and inches fore and aft, to be bolted with two Bolts in each of inch diameter, and clench'd, to have such Blocks placed for the main Topsail Hal- *Main Topsail Halyard-blocks* yards, the Shivers to be inches thick and Blocks to be inches in and out, and inches fore and aft, and to be fasten'd with two Bolts of inch diameter, and clench'd To have two Blocks for the fore Topsail *Fore ditto* Halyards, the Shiver to be inches thick, the Block to be inches long, inches in and out, and inches fore and aft, to have such a Block placed for the Mizon Jeers by the Mizon Mast, the Shiver to be *Mizon Jeer.* inch thick the Block to be Inches in and out, and Inches fore and aft, to be fasten'd with two Bolts of Inch diameter, to have a Block fitted Feet abaft the Main Mast, for the Main Topsail Clew-lines and *Topsail Clew lines* Bunt lines, the Shivers to be Inches, and Inches thick, to be Inches square, and fasten'd with two bolts to the upper Deck beams and have a head of Inches long to belay the Ropes to. To have two small Knees of Inches square, fitted with two Shivers of Inches *Main top Bowline Block.* thick fix'd on the Forecastle, for the main Topsail Bowline, and fasten'd to the after Forecastle beam with a bolt in each, and two Nails, with a head of Inches long to belay the Rope. To have such Conveniencies for the fore Lifts, *Fore Lift.* fasten'd to the beams with two bolts of Inch diameter, and clench'd, and nail'd

Shank-painter Chain nail'd with two Nails in each. To have a Shank-painter Chain of each side of Foot long, each Link to be Inches long, and the Bolt-staff that makes it Inch diameter, to have a Ring at each end of Inches diameter, equal in bigness, to have an Eye-bolt welded into one of the Rings of Inch diameter, drove through the Ship's side, and well forelock'd, to *Span-shackle for the Davit* have a Span shackle for the Davit, drove through the Forecastle-beam and upper Deck-beam, if they will suit, otherwise to have a Carling of Inches up and down, and Inches thwart fasten'd, for the Bolt to be drove through, and the Bolt-staff shall be Inches diameter both for the Shackle and Bolt, which Bolt shall be well and securely forlock'd in each Deck, to have *Chocks* Elm Chocks fitted on the Gunnel of Inches up and down, and Inches thwart, for the Davit to lay in, nail'd at each end with two Nails of Inches long, and every Hundred of them to weigh Pounds. To *Steps of the Sides* have Steps to come up the Ship side by, placed just afore the main Channel, to be Inches asunder, and Inches up and down, and Inches in and out, and Inches long, the upper Edge to lay Horizontal, and to be nail'd in every Inch distance with a Nail Inches long, that every Hundred of them shall weigh Pounds, to be imboss'd as Customary, and *Skids or Fendors* placed from the upper Wale to the Gunnel. To have Skids, or Fendors, on each side, placed opposite to the main Hatch-way Inches asunder, to be in and out equal with the Chestree, and Inches fore and aft, to be nail'd in every Inches, with a Nail of Inches long, and every Hundred of them to weigh Pounds, laying Hair Size under in every Seam. *Lining for the Bows* To line the Bow in the Wake of the Anchors going up and down, with Plank of Inches thick, and Inches broad, and Feet long, to place it from the Channel downwards, as Customary, to have a Piece between the Wales, and one Piece under the Wale of Inches broad, to have the Ship side well calked under it, and laid with Tar and Hair, and Hair Size in the Seams, to nail the [illegible] in every Inch distance with a Nail of Inches long, and every Hundred of them shall weigh Pounds, and all *Stopper-bolts* the Seams of this Lining shall be also well calked. To have Bolts to make fast the Stoppers to at every beam from the Hatch way in the Midships to the main Bits, the Rings to be Inches diameter, and the Bolt in every part to be Inch diameter, and well forlock'd under the beam. To have Ring-*Lashing for the Long-boat* bolts for lashing the Long-boat in every beam in the Wake of the Waste; the Ring to be Inch diameter, and the Bolt in every part to be Inch diameter, and forlock'd at the lower part of every beam, to have Ring-bolts *Other Lashing [illegible]* for lashing the Guns between every Port, opposite to the main Capstern and the bits, drove between the Ports, and of Inch diameter, to have Ring-bolts drove upon the Deck, for halling in the Guns, in such places as has no other Conveniencies, of Inch diameter, to have a large Eye-bolt drove on each side at the Forecastle, and Steeridge-beams, and well forlock'd, and *Clew-garnets Topsail Halyard* Inch diameter; to have Eye-bolts for the main and fore Clew-garnets, and standing part of the Topsail Halyards, of Inch diameter, well forlock'd; to have Eye-bolts for the main Braces on each side at the Tafferal, and one Eye-bolt for the Mizon Sheet of Inch diameter, to have an Eye-bolt of each side drove through the Spirkit-rising of the upper Deck, by the *Carved Work* main Hatch-way, of Inch diameter, and well forlock'd. To have Carved Work on the Stern, Galleries, Head, and in every place agreeable, and in Proportion to what shall be described in the Figure. The Work to be Cut in due Form and Fashion, to be Cut on sound and serviceable Elm or Firr Timber. *[illegible]* To Paint the Stern, Head, Galleries, and all the Weather Work, as usual on board of any other Ship, with a good bright Colour, well laid. When the Work is thorough dry, and to first size, and Times painted, to specify in particular what the Colour shall be, and whether shadow'd, or Carved freize. *Joiners* To Wainscot the Great Cabbin with Deal Foot long, to raise Pannels, *Great Cabbin* and imboss'd work with Glass of In the Stern and Galleries, Sash Lights; to have a Screen Bulkhead Foot abaft the main Bulkhead, with Sash

Sash Lights of Feet square; and the Wainscot shall be valued at a Yard, Stuff and Workmanship. to paint it with a bright Colour, once sized, and Times painted, to have a Lock on the great Door, Value Shillings, and other Locks on Pantries and Closets, with Hinges on the great Doors, and pair of Hinges on Lockers. The Galleries to be fitted within side with a House of Easement in each aft part, and Closets in the fore part, to pannel and imboss with Mouldings agreeable to the Great Cabbin, to have Cabbins at the foremost part of the Cabbin, half in the Great Cabbin, and half in the Steeridge, fitted according to the fancy of the Commander, but specified, to have a Bed-room between those Cabbins, in the Great Cabbin of Feet square, and the Work to be set off agreeable to the Cabbins, to have Cabbins in the Steeridge, and two at the Steeridge Bulkhead: All which shall be Feet square, and to be made fitting for Lodging, and Pantries, according to what is required. To close the outside with Deal, to have Settle Lockers, and side Cupboards, all fitted with Locks and Hinges suitable; that the Value of each Cabbin shall be judged at for Stuff and Workmanship, to have Lights in the Bulkhead Cabbins of Stone ground Glass of Inches square, of the Cabbins to be painted with a bright Colour, as aforesaid The Steeridge over head to be lin'd with Deal slit between the beams, having an imboss'd Moulding on the ends fasten'd to the beams The Round house and Coach to be Foot long from the Stern, to take out of that Feet for a Round-house, which is always various, either double or single, the Work to be wainscoted with Deal, and raised Pannels that shall be valued at *per* Yard square, to have Lights in the Stern of Inches up and down, and Inches thwart, of Glass to have Conveniencies for Lodgings fitted with twisted Bannisters, or other Ornaments as commodious, to have Settle Lockers, and side Cupboards, fitted with Locks and Hinges; to paint it with a bright Colour, as the Great Cabbin, to have Cabbins in the Coach fitted for Lodgings, like those in the Steeridge, to paint the Coach and Steeridge with a bright Colour, once primed with Size, and three times Painted, and lined over head, as was afore said, to have a Cabbin on each side at the Bulkhead of the Forecastle, fitted in every respect like those at the bulkhead of the Steeridge, to have Cabbins in the Forecastle, which shall each be valued at To have a Bulkhead at the Gun-room, fitted very well with whole Deal, and Door-way of Inches broad. to have a Cabbin for the Gunner, with Conveniencies for Lodgings and Apartments for small Stores, to have a Cabbin opposite to the Gunner's, fitted like the Cabbin at the bulkhead of the Steeridge, to have Cabbins in the Gun-room valued at each, to have Cabbins on each side on the Transums, valued at each, to fit the Gun-room in every respect convenient for the small Arms, and other Uses belonging to the Gunner, and to have a Table Feet long, and Inches broad, of whole Deal To have a Lazaretto forward Feet from the Stem, convenient, and in every respect commodious, for the use, and according to the magnitude of the Ship, and what the Commander, or whom he deputes, shall reasonably see necessary To have Conveniencies on the after Cockpit for the Steward, and a Lodging for him, Lodgings for the Purser and Surgeon, and a Slop room, Captain's Store-room, Fish-room, fitted in every respect according to what has been usual on board of such a Ship but as the respective Officers shall reasonably desire, also a Bread-room Feet from the Post measured on the Gun deck, lined with the Fish-room Feet long before, that the Cabbins Feet fore and aft, and Feet thwart, fitted as convenient and ornamental as the Gunner's Cabbin To have a Powder-room abaft of Feet square, fitted as usual, or as the Gunner shall reasonably desire, also the fore Powder-room to be fitted with great exactness for the Safety of the Powder, to be Feet from the Stem, measured on the lower Deck, and to have Apartments for the Gunner's Stores Feet from the Stem, fitted with Chests, and Filling-rooms,

and

and what can be thought proper and convenient for the more easy managing of the Powder, and all other small Stores. To have an Apartment for the Boatswain's Stores Feet fore and aft, and Feet thwart, to have a Sail-room Feet fore and aft, and Feet thwart To have an Apartment for the Carpenter's Stores Feet fore and aft, and Feet thwart. All which Rooms shall be intire, and convenient in every respect to lay the *Plummer* Stores with Safety, one Specie clear from another To have all Scuppers either well cast, or join'd, and sodder'd, with Lead, that every Foot square shall weigh pounds, well wrought without Flaws, or any other Defect, Pissdale Pipes to be Inches diameter in the bore, and every Foot to weigh pounds, the Bowl to be Inches in and out, and Inches fore and aft, and to be lined with such Lead that every Foot shall weigh pounds, to be one of each side, to have Funnels in the Houses of Easement in the Galleries Foot long, and Inches diameter at the upper end, and Inches below, and to be well sodder'd, to have Lead on the Brick-work of length, and Inches broad, of such Lead that every Foot shall weigh pounds, all Lead to be nail'd, as Scupper to have but Inch distance between Nail-head and Nail head, both within side and without and to have Tar and Hair laid under, Pissdale Pipes nail'd after the same fashion, and the Bowles and Funnels in the Houses of Easement, Inch between Nail-head and Nail-head, Lead of the Furnaces on the Wood ditto, to have Lead over the upper Stool of the Gallery, that every Foot shall weigh pounds nail'd as the Scuppers, and Tar and Hair under, and all other Lead which shall be found requisite or usual in Building such a Ship, shall be provided, and nail'd as *G[illegible]* [illegible] To have Stone-ground Glass that shall be valued at *per* Foot, laid in with Putty; and the Number and Quality of Lights that shall be found usual, if required, shall be found and provided as good, although not specified *C[illegible]* in the Contract To drive into the Seams, from the Keel to Seams upwards on each side in the Wake of the Bulge-water, Thread of spun Hair, Thread of well spun white Oakam, and Threads of spun black Oakam, and from thence to Seams upwards Threads of white, and of black, and from thence to the lower Wale, of white, and of black. If the Wales are double Wales, then drive of white and of black, between the Wales, of white and of black, Seams above the Wale of white, and of black; from thence to the Channel Wale of white, and of black, between the Channel Wales, and one Seam above them of white, and of black, from thence to the Top timber head of white, and of black, the lower Deck to be calked with of white, and of black, the Spirkit-rising with of white, and of black, as usual, the upper Deck to be calked with of white, and of black, the Spirkiting with of white, and of black, all the other Quick work, or Weather work, to have of white, and of black, that is, the Forecastle Deck, and Quarter Deck, Poop Deck, all Planshcers, and about the Timber-heads, and every part of the Ship that is exposed to the Weather, or for preserving any Goods or Utensils, shall be made as firm, and dry, as any part of the Plank, calking all Trenels without board, and wedging of them within side, the Trenels to be mooted as high as the Channel-wale, to calk all Rents or Shans, and nailing of them in Workman-like manner, and with such a Proviso, that if it shall be observed, or there is any manner of room to believe, that such a Quantity of Oakam is not sufficient to fill the Seam, then it shall be Lawful to cut out pieces in divers places, to see whether the Oakam is bottom'd, and the Seam fill'd, and if it's found otherwise, then the said Ship shall be calked over again, till the Seam is fill'd, and the Oakam at the bottom, to pay every Seam with clear Pitch (as the Work is calked), that a barrel of Pitch shall be produced from barrels of Tar, to bream or melt all that Pitch off again, and pay or cover the Ship's bottom from the Keel to the lower Wale with to black all the Wales, and between, and one Strake above, with Pitch, that every barrel shall be produced from

from barrels of Tar; to pay the upper Work to the Sheer Rail with Rozin mix'd with Tallow, that to every Hundred of Rozin shall be put Pounds of Tallow; the upper Decks, Quarter Deck, Forcastle and Poop, to be well Tar'd, and all other Weather work to be Painted, as aforesaid; to find the standing Masts, as Main Mast, Fore Mast, Mizon Mast, and Bowsprit: The Main Mast to be Yards long, and Inches in the lower Partners, to have Oak Cheeks of Foot long, and Inches in and out at the Head; to have Trusle-trees and Cross-trees in due proportion, and the Mast to be wrought in every respect as usual for a Mast of such a Diameter and Length; the other Masts to be made in proportion to the Main Mast in every respect. To do and compleat every individual piece or part of Work which is found necessary to be done to compleat the Ship, and make her fitting for the Sea as to the Hull of her, without any Equivocation, as any Ship is or has been done of the like Magnitude, and for such a Voyage or Use. And if it shall happen in the Term of Building the said Ship, that any part of the Premises should be found improper for the Use, then the same shall be alter'd at the Owner's Cost, with such a Proviso that the Builder shall alter it, both as to Materials and Workmanship, according to the currant Price for either, or as the Owner could have it done in another place. And the said *C. D* for himself, his Executors, Administrators and Assigns, doth Covenant and Grant, at his or their proper Cost and Charges, to find and provide all manner of Iron work, of the Iron, or what shall be equal in Goodness, as Spikes, Nails, Brads, likewise all Timber Plank, Deals, Trenels, white and black Oakam, Pitch, Tar, Rozin, Hair, Oyl, Brimstone, Lead, Tin Plates in the Wake of the Fire-place, and all other Materials whatever that shall be requir'd to perform the Premises, or expended about making every piece, and parts of pieces herein mentioned, good and substantial work, and compleat and finish the Ship, as aforesaid, in every particular with Workmen, and to pay and discharge all sorts of Workmen which shall be requisite, and to re-enter Artificers again at pleasure, only with such a Caution, that the said Ship shall be perfectly Compleated, as aforesaid, and Launch the said Ship, and Deliver her safe into the hands of the said *A. B.* (without any manner of Incumbrance) or some other proper Persons that shall be duely authorized to receive her, at Floating, at or upon the day of which shall be in the Year of our Lord Otherwise, for every Week that the said Ship shall continue on the Launch, and not safely Deliver'd into the hands of *A. B* or some other fit Persons, fit and compleat, as was aforesaid, the said *C D.* shall allow unto *A. B.* the Sum of which the said C. *D* doth bind himself, his Executors, Administrators and Assigns, to allow unto the said *A B.* his Executors, Administrators and Assigns, out of the Sum of which shall be allowed unto the said C. *D.* for his last Payment. And it is further agreed, That the said *A B* shall have Liberty to appoint such Person or Persons, as he shall see fit, to inspect and oversee the Building of the said Ship, which Person or Persons shall have free Liberty at all times to Discharge his Duty therein, without any Lett, Hinderance or Molestation, and if at any time during the Building of the said Ship, there shall be found and discovered any individual matter contrary to the true intent and meaning of this Contract, either in Dimensions, Proportions, Measure or Scantling herein expressed, or otherwise what may be observed by the said Person, in other Ships of the said Magnitude and Use, that may in Reason be taken for a Sample for the said Ship, as is here specified, or that any unsound, or unsufficient Timber or Plank, or any other Material whatever, or that any neglect in the Manager, or any of the Artificers under him be found, or observed, to be either in Goodness or Quantity that may be any ways prejudicial to the said Ship herein mentioned, that then the said Overseer shall give due Notice thereof unto the said *C. D* or to his Deputy, or Foreman Upon which Notice it shall be amended, and effectually remedied, at the sole Charge of the said *C D* his Executors or Assigns, reforming all and every such Defaults And the said *A. B.* for himself, his

Hh

his Executors, Administrators or Assigns, shall and will well and truly pay, or cause to be paid, unto the said C. D. his Executors, Administrators or Assigns, in Sterling Money of *England*, the full and just Sum of in manner and form as follows: That is to say, the Sum of within Days after the Sealing and Delivering this Contract; the Sum of when the Floor shall be bolted, the Sum of when the Foot-hook shall be fast in the said Ship, the Sum of when the Orlop Beams are fast, and Foot-waleing in the Sum of when the lower Gun-deck is fasten'd with Knees, and both that and the upper Deck is laid and compleat, the Sum of when the Quarter-deck and Forecastle Beams are all fast, and the Work compleated in due course to them Parts, and the Remainder, which shall be due when the said Ship shall be delivered, as aforesaid Only in Case of Default, as was afore-mentioned, to have a Draw-back, or Stopage, for such Non-performance, in Proportion as was before specified And to the end the several Sums of Money, hereby and herein mentioned and contracted for, and agreed to be paid to the said *C. D.* for and towards the Building of the said Ship, may be effectually laid out; so that if in Case the said *C. D* should depart this Life, before the said Ship shall be built, or any other Inconveniency or Incapacity should happen to the said *C D* then that the said *A B* may in some manner be secured for such several and respective Sums of Money, which shall be paid unto the said *C. D.* The said *C D.* doth Covenant, Grant and Agree, to and with the said *A B* that the said *C. D* shall give due and effectual Notice unto the said *A B.* or his Overseer appointed for that purpose, when any Timber, or Plank, or any other Material, is brought to the Place where the said Ship is Building, declaring that such Material was purchased, bought and provided, for and toward the Use of Building the said Ship, and for no other Use whatsoever. And that it shall be Lawful for the Person appointed to survey the Building of the said Ship, immediately upon the bringing of such Timber, Plank, or any other Material, into the aforesaid place of Building the said Ship, to make the said Materials, as the proper Goods and Merchandize of the said *A B.* and so it shall be adjudged from thence forward, notwithstanding the said *C. D.* had Contracted for it in his own Name And finally, for all such Sums of Money that shall grow due, by Vertue of this Contract, the said *C D.* is content to accept of the said *A. B.* or for Payment. In Witness whereof, to one part of these present Indentures, the said *A. B.* or *C. D* hath set his Hand and Seal, in the Day and Year first above-written.

C D.

Sealed and Delivered
in the Presence of

And this has been a standing Custom for Contracting by such Indentures, for Building new Ships, both in the Publick Service, and also for the Merchants, altho' I have been abundance fuller in Particularizing the Nature, and necessary Cautions, which ought to be minded in Building a new Ship, yet notwithstanding will not allow my self to be perfect, in laying down every individual Matter that ought to be put together, to make such a Machine compleat: I shall therefore shew some Reasons why such Indentures (or indeed it may be as properly call'd a Guide) ought to be made, as full and Particular as it possibly can be made; and shall also give some Directions how it may be made so

First, It will be of Use and Service to the Builder, or Undertaker, since it will hinder any Disputes that often happen between the Builder and Owner. That there shall be no Heart-burning, or Reflections happen, but the Builder seeing it fairly inserted what he ought in Justice to do, and effectually doing of it, the Owner fairly seeing that he has a Penny-worth for his Penny, will not in Reason

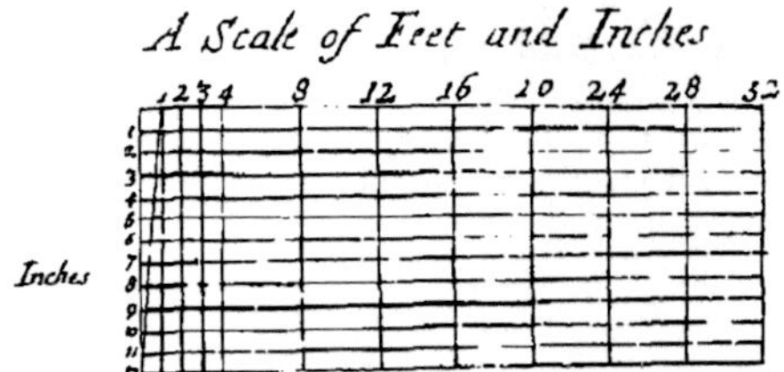
A Scale of Feet and Inches
1 2 3 4 8 12 16 20 24 28 32
Inches
1 2 3 4 5 6 7 8 9 10 11 12

Fig

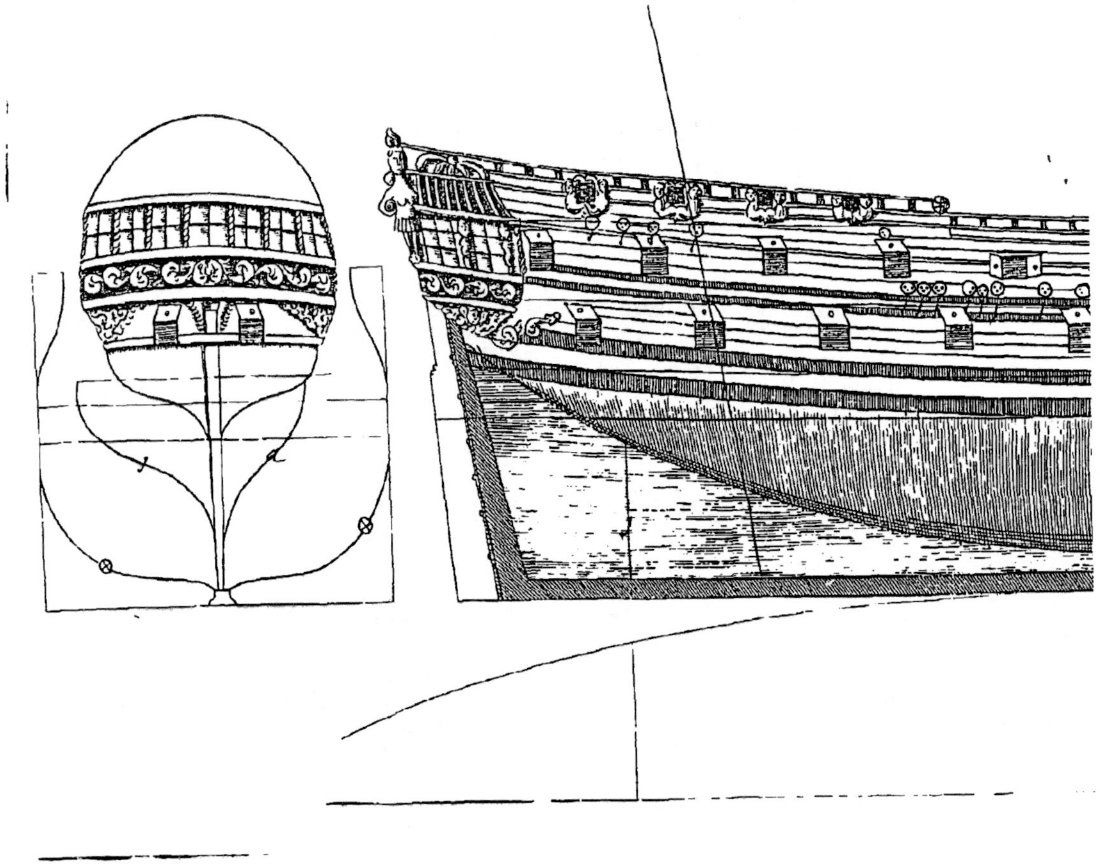

A

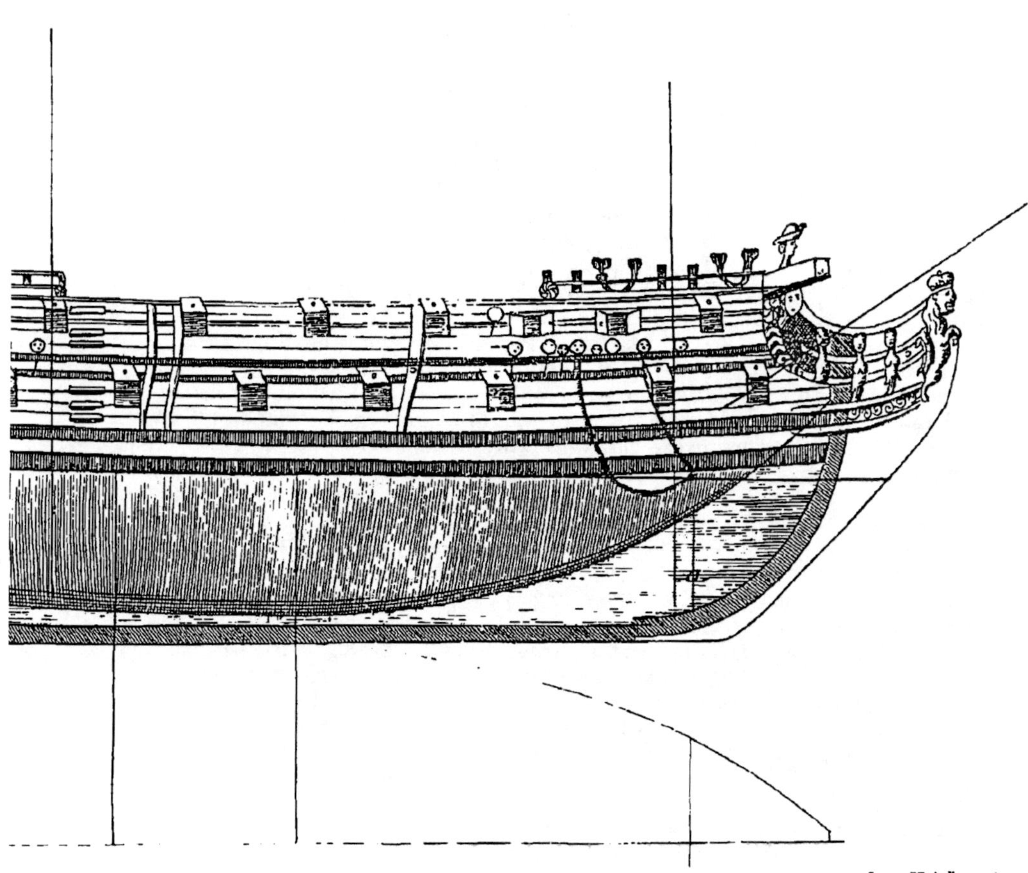

Sutton Nicholls sculp

ſon deſire any more, but the Buſineſs will be carry'd on ſmooth and gradually, without any rubbing or diſcontinuance.

It alſo being ſo plain and palpable a Guide, that in Caſe the Builder is indiſpos'd, or at the *Exchange*, as it often happens, and his Foreman in the Country Purveying, or in any other Buſineſs; ſuch a particular Direction will be able to capacitate the meaneſt Servant to direct the Buſineſs, and carry on the Building of the ſaid Ship in every particular Part.

It will be alſo of Uſe and Service to the Owner, ſince it will be a Guide for the meaneſt Shipwright, and make him effectually able to ſurvey and inſpect the well performing, and building any Ship. It will ſhew him what he can lawfully Demand to have done, without having any Cavilling, or needleſs Diſputes. Neither ſhall it lay at the Pleaſure, or honeſt Part of a Builder, or his Deputy, to pinch a Penny-worth of Workmanſhip, or Materials, out of Sixpence, and perhaps to the quite Ruining of the ſaid Ship, but that the ſaid Machine ſhall be duly proportion'd and wrought in every particular throughout, and to the effectually finiſhing of the Work ſo contracted for.

I ſhall therefore from theſe, and ſuch Conſiderations, ſhew how an Indenture, or Contract, may be drawn in a true Method, both for the Eaſe of Builder and Owner: That it may as directly guide them, as the Alphabet to greater Learning, or any direct grand Road will guide you to a Town or City.

It may be obſerv'd in this, and moſt other Contracts for Ship Building, That they are not made in due Courſe, or ſucceſſively leading you to the Building of the Ship, but what Part may be in Hand to Day, ſhall follow another Part in the Contract, that was done a Month or two ſince, ſo that a Man of indifferent Learning may be puzled to find his Leſſon, and whilſt he looks for a Hog, may find a Pig; therefore it would be highly neceſſary to draw a Contract, and mention the Parts directly, as the Ship is put together, or as near as poſſible, without either puzling the Manager, or the Scribe.

Then to begin, and give you a Method, The Keel being firſt fitted with a falſe Keel, then the Stem, and the Parts belonging to him; not deſigning to mention every Particular over again, but only to ſhew a breviate of the Method. The Sternpoſt and Parts Dead-wood afore and abaft, the Floor-timbers, Foot hooks, Toptimbers Hawſe-pieces, and every individual Part of the Frame; altho' it is often ſeen, That the large Ships has not the Framing compleated, before ſome Plank is work'd both within and without: However, the Performance of it being various, according to the Fancy of the Manager, I ſhall not mention it, but proceed to the Plank without Board, from the Keel to the Toptimber Head, without minding the Plank within, altho' it is always found to be done near as high as the lower Deck Clamps, before the Plank is compleated without Board; then to Plank or foot Wale within Board, and all the Riders Steps and Crutches, and Breſthooks: Then the Orlop Beams, lower Gundeck Beams, and that Deck compleat, the Spirkitriſing and Clamps between the Decks, and then the next Deck compleat, then the other Spirkitriſing and Clamps; and ſo ſucceſſively every Deck, till you are up to the Toptimber Head, and then proceed to finiſh in Courſe, but firſt to calk her. Then to the finiſhing all without Board, as Head, Stern, Galleries, Channels and all Rails, with every individual Planſheer and Gunels: Then the finiſhing all in the Hold; and ſo ſucceſſively between every Deck upwards. Then Joyners Work, Blockmakers Work, Carvers Work, and Painters Work, ſince it may be obſerv'd, That the Plummer doth little more than make his own Work, and the Shipwrights and Joyners put it into its Place. Alſo the Glaſs is put in by the Joyner. The Tin Plates may alſo be nail'd on by the Ship wrights: Then the Maſts if found by the Builder, and if there be any particular Ship that is approved on, to be taken for a Sample or Precedent, ſhe may be particularly mention'd; provided you are ſure that ſuch a Ship may continue by you, when you want ſuch a Sample; or that every particular Piece or Work can be eaſily laid to the View, at all Times, otherwiſe it will be abundance better to mention every particular Jobb. Of which I ſhall give ſome Reaſons, as follows.

Some

Some Confiderations *or* Cafes, *which may happen in* Ship-Building, *and* Refiting *and* Hiring Ships.

Some Part in a Contract put in and some left out

IN Cafe a Perfon Contracts for building a new Ship, of fome certain Dimenfions; and after the Indentures are drawn, fign'd and feal'd, it be found, That amongft abundance of Dimenfions, Scantlings, and other Particulars fpecify'd in the faid Indenture, there fhould happen to be feveral Materials highly neceffary, to be put into the faid Ship, left out, and not mention'd in the faid Indenture; only that fhe fhall in every refpect be built and perform'd, as fome certain Ship, or any Ship that ufes the fame Voyage, that our Ship is defign'd for, and alfo equal in Magnitude

Whether the Builder can be oblig'd to do the faid Work, that is not mention'd in the Contract; but may bring the Owner a Bill for doing the fame, amongft other Contingencies, and oblige him to pay fo much more than the Money allow'd by Contract

It feems to me reafonable, That the Builder cannot be oblig'd to do any more than what is mention'd; and if he makes every Particular Part, which is mention'd in his Contract, equal and agreeable to the Ship that is approved on, to be taken for a Sample, it is as much as can be defir'd of him, for who can affirm, Whether fuch Work which is requir'd to be done by Precedent, was done in the other Ship, at the Charge of the Builder or Owner? From which I am of Opinion, it would bear a Difpute, and would be as well to mention nothing of Parculars in Contracts, as not to do it full and compleat.

Overfeer Dilatory

In Cafe an Overfeer be plac'd and appointed to furvey, and infpect into the Building and Goodnefs of both Stuff and Workmanfhip, that any Ship is to be perform'd with; and it happen that the faid Overfeer be Dilatory, and that the faid Ship, after launch'd, and receiv'd into the Care and Charge of the Owner, proves Defective in divers Places, either in Workmanfhip or Materials, or both.

Whether it be reafonable for the Builder, to make good this Work at his Charge, or to be done at the Owner's Charge?

It feems unreafonable to me, That the Builder fhould be at any Charge, fince the Owner wholly confided in his Overfeer, to look into the Performance of the Building; and, That the Builder doth his Part in finding Men and Materials, anfwerable to the well liking of the Overfeer, fo plac'd to infpect.

Overfeer removed

In Cafe an Overfeer fo appointed, fhould have fomething happen to remove him from the Place, fo that he could not ftay or continue the Building of the Ship.

Whether it be reafonable for the Owners to place another. Or, That the Builder is obliged to ftand to fuch an Infpection

Since there is a vaft Difference in Men, both for Temper, Judgment and Infpection, the Builder cannot be oblig'd to be accountable for fuch a Survey, unlefs it was mention'd before in the Contract

Failing of a Builder

In Cafe any Cafualty fhould happen to a Builder, either by Death, or otherwife, he fhould be render'd uncapable to perform his Contract, and, That either after receiving the firft Payment, or any intermediate Payment, he fhould happen to fail, and not be able to compleat, to the Extent of the Money he has receiv'd

Whether the Owner can feize upon his Ship fo contracted for, and as much of the Effects of the faid Builders, as will make up to the full Value of the Money he has paid to him?

It feems reafonable, That the Owner may take into Poffeffion what he had actually made his own, according to the Tenor of his Contract, before the failure,

Fig

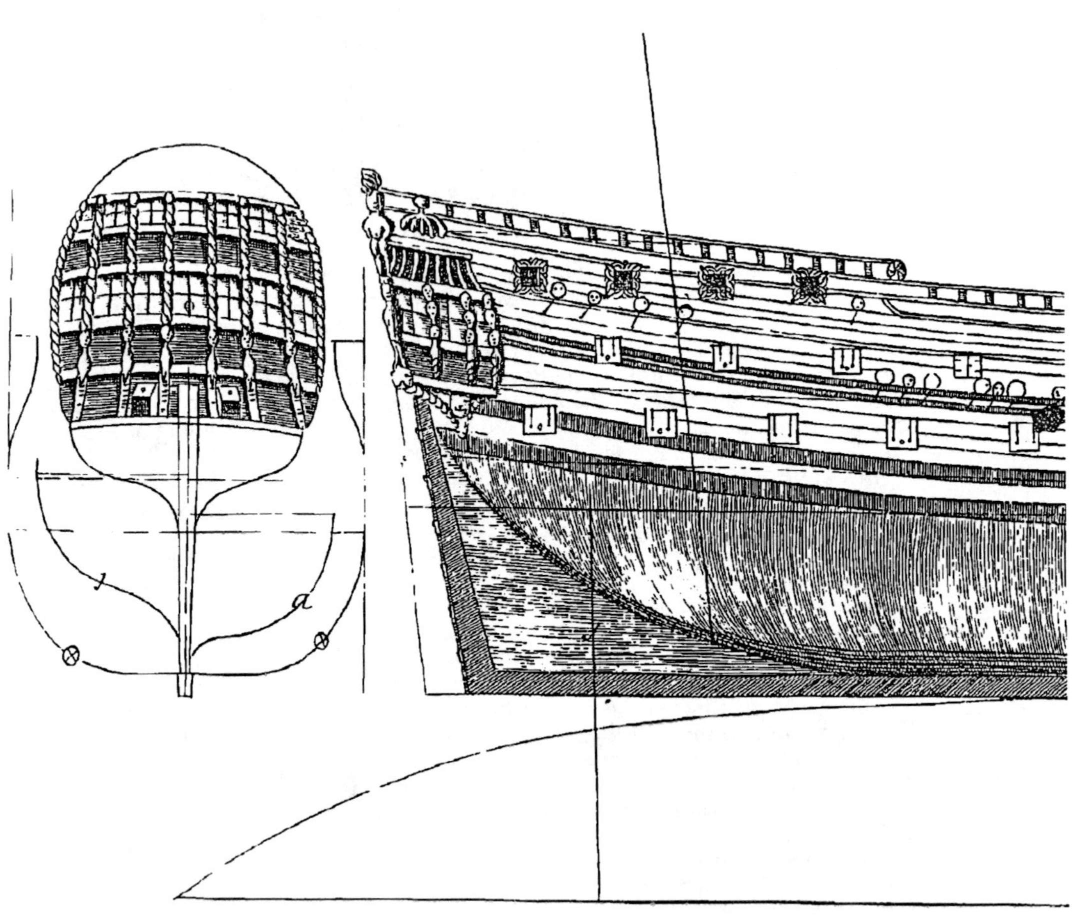

B

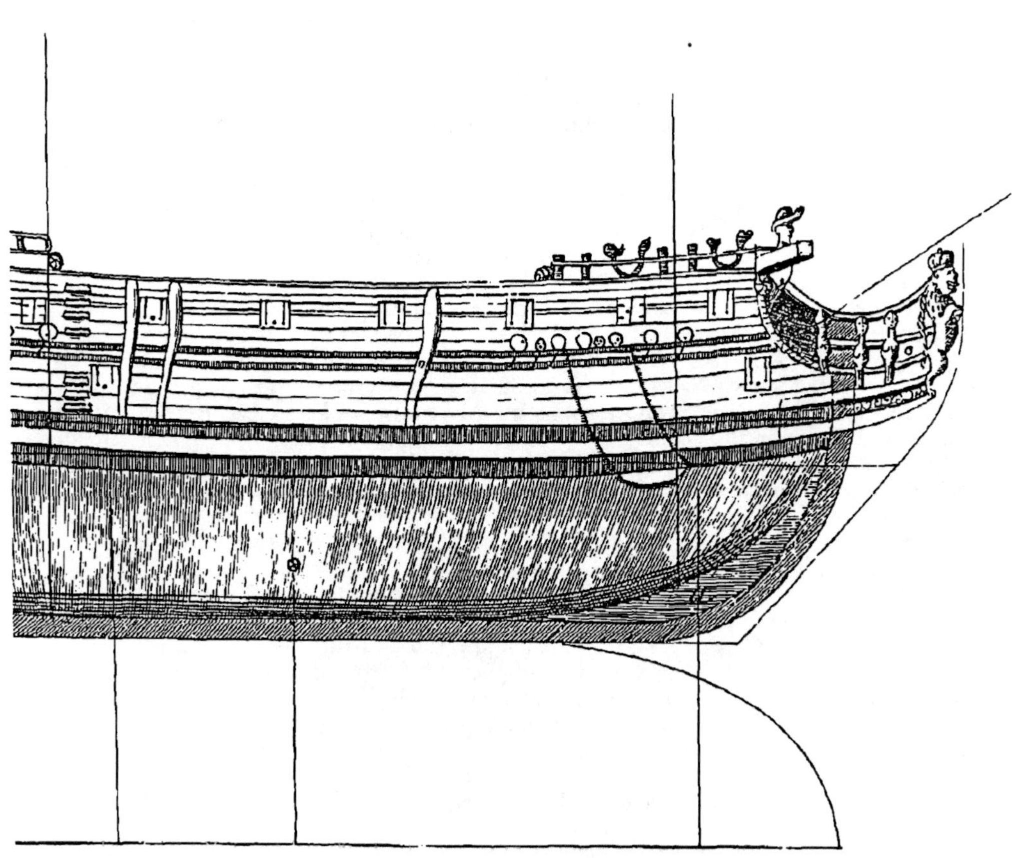

Sutton Nicholls sculp

lure of the said Builder; and must come upon the Executors of the Builders, to make good the other Part.

But supposing there may not be Assets left; and, That the Place which the Ship is erected on be sold, and put into the Custody of a Stranger; Shall such a Stranger be oblig'd to give Liberty for the Owner to build his Ship there, without farther Consideration? No, That cannot be reasonable; but the said Stranger may make what Bargain he pleases with the Owner, which if the Owner dislikes, he must take his Ship from thence, let her be in what Condition she will.

Sh[illegible]

In Case the Ship comes to any Casualty in Building by Fire, so that she be totally consum'd; Can the Owner come upon the Builder to make her good, and put another Ship in the room of her?

I cannot perceive the Indenture obliges him to it, provided it be not found the Builder did it, or order'd it to be done.

And provided such an Accident happen, just at the Time of some Payment; Cannot the Builder recover such a Payment, altho' the Ship is wholly consumed?

It seems reasonable, That the Builder shall receive to the Value of what Work is done, altho' it doth not amount to another Payment. For the Builder cannot be accountable for such Casualty, unless a Consideration be made for Insurance.

The Owner desires some of his Acquaintance to [illegible] on his Ship.

In Case the Owner should desire to have three or four of his Acquaintance, as Shipwrights, imploy'd in the Building of his Ship; and that by their Insufficiency, some valuable Materials that's to be plac'd in the said Ship, be made unfiting for Service, by the Judgment of the Overseer; Shall the Owner be at the Loss, or the Builder?

Since the Builder had his Liberty, whether to imploy them Men, or any other, it seems reasonable for him to bear the Loss, and not the Owner; but if he was oblig'd by Contract to imploy such Persons, without there was a Clause in the Contract, for the Owner to bear the Loss, the Builder must come upon the Men, for spoiling his Timber, or other Materials, if he expects Recompence; and not upon the Owner.

Men deficient, not liable to bear the Loss.

Neither doth it seem very agreeable for the Builders, or Head Manager, in such a Matter, to recover, or so much as stop any of a Workman's Wages, for Insufficiency, in wasting or spoiling of his Timber, or other Materials, since when any Person applies himself to a Master for Imployment, it lyes in such a Master's Breast, whether he will or not; and if he be a Stranger, and never experienc'd to the Place, such a Master ought either to inspect, and watch the Ability of his Journey-man, or set some other able careful Person so to do; otherwise ought to sit down and content himself in bearing the Loss, which may happen by such a Persons want of Judgment or Craft. But if it can be any ways made out, that such a Journey-man had spoil'd any Material through Willfulness, he ought in all Reason to make it good, and pay the full Value of the Goods so wasted, or otherwise, if a Master puts in such a Clause in the Entry, of such a Journey-man, to pay for all the Stuff he wasts or spoils, either by Ignorance or Willfulness, then the Journey-man cannot be angry to comply with what he has promis'd.

Overseer ill-temper'd.

In Case an Overseer, out of ill Temper, should be so rigid as to refuse several Materials that are provided, and ready to be wrought in the said Ship, and it should plainly appear that the said Goods should prove sound and serviceable, and every way fitting for the Use it was design'd for, must the Builder be oblig'd to stand to such an unwarrantable Disappointment and Loss?

If the Owner is govern'd by the Overseer, I cannot perceive how he complies with his Contract if he denies it, since he has bound himself to accept of reforming all Defects at the Request and Notice being given him by the said Overseer. Notwithstanding I am of Opinion, that upon an able and sufficient Survey, taken by any certain number of Master Workmen, of the said Materials, and it be allowed by them that the said Goods doth in every respect answer the Contract, both in Quantity and Quality, that the said Builder may recover the full Damage, he has sustain'd by the said Overseer's casting his Materials, of the Overseer, and not of the Owner.

Owner uncapable. In Case any Owner, after he has sign'd his Contract, and the Ship begun, he should be by some Means or other render'd uncapable to comply with his Payments, but after the first and second Payment, should neglect, and not pay any farther; the Builder not knowing the Fault, or mistrusting his Money, should proceed and finish the said Ship; Shall the Builder detain the said Ship, because she is partly paid for, and partly not paid for?

It seems more feasible for the Builder, in such a Case, to forbear proceeding any farther, at the first Failure.

Ship stand[illegible] But then supposing, That there be no Remedy, but the Ship should stand for want of Payment, a considerable Time; Shall not the Builder have some Recompence for the Incumbrance?

It seems very reasonable he should, altho' it be not mention'd in the Indenture, since the Contract is not comply'd with, the Builder ought either to have so much a Month according as it may be valued by Judgment, or otherwise, according to the Loss he can make appear he sustains, by the Hindrance he receives, in making room to build other Ships

Owner alters after the Contract drawn. In Case that after a Contract be made, sign'd, seal'd and deliver'd, and the Ship begun, the Owner out of some Perswasion or other, desires the Builder to alter his Ship, either in the Materials or Dimension, as to make her broader, longer, deeper, higher; or to work in some Places his Timber, or Plank, or any other Material of larger scantling, than what is mention'd by Contract, and the Builder is very willing to comply, Shall the Builder be oblig'd to do this Extra-work, which is found to be of greater Value, without farther Consideration, than what is specify'd in his Contract?

Or upon the other hand, Will it cause the Contract to be void, and give the Builder Liberty to bring in a Bill of Charges, from the Beginning of the Ship to the finishing of her?

It seems unreasonable for the Builder, to be oblig'd to do any thing more than what was mention'd by Contract, without swelling the Sum of Money so mention'd, as well as to make the Timber any bigger, and so of Consequence, so much the more chargeable to purchase But that the Builder may bring in an Extra-bill, for what ever he can prove to be order'd by the Owner, that has swell'd his Charge, either as to Workman's Wages, or Materials; and in Justice ought to be paid

But upon the other hand, I cannot perceive it any ways reasonable, for any Builder to heave up a Contract, for what he doth voluntary: Or, That his engaging to perform (or alter) one Obligation, will dissolve his Obligation he stands in, to make good another

[illegible] to the Builder's Advantage. In Case the Owner is perswaded, and desire the Builder to alter his Contract, in some particular that will be found advantageous to the Builder, Shall the Builder be oblig'd to make a draw back, and allow the Owner what fairly appears he saved by such an Alteration?

Except the Owner at the same Time brought the Builder under such an Obligation, to allow him such a Sum, as appear'd he should gain by such an Alteration; since it seems, That the Owner accepts one in lieu of the other: As if a Man should accept of five Pounds for five Guineas. And so much for the Building of New Ships And I shall now proceed to consider what may happen in repairing Old Ships.

Ships Rebuilt. In Case any Owner should have a Ship that has been worn, and for either the Years she has been used, she becomes dangerous to traffick at Sea, or otherwise, having some bad Faculty, the Owner resolves to lay her by, and not make any farther Use of her, and happens to light of a Builder, that will build him a New Ship, in Barter for his Old, and some other Considerations, equivalent to the Price of such a New Ship.

A Contract being made, it is agreed, That the Owner shall have a New Ship

Old Ship to Pieces, it be found, That ſhe has a great deal of good ſound Timber in her, that will ſerve in the New Ship, upon which the Builder orders it to be wrought in the ſaid Ship, but the Owner refuſes to have it put in, upon the Word New Ship; and this Timber being old, he objects, as not having his Bargain.

Now, Whether the Word New Ship, is deriv'd from the Workmanſhip, or Material, or both is firſt to be conſider'd? And after, Whether it is reaſonable, That the Builder ſhould be hinder'd, in putting ſuch Timber, that is in every reſpect as good as any other Part that he doth put in?

The Word New being general, is in ſome meaſure meant for that which has not been, and in that Senſe, the Timber that was before uſed, ought to be hove out, and not uſed again: In another Place it means Freſhneſs, or of late Time.

It is reported, That Oak Timber comes not to a full growth under 100 Years, and ſtands 100 Years at that ſtay, and is alſo 100 Years decaying, which together is 300 Years

Timber being a matter inanimate, contrary from the Nature of Animals, Timber being tendereſt, and more pliable when decaying than in its Youth; ſo that it may be as well meant, to have no old decaying Timber, as to have all new Timber in any Ship. And altho' it doth not ſeem unreaſonable, for a Builder to put in ſuch Timber, as is ſound and ſerviceable, altho' it has been uſed; yet I cannot ſee, what room he has for it; without its mention'd in the Contract: Or, That the Owner will conſent to have it put in

And therefore, it would be very proper to particularize ſuch Things, to avoid Diſputes, and would be much properer for the Owner, if he has the leaſt Miſtruſt, that there is a great Part of his Ship ſound and ſerviceable, and fitting for to uſe in the Ship, he deſigns to have built; to make it in his Contract, That the Builder ſhall allow him for every Piece, that is found ſo fitting for Uſe, and put into the ſaid New Ship again, the full Value of a Piece of new Timber, that would make ſuch a Piece that is ſo uſed; and that to be abated out of the Sum of Money, that a New Ship, of the Magnitude he deſigns to have built would come to; only the Builder to be conſider'd, for pulling the old Ship to pieces, and ſaving the ſaid good Timber, and making it ſerve again.

In Caſe an Owner has a Ship to refit, and for the Purpoſe, would have her dock'd, as it's term'd. A Place like a Pit, with Gates convenient, to make it a dry Dock, and keep the Water from coming in *Ships Dock'd and ſpoil'd.*

The Owner only makes a verbal Bargain, to have the Uſe of ſuch a Place, and is to give the Builder, ſo much a Spring, or between the Full and Change of the Moon; and either to fit her himſelf, in every reſpect, or the Builder to do it, and ſuch a fitting allowed to by him at the Market Price, or according to the Cuſtom of the Place ſhe is fitted at

The Ship being dock'd, and the Gates ſhut upon her, as ſecure ſeemingly, as upon any other Ship, it happens by ſome Caſualty, or other, the Gates are blown open, as it's term'd; and by which Means, or ſome other, the Ship is much damnify'd; ſo far, that it will coſt conſiderably to make the Damage good, Ought this Damage to be at the Builder's Charge, to make it good, or at the Charge of the Owners?

I cannot perceive the Builder to be in any Fault; but will be as great a Sufferer as the Owner, in giving Occaſion for to hinder others from bringing Buſineſs to his Yard, or Place of his Livelihood

But in Caſe it doth appear, there ſhould be ſome ſmall Neglect, either in the ſhoring the Ship, or laying Blocks under, to receive her Keel; Shall the Builder be damnify'd for ſuch Neglect? Yes, as was aforeſaid, in begetting an ill Name, and hindering his Buſineſs, and not otherwiſe; ſince it cannot be expected, that ſuch a Gentleman that owns ſuch a Place of Buſineſs, that is valued at one or two Hundred a Year; or that Rents ſuch a Bargain, and perhaps deals by the Way of Trade, for ſeveral thouſand Pounds Yearly beſides, can, or will be at the doing of every little petty Piece of Work. No more than a Commander of one of the Owner's *Builder in Fault*

Ships

Ships, will look conſtantly over his Sailors, that they do their Buſineſs as they ſhould do.

But if it be fairly prov'd, That the Dock, or Gates, is not ſufficient to receive ſuch a Ship, as a Builder perſwades the Owner to let him repair, in ſuch a Caſe, it looks reaſonable, That the Builder ſhould make good the Damage the Ship receives, by ſuch his pretending to provide, what he abſolutely knows is not in his Power to perform. Notwithſtanding I am of Opinion, That the Owner would recover nothing of the Builder, for making good the Damage he receives by Caſualty; except he obliges the Builder by Contract, and allows him ſome Conſideration to preſerve his Ship from Caſualties or Accidents. No more than any Tenant could recover of a Landlord, that lets him a Houſe, and after he has got his Goods, in the Rain, or one ill Property or other, damnifies all his Goods: Since they might have experienc'd, or inquir'd into the Goodneſs, or Fitneſs of ſuch Places; or choſe whether they would have made uſe of them or not. And it would be highly neceſſary for any Owners of Shipping, to have an able Shipwright, hearty to them, to aſſiſt them in ſuch Undertakings, and ſee into the Goodneſs of ſuch Places; it would pay the Charge of ſuch a Survey.

Ships Lengthned In Caſe that after a Ship be taken into a Dock, and it be deſir'd by the Owner, or Commander of the Ship, That the ſaid Ship ſhould be lengthen'd, in the middle, or at either End, and only by a verbal Order, he lets this Jobb to the Builder to do, for ſo much Money. Then if in lengthening in the Middle, and drawing one Part from another, it ſhould happen, That the Parts ſhould be put ſo much out of Order, that they could not be put to rights again; and this not ſeen, till the Ship comes afloat again. Or, That by not conſidering the Extralength of what the Ship will be after alter'd, to what ſhe was before; the Plank Wales, and Foot-waleing be not wrought proportional to that increaſe of Length; but that the Ship proves Hog-back'd, or Camber-keel'd, as it's term'd, or otherwiſe ſo much diſorder'd, that it proves very prejudicial to the Owners, ſhall the Builder be oblig'd to make Reſtitution for ſuch a Neglect, or, for ſo ſpoiling a good Ship?

If there is no Contract drawn, nor ſcantling mention'd, or Directions given, by way of ſome able Shipwright, as an Overſeer, to take a particular Care of ſuch weighty Matters; I cannot perceive, how ſuch Damage can be made good by the Builder, ſince it's very probable, That he might act to the beſt of his Genius; or, That perhaps leave it to a Foreman, and let out the Workmanſhip to ſome labouring Men, as are term'd Takers: And in another Caſe, not conſider the Extra ſtrength that will be requir'd, in adding Length to Shipping, but believes if he works the ſame Scantling as was before wrought, he doth his Duty.

Or in lengthening a Ship forward, to place a Stem of one Side, or not to make the Bows one like the other, ſo that the Ship ſhall ſteer to one Hand more than to another. Or in lengthening Abaft, to place the Poſt of one Side; ſo that the Rudder will effect the Ship more, being put over one way, than by putting it over the other.

All which bad Faculties, may be of dangerous Conſequence; and yet the Builder excuſable in ſome Meaſure from being damnify'd.

Ships ſhortned And alſo in ſhortning a Ship, there may be ſuch Errors committed, That may prove of the greateſt Detriment to the Ship; and yet, the Owner muſt, or at leaſt had as good be contented, as to expect Satisfaction of the Builder, without he had bound him to it, ſince it will, as was aforeſaid, be hard enough upon the Builder, to have the Diſgrace, and be a Means to hinder him in his Practice, by imploying ſuch Perſons that will not take Care of his Work.

Builders doing Jobbs without Lumping In Caſe the Builder has the Liberty to do ſuch Jobbs without Lumping of it, as it's term'd, or doing the whole for ſo much Money; but has that Liberty to make out a Bill of Contingencies, and charge every individual Material that is found neceſſary, as well as every Man and Boy's Labour that acts upon the Work.

And it appears, That he has uſed a great deal more Materials than what was really needful, and taken out ſeveral Pieces of Plank and Timber, that might have ſerved again, as well as that new Timber, which he puts in, Can the Owner

Owner come upon him, or recover Damage of him for so doing ?

If the Builder doth such Jobbs by Verbal Agreement, and not bound by Contract, to shift no more Stuff than what shall appear needful by a Survey of a certain number of able Shipwrights, it seems as if he was left to his Liberty, to use the best of his Skill and Judgment, and therefore since no Mortal can dive or penetrate into the Secrets of another, it may be in some measure allowed to be his Insufficiency, and not wilfully done to make a penny of the Owner.

Upon the other hand, if the Builder, being left to his Liberty, should rate his Materials higher than what the Market Price is, and the Customary Value of such Materials, in some other places lying adjacent to his, Is it reasonable that the Owner should be obliged to pay for such an Extortion ? Notwithstanding, I cannot perceive how he can get clear of it For who can desire a Man to sell cheaper than he buys ? And who knows another Man's Method of Dealing, and what Disadvantage the Builder met with in obtaining such Materials ? And since the Value of all Materials may be easily known, it will be much better to have some punctual Agreement for both Stuff and Mens Labour

In Case an Owner has a Ship which requires to have her Keel taken out, and another put in the room of it, or a False Keel, where, in either of the two, there will be required abundance of Shores to hang the Ship up from the Ground, and the Builder charges the Owner with the Value of all these Shores, or some Considerations larger than what can reasonably be expected the Value of using them can be thought to be worth, Shall the Owner be obliged to pay the Builder according to this his Valuation, or according to the Prime Cost ? *Ship [illegible] her Keel [illegible]ed*

It seems to me that the Owner is obliged to pay the Builder the full Value of the Shores in the first place, or what he will charge for the Use, which if the Builder believes to be unreasonable, he may take the remainder of the Shores into his keeping ; since it seems to be hard on the Builder to provide Materials for every Jobb that may happen to a Ship, and have his Materials return'd upon his hands.

Since it may happen so, that such a piece of Work may not happen to that Builder in some Time after, that such Materials that he is obliged to provide for doing of that Jobb, may not suit another Jobb, so that they will not be only an Incumberance, but so much Money lying dead.

In Case an Owner bargains with a Builder verbally, to do a certain piece of Work, either in New Building, or in some large Reparation, and the Builder provides Materials for doing the same, and after such a Provision is made the Owner's mind changes, and will not have the said Work done Can the Owner be obliged to stand to the Loss or Damage the Builder sustains by such a Disappointment ? *Verbal Bargain*

If the Owner had given the Builder Earnest for doing such a Jobb, it would have been part of his Pay for doing of such a piece of Work, and in all Reason ought to lose it, let it be as much as it will Notwithstanding, I cannot perceive how the Owner can be obliged to make good the whole Disappointment the Builder sustains by his being too forward. *Failure in the Owner*

For first, the Builder, if he design'd to secure himself, should have had an Indenture drawn, to have bound the Owner to fulfil his Agreement, and not only so, but there should be mention'd a certain Forfeiture, in Case it be thought advantagious for either Party to forbear engaging, and not only so, but the Builder may choose whether he will be so very forward in providing Timber, and other Materials, any farther than to the period of every Payment : Only observing by the way, that the Builder may have some Disappointment that way, since the Advantage and Disadvantage in obtaining Timber, and other Materials, will be always various, and at some times much cheaper in obtaining than at another time

Upon the other hand Set the Case there be a Contract drawn, and a Builder obliges himself to fit one, or several Ships for a certain Owner in such a time, and it be also mentioned what Emergency requires it, that he is to take in, and carry some where beyond Sea, a certain Parcel of some Commodities, and upon the Non-performance of which he forfeits such a Sum of Money, it will be very barbarous for the Builder to disappoint the Owner.

Failure in the Builder.

But since Self-interest is an inherent Faculty, it being the Builder's Trade for Bread to engross Business, and perhaps at first, by a single View, believes he is able to perform what he has undertook, but by making a more thorough Calculation, he finds himself not able. And then it would be really very ingenious in the Builder either to tell the Owner, or imploy more Hands, and also get more Places convenient for doing the same

However, he hopes the Owner's Case may not be so desperate, but the Time given may be put off, and removed to a farther Season, and so of course when the Time comes the Ships are not in a Readiness

Upon which the Owner is sued upon his being bound by a firm Agreement to forfeit a certain Sum of Money to the Merchants, if he has not so many Ships ready of such a Magnitude, and every way in a Condition to sail, if wind and weather permit, at such a certain Day: The Owner being forced to pay his Forfeiture, and considering that he has a firm Contract upon the Builder to fit the Ships against the Time, and the Emergency mentioned, and still he Failing of his Promise, hopes he may recover his Cost and Charges again from the said Builder

Whether the Builder (as making a Contract to fit the Ships at such a certain Time, and Failing) is obliged to make good the Owner's Loss, or not?

It must be allowed that the Builder lyes under a great Fault, and in strict Justice ought to pay the Owner for what he can Reasonably prove he has Lost: But I cannot perceive how the Owner will recover any more than what the Hire of such a Ship, or Ships, will amount to, in the Time that he is short of Fitting of them, above the Time that he was bound to do it, except he had bound himself in a certain Forfeiture, as the Owner did. And therefore in such Cases it would be very proper for the Owners to consider first, what their Ships Repairs will be, and then make a nice Calculation, being assisted by some able Shipwright that's hearty to them, that so they may be sure, and preserved from Damage

Workmen shifting Work spoil more.

In Case a Workman in shifting some particular pieces of Work, and in taking out and putting in one piece spoils another, whether the Owner, or Builder, shall stand to the Loss?

This is a Case that often happens; and not always by Carelesness, but sometimes by the Defects which are secretly incident to Shipping, and not only from that, but sometimes for want of Conveniency to get the new parts into their places.

As in Case there be a Plank, or several Planks, to shift without board, and it happens that the Edges of such Planks you are to shift weakens outwards, that is, the Plank is bigger within side than without side, which is a Property that cannot well be seen (before experienc'd by the Workman) and in Ripping or Setting out such Plank (as it's term'd) with Wedges, the Planks joining to it are squawl'd, or tore, and of Consequence spoil'd, and obliged to be made new.

Since the Method prescribed in setting out such Work, both for Quickness, and saving the Old Stuff, is the most suitable to the Use, I cannot perceive how the present Builder, or Workman, can be so much as blamed, since the Fault lyes upon the building of the Ship in the first place, or perhaps in shifting of some particular Work afterward.

In another Case Let it be that here is a Plank to be shut in, and the new Piece not being directly shaped to its work, but must be pent, or bended to the Hole, either flat ways or edge ways, and in making provision to do the same, by straining the Plank next to the Hole, that is spoil'd.

In one respect it must be own'd a Fault, because there might been got a piece that would exactly shut the Hole up, without wrenching or straining

ſtraining the Work adjacent, but then perhaps the Value of ſuch a Piece would been double ſo much as the Piece which was made uſe of

As firſt, in a Bow or Buttock Plank, if the Piece grows naturally to the Work, it muſt be cut out of principal Compaſs Timber, which in all likelyhood might been double the Value of the Plank that would do ſuch a Service, and might have given the Owner occaſion to find fault with the Builder's Bill of Charges, and ſcrupled the Payment. *Bow or Buttock*

Or otherwiſe, that there might not be a Piece in the Yard that's more proper for the Work, than that he has took; neither can he obtain ſuch a Piece that would exactly do, without delaying the Reparation of the Ship, and continuing her in his Dock a conſiderable time longer than what is really requiſite, and what may be charged on the Builder for as great a Fault as any other. Which Caſes ought to be throughly conſidered, and conſulted continually, between the Builder and Owner, or any Perſon that he appoints to over-ſee the Work.

In Caſe there be ſeveral pair of Standers on a Deck, and it be found requiſite, for the good of the Ship, to have them over-ſet, as it's term'd, which is to take them from their places, the Standers being obſerv'd to be ſound and ſerviceable, and in every reſpect as good as new, and ſo allowed to ſerve again, in order thereunto they are requir'd to be taken off whole; but notwithſtanding in unbolting and taking off, ſome of them are broke Shall the Builder be obliged to make good the Damage? No, it ſeems unreaſonable he ſhould, for ſuch Accidents may happen, and not by Careleſneſs neither *Standers.*

For ſuch parts may be made very difficult to be removed, and yet not one whit the better for the Ship, nor any thing the ſtronger faſten'd, beſides there may be Defects in ſuch parts, and not viſibly appear. And ſet the Caſe it be by the Inſufficiency of the Workman, or otherwiſe, the Careleſneſs of him: Why then it ſeems unreaſonable that the Builder ſhould ſtand to the Damage; and if the Workman is put off from the Work, it's all the Owner can well deſire But if he is continued, it ſeems very Reaſonable that the ſaid Workman ſhould ſtand to the Loſs of every Material he ſpoils for the future, provided ſuch a Bargain be made And therefore in ſuch Caſes an Overſeer, that's hearty to the Owner, would be there requiſite

In Caſe there ſhould be a Stem, or a Stern-poſt, to be ſhifted, and it be found that in ſhifting the ſame there ſhould be a great deal more Plank ſhifted, to put this Poſt or Stem in, than what can Reaſonably be allowed requiſite: Ought the Owner to ſtand to ſuch a waſte? *Stem, or Post*

Theſe are intricate Caſes; for Stern-poſts and Stems are very troubleſome to ſhift, and requires very good Judgment to perform ſuch pieces of work, and therefore it would be very proper for both Builder and Owner, if they deſign to make themſelves ſafe and eaſy, to have a Survey, and allot what ſhall be taken out, or done, in ſuch intricate and dubious Jobbs.

Not but that it muſt be allowed contrary to all Reaſon, for any Builder, after he has got an Owner's Ship into his Dock, immediately to cut and ſlaſh her to pieces, on purpoſe becauſe he will make an Advantage in doing of the Work again, neither will any Man of Senſe preſume to touch a Ship in ſuch Caſes without poſitive Orders.

But if an Owner ſhall leave the Fitting of his Ship to a Builder, with ſaying, Mr *Builder*, Take my Ship into your Dock, and do ſuch and ſuch Work, according to what Voyage he deſigns to ſend her on, or otherwiſe according to the Condition of the Ship; or to ſay, Shift ſuch a Deck, or my Stern-poſt, or my Stem, or any other material Jobb Why then the Builder muſt needs be wrong, and ſtand directly againſt his own Intereſt, if he ſhould ſay to the Owner, How muſt it be done? Or how ſhall I do it? For if the Owner can tell as well as the *Builder*, he will have no occaſion to be at the Charge of Hiring a *Builder*, and paying him a large Salary for taking Charge and Care of Fitting his Ship. *Owner leaving the Fitting of his Ship to a Builder*

And

And therefore if the Owners expect to be made safe and easy, they should be very well inform'd before they suffer their Craft to be deliver'd into the Care and Charge of a Stranger: For if the Builder is either Careless, or Insufficient, he may be blam'd, but not harm'd, if he doth this Owner's Work as well as he has done others.

Owner uncapacitated upon a Ship's being ready to go out of the Dock.

In Case that after a Ship is fitted, and just upon being put out of the Dock, the Owner is render'd Uncapacitated, or Bankrupt, the Builder knowing it, refuses to let the Ship out of the Dock, but detains her, although she is fit and ready to proceed on her Voyage: Can the Builder stand by such a Proceeding? I cannot perceive him safe in it, and may be lyable to stand to the Loss the Owner sustains by such a Stopage.

For the Ship being the Owner's, the Builder has nothing to do any farther but to fit her, and make her in a Capacity to proceed on some intended Voyage; which cannot be performed till he has let her out of his Dock again, neither can his Payment be due till she is let out again, since Docking and Undocking may properly be reckon'd as part of the Refitting. So that if the Builder had every piece of Stuff by him, that he had shifted, and would be at the Charge of taking out his New Timber again, and put the Old in the room of it, as well as it was before he took the Ship in hand, I cannot see but that very shifting his own Work would bear a great Controversie, for it might easily be proved to be of an ill Consequence, to have Work fastened, and unfastened, so often.

Owner to force the Ship out.

But provided the Owner, or some other concern'd at that juncture, was resolved to force the Ship out of the Builder's hands; in order thereto they force open the Dock Gates, and take the Ship out. This, I am of Opinion, would be very well for the Builder, provided those that took the Ship from him were able to pay him his Charge of Fitting the Ship, and make good the Damage he might sustain by such a Force.

Careening.

In Case an Owner would have his Ship Careen'd, and afterwards to have his Mast taken out, and put in again.

In order thereto he agrees with a Builder, or Yard-keeper, to supply him with all necessary Implements, both for the Careening Gare, (as it's term'd) that is, what Materials will be wanting to secure the Masts; and also all manner of Utensils that may be wanting to do some certain Jobbs that he expects will be wanting to be done to his Ship. As let it be a false Keel to be put on, and the Ship to be bream'd, and paid, or cover'd over with a Coat of Stuff, of some sort of Ingredients.

And because Careening is such a work as requires very good Management, since every Ship will not suffer to be hove bottom out, or at least lye any considerable time when her bottom is hove out without hazarding the Foundering of the Ship, the Owner desires every Thing that the Builder can imagine to be requisite for doing the Work as he mentions to him, and expects will be requir'd to be done to his Ship, to be in as great a Readiness as he can possibly make them: Upon which the Builder provides every Material he can think of, and brings them upon the Floating Stages, that he has for that purpose, by the Ship, and what the Workmen are to stand upon to use the said Materials; but not expecting any Casualty, never shews the Owner what he has provided, and in what Readiness he has put every Thing in.

[illegible] Materials, and they are lost by Casualty.

First when the Ship's Keel is hove out of the Water, it's found that the False Keel is in a very good Condition, and not at all requisite to be shifted, so the Owner desires the Builder to forbear making any farther progress in shifting the said False Keel: And after, by some Mismanagement or other, the Ship breaks her Tackling, and rises, by which sudden Surprize, all the Materials which the Builder provided is lost, some sunk, and others drove away on the Stream: Who shall bear the Damage?

It's very Reasonable that the Owner should be at the Damage: For the False Keel is a very plain Case; it was provided by his Order, and brought in every respect as near to the Work as it possibly could; which if it had been tryed, and not fitted, then the Builder ought to have got another, and made a Keel suitable, and not made a shew of such a Material only, but since it was provided, and brought to use, the Owner ought to be at the full Value for the Plank, as if it had been used.

For the other Materials, that is not quite so visible; for if the Builder was resolved to secure himself, he should have desir'd the Owner, either to go himself, or have sent some other, as he would trust, to see every Utensil, and take an Account of the Quality and Quantity of each Material; and also, That they was actually carry'd on the floating Stage fitted for the Purpose.

But since this was a Casualty, Should not those that were concern'd, been at the Damage? *[illegible] in the Sailers*

The Use, in such Cases, is for the Sailers and Riggers, to fit all the Rigging and Tackles, which if the Fault lay there, it might be done, and yet as much Care as possibly could be apply'd by the Manager; for in new Hemp, it has been often observ'd, That great Defects it has caus'd in the Cordage, and yet not visible, and in a Pin of a Block, or the uncertain moving of a Capstand, or perhaps by the Carelesness of the Men, that holds on the Hawsers at the Capstand, or ten thousand little Cases that may happen, and yet not materially a Fault in the Manager.

But as it sometime happens, That the Ship when her Bottom is near out of the Water, she oversets, making almost an intire Revolution, without she has something to prevent it, as what is term'd a relieving Tackle; Shall the Manager suffer for this Fault, if the Owner desires to have such a Preventer? The Manager is in a great Fault, notwithstanding the Owner might have hinder'd the Manager to have careen'd his Ship, before such a Preventer was got ready, neither will a Manager make any Assurance from Casualties, without a Consideration.

But in Case all Things are done Right, and to Satisfaction, and the Builder in making out a Bill, charges the Owner with the Prime Cost of divers Materials: As the Shores for shoring the Mast, also the Out-lickers, and Shoals for them: All Shores under them, and some other trivial Materials Shall the Owner be oblig'd to pay for them, according to the Bill of his Charge? *[illegible] in a Bill.*

This Case seems to be like the Case concerning shifting a Keel: For it may be, That the Builder may not do such an uncommon Jobb as Careening, which none would have done, except in Case of Necessity, when a Dock cannot be obtain'd, it being much dearer, and of greater Disservice to the Ship, than a Dock.

And therefore, I cannot perceive it very unreasonable, for the Owner to pay the Builder the full Value of the said Materials; but then they are the Owner's, and he may make what Advantage he can of them And in all such Cases, it will be very proper for the Owner to come to punctual Agreements, before he proceeds.

In Case an Owner speaks, and agrees with a Builder, or a Mast-maker, for a Suit of Masts, and in the Bargain they make, the Mast-maker is to make them in every respect, according to custom, having the Dimensions given him in every Particular. He is also to do his Part; and after they are ready to launch them safe out of his Mast-yard, and bring them on board of the Ship; and having the Assistance of the Boatswain, and Ship's Crew, or a Number of Men, sufficiently strong to get them into the Ship, the Mast-maker is to set them, and see them fit in their Places *Mast maker.*

And the Boatswain in slinging of them, or making them fast in Tackles, in order to heave them in; and in hoisting of them, something fails, the Mast falls down, and is broke to pieces; *Boatswain [illegible]*

Ought the Mast-maker to bear the Damage or the Owner? For the Mast-maker seems to oblige himself to get the Masts in, and make them fit in their Places

It's true, the Mast-maker seems to oblige himself to get the Masts into their Places, and if he had also bound himself to hire Men, and to do the Sailers Labour, it would seem very feasible he should stand to the Damage

But in the first Place, he mentions to do his Part, which according to a general Observation, is no other than to make the Mast fitting, and to see that the Steps, and Partners, for each respective Mast, be proper, and fit to receive them; for the Tackles and Lashings, are quite beside the Mast-maker's Sphere, and cannot be any ways consider'd as the Mast maker's Business.

Besides, The Owner in promising to let the Mast maker have the Assistance of his Boatswain and Ship's Crew, looks in all Probability, as if he discharg'd the Mast-maker of the least Care of Casualty, which might happen to the Mast, in heaving or hoisting into the Ship, only to make them fitting for their Places when they are got in, and perhaps to drive a Wedge or Cleat to make fast the Lashings.

Boat-builder In Case an Owner bargains with a Boat-builder, to build him one Long-boat, of such a certain length and breadth, and depth, and a Pinnace of such a certain length, breadth and depth, and a Yawl or Cock-boat, mentioning the said three Dimensions also, and withal, intimating the Goodness of the Materials, but nothing as to shape, and when the Boats are built, and launch'd, it be found, they are not fit for the Use that the Owner design'd them for.

Shall the Builder be oblig'd to take the Boats again, and the Owner be clear'd of his Contract?

If the Boat-builder fulfils his Agreement, and builds the Boats agreeable, in the Particulars that's gave him; altho' they be directly contrary in other Properties, which the Owner design'd, I cannot perceive, but that he will be oblig'd to pay for them accordingly, either to the customary Price, or according to the Price they agreed for.

And therefore, it would be much properer for the Owner, in such Cases, to particularize the Shape, as well as length and breadth, and not only to say, I will have such a Boat, built very full, or in a Medium, or very sharp, but to have an exact Figure made of the Boat, which will be able to guide him: Or otherwise, That a Boat of such a length, breadth and depth, shall carry so many Tuns, and have so many Inches Free-board, as it's term'd, which Method, although it would require a little more Charge, it would positively guide both Owner and Builder, one, in knowing what he has for his Money, and the other, in knowing what he sells; and also be an exact Guide for him to do the same again.

Rope-maker In Case an Owner agrees with a Rope maker, to find him as much Cordage as would rigg his Ship, both standing and running Rigging, also Cablets, and Cables, intimating how many Cables; and the Rope-maker knowing the size of the Ship, obliges himself to find every Part of such Materials, agreeable to the size of such a Ship, of the like Magnitude; and in rigging of the Ship, the Owner either out of Fancy, or Information, finds that the Rigging, in several Particulars, answers not the size of some Ship of the same Magnitude, that he takes for a Precedent; upon which, he complains to the Rope-maker, and withall, desires to have such Parts of his Rigging shifted

Upon which, the Rope-maker examines, and finds it to be as the Owner has reported it; but believing himself not directly obligated, to stand to the Sample of one particular Ship, looks farther, and finds several other Ships, that's rather bigger, has less Rigging than any that he has put into the Ship he is actually Rigging.

Shall the Rope-maker be oblig'd to shift the said Rigging, as the Owner desires to have done, upon such a single Sample?

If there had ever been a Standard for Rigging a Ship; that a Ship from either length, breadth or burden, should have her Rigging in every particular, sized from such Dimensions; and that such a Ship as the Owner pitch'd upon, be found to be rigg'd by such a Standard, then it seems very reasonable the Rope-maker should be guided by that.

Rigger But since rigging, as well as several other Matters, is perform'd so very various, that it is chiefly done by the Fancy of the Manager, where it doth plainly appear, That some Ships, that's 100 Tuns less than another, shall have their Rigging bigger,

bigger, and more of it, than shall be found on board of the large Ship, it cannot be expected that the Rope-maker can be oblig'd to find Rope, according to such promiscuous Management.

But set the Case, That this Ship is rigg'd, in every respect, to the good liking of the Owner; but in the Progress of the Voyage, it be found, That either through the Badness of the Hemp, or the Neglect or Insufficiency of the Rope-maker, or perhaps in selling of the Owner twice wrought Yarn, in lieu of new, the Shrowds brake, or the Cables part, and perhaps the Mast carry'd by the Board, or the Ship drove a Shore and lost; Shall the Rope-maker be liable to make good the Damage?

It is undeniably a great Fault in the Rope-maker, and scarce pardonable; but I cannot perceive, How he can be oblig'd to make good the Damage; since the Owner had his Liberty, to have plac'd an Overseer, to look into the good Performance of the Material, for the Rope-maker will not be wanting to make a Penny by his Commodity, and perhaps in buying Hemp, he may have damnify'd Goods amongst that which is not so.

In Case a Block-maker obliges himself to find Blocks, sound, serviceable, and agreeable for the Use of rigging such a Ship, as is to be rigg'd; and not corresponding with the Rigger, but sends Blocks as usual, according to the size of the Ship; and in rigging it be found, That some material Blocks are too small, and some too large, but the Rigger, willing to do his Work as quick as he can, cuts some to make them larger, and others he makes use of, and straps them, which are really too big, the Owner, or Commander, upon over-haling his Rigging, finds it so, goes to the Block-maker, and tells him that he must change his Blocks. *Block maker.*

However, I cannot perceive, the Block-maker oblig'd to comply; for they should have sent them before they had defac'd them. For altho' the Master, Commander or Owner, did not actually take and receive such Goods into his Custody, notwithstanding his bespeaking them; and the Workmen that he employ'd to use the Blocks, took them, and used them for the very Use they were design'd for. *Block maker.*

May not the Workman be oblig'd (that's to say, the Rigger that defac'd the Blocks) to pay the Damage? No, For it's like he knew no better, but that they were design'd to serve for the Use that he put them to.

In Case a Rigger agrees with an Owner, or Commander, to rigg his Ship, for so much Money, the Owner to find every Material proper for the Work, only the Rigger to do the labouring Part, and it appear after the Ship is rigged, That the Rigger has made use of a great deal more Rope than has been usual in such Cases, for rigging such another Ship, that her Masts and Yards is in every respect equal to ours, Can the Owner oblige the Rigger to make Restitution for such a Waste? *Rigger.*

If it be Insufficiency in the Rigger, it will appear by the Ends that will be sav'd, and swep together by the Ship-boy, and then it cannot be reasonable for the Rigger to pay for his Ignorance; since the Owner might have chose whether he would have employ'd him or not. But if it can be prov'd, That the Rigger has cut the Rigging to waste, in order to make a Penny of it, it's but little better than Robbery.

But in Case the Rigger places the Rope wrong, some in the Places that others should be put, and others in their Places, and the Owner observing it, will have them shifted; Is the Rigger oblig'd to do it, without farther Consideration?

It cannot be, according to the Tenor of his Agreement, if he fail in doing of his Work, according to an experimental Rule. And I am of Opinion, An Owner may forbear paying of him, til he compleats his Work, according to what he undertook.

But in Case the Rigger has spoil'd some of the Ropes, by cutting of them to short, Shall he be oblig'd to make them good? It seems reasonable he should, but in the first Place, If he is Poor, and not able, there can be no more expected of the Cat than her Skin; besides, it would be very proper for all Owners, either to obtain a Man which they are sure is honest, and able to perform such Services,

Services, which they intrust him with, or to be contented to stand to the Loss they sustain, by the Ignorance of such a poor Man, rather than to ruin his poor Family

Sail-maker In Case a Sail-maker agrees with an Owner, to make a Suit of Sails, for a Ship of that Magnitude which his Ship is of, but either by Mistake, one way or ther, when the Sails are bended to the Yards, they are found either too square, or not square enough to spread the Yard; also the same Error deep-ways, or that they are not well shap'd; Shall the Sail-maker be at the Charge in altering them? If the Sail-maker made it in his Contract to alter the Sails, till the Owner lik'd them, I cannot see how he can be free from the Breach of such an Agreement, if he refuses to do it, but otherwise I am of Opinion, he may refuse, since the Owner ought, if he expects to have his Sails nicely fit, to make exact Patterns, and give the length of his Yards, from Cleat to Cleat; also the length of the Masts, as they stand rigg'd to the Sail-maker; and oblige him in every Particular, both as to the lengths, bigness and shape; and also to the Goodness of performing his Work, as well how many Stitches he shall make in every Yard, in either round or flat Seams, and also in the Bolt-ropes; and in such Cases, nothing can make a better Sample than a Draught drawn by a Scale, for taking the lengths, and bigness, and also to see the Shape.

Anchor-smith In Case an Owner agrees with an Anchor-smith, to make him so many Anchors, according to what he designs his Ship shall carry, which being one of the most material Cases, ought to be very carefully look'd into, since upon the Goodness of such a Utensil, the safety of both Ship and Goods, nay, and Mens Lives also doth depend.

The Owner gives the Weight of every Anchor to the Smith, and desires they may be made by such a Dimension; that according to Custom, every one shall weigh so many Hundreds, and Pounds, according to the Weight he has gave to him

The Smith complies with the Owner's Demand, to some few Pounds, which is seldom scrupl'd in such a Piece of Work; the Shape is also lik'd, and the Anchor taken from the Smith, and carry'd on board the Ship, and put into its Place; but the first Time its us'd, in heaving, a tolerable Strain, the Anchor breaks.

Shall the Anchor-smith bear the Damage? Or in Case he is not paid, Shall the Owner be able to stop the Payment? No, For the Anchor is properly the Owner's, at the taking of it out of the Smith's Shop, neither shall the Owner try the Anchor, without he makes it in his Agreement, what strain shall be applyed to prove the Goodness of the Anchor, tho' it would be highly necessary, for such a Custom to be made use of· It would not only be a Means to make the Smith very careful in working the Iron, but also prevent the Casualty that has often happen'd to Shipping, by the bad Management that has been in making of such Materials.

And such an Undertaking may be very easily comply'd with, and not very chargeable; provided it was made general, and every one help'd to pay for the Engine.

Merchant-Ships. In Case there be a Merchant, or several Merchants, that has some certain Commodities to carry beyond Seas, and that they make an Agreement with an Owner, or several Owners of Shipping, to take their Goods on board, at such a certain Time, and carry them to such and such Places, according to their Traffick, and perhaps they may mention what number of Guns they expect to be carry'd by each Ship, and the Number of Men, also the Magnitude of each Ship.

But at the Time appointed, when the Goods are to be receiv'd on board, the said Ships are not found any ways capable of carrying the Goods, which being debated, the Merchant believes himself much wrong'd, by being disappointed of having his Goods carry'd, according to the Time and Season, of the usual want of such Commodities at the Places they are to go to, and therefore expects Satisfaction.

The

The Owner on the other ſide, believes himſelf to receive the greateſt Injury, in having a diſappointment of the Imployment of his Shipping, and himſelf perhaps innocent in ſome meaſure of the Merchant's diſappointment, beſides the Sum of Money laid out to fit his Ship, and the Ship (as we term it) laid by the Walls.

But perhaps the Goods are received on board, and the Ship proceeds to ſail on her Voyage, and in the Paſſage the Goods are damag'd ſo far, that it proves a great Loſs to the Merchant. Or perhaps the Maſts being defective are hove by the board, by which means the Ship is taken, and made a Prize to the Enemy.

Or the Anchors and Cables give way, and the Ship by that means is drove on the ſhoar, and all Loſt, or Shipwreck'd.

Or in not carrying the Complement of Men according to the Bargain, the Ship is Loſt for want of Help.

Or the Guns and Ammunition being not fitly adapted to the Uſe, the Ship is not able to defend herſelf againſt a Force which ſhe might eaſily clear herſelf of, were the ſaid Guns and Ammunition put into a method, according to the Uſe or Cuſtom that ſuch Utenſils ought to be.

And in all or ſeveral of theſe Caſes, Whether ought the Owner or Merchant to ſuffer?

Firſt, In Caſe the Ship is fairly proved not to be capable of receiving the Merchant's Goods on board, according to the Agreement; Ought the Owner or Merchant to bear the Loſs?

In my Opinion, the Merchant was ſomething ſhort in providing Goods, and abſolutely depending on Shipping to Tranſport the ſame, only upon the bare word of an Owner, which perhaps knows as little what Ships are capable of doing ſuch and ſuch Services, as the Merchant himſelf: And therefore it would have been very proper for the Merchant to have ſent an Able and Experienc'd Man, that was thoroughly knowing what the Ships were capable of, to acquaint him how the Caſe ſtood, that his Dependance had been ſure and firm.

But for the Owner's part, he cannot think much of being diſappointed, if it's fairly proved his Ships are no ways qualified for what he promiſed them for. And therefore it will not be at all unreaſonable for both Owner and Merchant to ſet themſelves down, and be contented to bear the Loſs they have in ſome meaſure brought on themſelves.

But in Caſe the Goods are received, and in the Voyage are damnify'd to a high degree, Shall the Owner or Merchant ſtand to the Loſs, or ſhall the Ship's Crew?

I cannot perceive yet that the Owner is much more in a Fault than the Merchant, ſince the Merchant might have had a Survey of Able Shipwrights, which if the Owner had refuſed, he might have left that Owner's Craft, and gone to another that would have endured a Survey.

The Survey might have inquir'd how old the ſaid Ships were, what Voyages they had been, what material Repairs they had received ſince they were built, and then might have ſurveyed the Goodneſs of the Ships throughout; as, the Thickneſs of the Decks, the Firmneſs of the Sides above water, and how the Oakam ſtands in the Seams, whether there's any ſign of the Knees or Standers working, what condition the Maſts, Yards, Rigging and Sails are in; alſo, to the Guns and Ammunition, and alſo to the Ship's Crew.

Beſides one would think, that if the Owner deſigned to ſecure his Ship, or ſet any value upon her, he would be as nice in fitting her well out, as the Merchant would be to have her. So that if the Ship be Loſt, or any Caſualty happen to her without any under-hand dealing, but for want of Skill or Judgment, I cannot perceive how the Owner can be damag'd. For if the Merchant loſe his Goods, the Owner loſes his Ship, (if ſhe is loſt), but if the Ship is ſafe, and the Goods damnified, here is a Fault ſome where.

The Merchant expects Satisfaction, and upon which endeavours to obtain it from the Owner of the Ship, in promiſing a Ship fit to carry the Goods, and ſhe proves otherwiſe, the Owner lays the blame on the Ship's Crew, and expects the Recompence to be stop'd out of their Wages: Whether or no the Damage can reasonably be placed upon the Crew?

Owner putting in a Commander. I shall state the Case as follows. A certain Owner has a Ship built and compleated in every particular, and designs her for some certain Voyage, upon which he bestows the Command of the said Ship upon some Friend or Relation of his; or otherwise, one that will come in as a joint Partner with him.

And this Person is placed absolutely to Command, Appoint and Order this Ship as he shall see fitting, as soon as ever she is out of sight (as it shall be term'd here) of the Owners and Merchant: Only with this Proviso, That the said Commander doth in every respect take Directions from the Owners, and Trade from Port to Port, according as he is order'd by them on their Business, without any manner of Fraud or Molestation to the said Owners, or their Craft, and at the Expiration of the Voyage, to produce a Journal of his Proceedings, in Case there should happen any Disputes.

Commander shipping his Crew. However, this Commander not being able himself to sail this Ship without Help, he desires a certain number to assist, which he terms his Crew.

Mate. First, he has a Mate or two, according to the Magnitude of the Ship, which Mates are to assist him in Case of Sickness, or Death: They ought to be fitly qualified to navigate the Ship, in order thereto, they ought also to keep a Journal, and an Exact Account of the Ship's way, that they may be able from Day to Day, exactly to know in what Latitude, and Longitude, the Ship is in; they also are to stow the Hold, and carefully to have an Eye on the Actions, and Transactions, of every individual Person that belongs to the Ship's Crew.

Gunner. In the next place you have a Gunner, which ought to look after the Guns, to see into the Nature and Condition of each, that he may have Powder and Shot, and every other Utensil fit and convenient for to Charge and Discharge, and use the said Guns for Defence against any Enemy, according to the Allowance which is alloted him by the Owners.

Boatswain. Next you have a Boatswain, which ought to have an Eye on the Rigging, Sails and Blocks, to see that every part is fitly adapted to the use, and that he has sufficient of every Utensil to supply the wants of what may happen to be amiss in the whole course of the Voyage, to see the Cables securely bent to the Anchors, and the Shrowds well sized, and that they may not be rub'd, or wore, by one Rope chafing against another, but to apply proper Provision to prevent any Casualty to either Masts, Sails, or Rigging.

Carpenter. Next you have a Carpenter, which ought to look after the Fitting of the Ship, to see that every Thing that's necessary and convenient for the good of the said Ship be done well and safe, that every part of the Ship be calked tight, both for to keep the Goods dry, and also Mens Lodgings, to see that the Masts and Yards are fitted in every respect proper and convenient for the Use, that the Boats are also fitly adapted for the Use the Owner designs the Ship for, and that the Anchors be well stock'd, to see that he has a convenient Quantity of Sea Stores of every sort, that may be proper to supply the Want and Casualties that may happen both to the Ship, and every other material wooden part belonging to her; also that he has help enough to keep the Ship in a proper Condition, and that such a Crew have a sufficient parcel of Tools proper and convenient to perform any Piece of Work that may be requir'd to be done. But especially that he minds his Pumps, Rudder, Ports if any, and Chain Plates, which are material parts of his Charge, also the Capstands.

That the Pumps, whether Chain or Hand Pumps, be in a very good Condition, well set and well fitted with Brakes, or Winches, and every thing else that has been customary for a Ship of the Magnitude to be fitted with, well Leather'd, either as Boxes or Chains, to see that his Rudder Irons be firm, and not too much worn, but be of sufficient substance to agree to that extraordinary strain, that always will attend such a Material; also that the Chain Plates be firm, and not too much worn, and also, that the Capstands be firm, and not decayed, well fitted with bars, or handspokes for Windlesses.

There

There may be several other Officers of a less Account, but these mention'd being those that materially manages such a Machine, I shall place all the rest in the general amongst the Ship's Crew; and proceed to shew some Cases which may happen, and the Reasonableness of placing them on the proper Persons, whose sphere it happens to fall under: Only observing, that all such Officers are directly under the Government of the afore mention'd Commander.

At the beginning of a Voyage it's a general Custom for the Commander to ship, as it's term'd, or hire all his Crew, and to give them so much Wages, according to the Quality of the Person, and what he may be shipped for: However this Agreement is various, according to the Custom of the Place you sail from; as at some Places, the Men are Hired by the Voyage, that is, to give the Persons so much Money at the Return of the said Ship they sail in, when she is unloaded, and secured at the very Place she belongs to, or where you first was ship'd on board her. But the more general way is to be Hired by the Month, which is to have so much *per* Month, and Victuals proper and convenient is always found at the Owners Charge. *Voyage beginning*

It happens that in the Passage either out or home, that by the Unskilfulness of the Commander, the Ship is run ashoar without giving any warning, upon which the Ship's Crew leave her, and being gone, the People living near the Place come on Board, and plunder her, and carry away the Goods, the Weather proving fair the Ship is got off, and saved. *Ship in a Boat*

Shall the Owner, or Ship's Crew, bear the Loss, or shall the Merchant? As the Saying is, *Skin for Skin, and all that a Man has, he will give for his Life.* The Crew by surprize were glad to get away in their Boats, or by some other parts of the Ship's Utensils, whilst they had that Opportunity. The Crew did their Duty whilst they were aboard, under the Command of their Commander; and it seems that the Ship was lost by Unskilfulness, which is a Misfortune upon both Owner and Merchant, that they could not be Judges of the Ability of the Commander.

However, if the Commander doth continue aboard of such a Ship, I cannot perceive how the Men dare to leave him, without expecting to suffer the Loss which is sustain'd by their disobeying of Command, and forsaking their Duty, but if the Commander leaves the Ship first, I cannot perceive the Crew in any Fault to follow his Example. Notwithstanding, as in divers Cases it happens, for a Ship's Crew to presume to carry away a Boat from a Ship, which in my Opinion must be of a dangerous Consequence, and little better than Felony, for it may be proved, that if that Boat had continued on board, she might have been of Use and Service to have saved the Ship, which on the other hand may be lost purely for want of such a Utensil. *Commander leaves the Ship*

But in Case the Carpenter should be remiss, and not minding his Pumps, there should be so much Water in a Ship, that doth damnify great part of the Goods, and it being found at unloading, Shall the Ship's Crew be lyable to pay for such Damage? It doth not seem Reasonable they should, except they had denied Pumping when the Commander had ordered them. *Carpenter remiss*

Shall the Carpenter singly bear the Damage? Yes, if he had not complied with Pumping the Ship, according to the Direction of the Commander. For it is a breach of his Duty, he forfeits his Wages in not doing what he hired himself to do. *Pumping*

But in Case the Carpenter has complied, and pump'd the Ship in course, shall the Commander be at the Loss, sustain'd by such damag'd Goods? If the Merchant has laid a Duty incumbant on a Commander to sound what Water is in the Hold at such and such Times, and obliged him to pump the Ship, at having so many Inches Water, at the Pumps. Otherwise if it shall happen, and fairly be proved, that such Leakage shall suddenly happen, it is a Casualty caused by the Turbulency of the Seas, and in such a Case the Ocean ought to bear the Loss, if the Merchant knows how to make it, which is term'd, Protesting against the Seas.

But

Calking. But in Caſe it be proved, that the Goods are damnified for want of Calking the Decks or Sides of the Ship, ſhall the Crew bear ſuch a Damage? No, it ſeems unreaſonable they ſhould, for the Fault is directly laid out of their ſpheres, except the Carpenter's.

Then ought the Carpenter ſingly to bear the Damage? It is really a Fault in a Carpenter to neglect his Duty, for ſince he ought to be a better Judge than the Commander, when the Ship requires to be calked, he ſhould have acquainted the Commander, if he had not Liberty to do his proper Buſineſs without acquainting of him.

Notwithſtanding it's but a Breach of being Remiſs in his Duty, and what the Carpenter cannot think much of being branded with ſuch an ill Name, but however it's not diſobeying Command, and refuſing to do what he ſhip'd himſelf for: And therefore I cannot ſee the Juſtice of placing the Damage upon the Carpenter.

Then ſhall the Commander bear it himſelf, for there is no other that it can well light on? If the Owner had obliged the Commander to calk the Ship, or rather order'd the Carpenter to do it, and it had been neglected, the Fault might have been charged wholly upon the Commander; but otherwiſe it muſt be imputed to the Commander's Ignorance. And in ſuch Caſes it would be very unreaſonable he ſhould ſuffer.

Then ſince the Commander and all the Crew ſeem to be clear of the Damage, it reſts now between the Merchant and Owner. And which of the two ought, in the ſtricteſt ſenſe, to bear the Loſs?

It ſeems very hard for a Merchant to pay the Owner Freight, and to have his Goods damnified, as much as for a Tenant to pay Rent for a Houſe that he cannot ſecure his Goods from ſuch Diſaſters.

Parallel between a Ship and a Houſe. I have obſerved it a general Saying amongſt Tenants, that if the Landlord will not make his Houſe Wind-tight and Water-tight, they would not pay their Rent. But then I preſume, they muſt acquaint the Landlord with the Faults, and ſhew 'em to him, before they can make ſuch Refuſal, which if he denies, I am apt to believe they may remove their Goods out of the ſaid Houſe, only paying for the Time they liv'd in it.

But our Caſe in Tranſporting Goods by Sea is ſomewhat foreign from the other: For here a Merchant puts a Parcel of Goods on board of a Ship, and ſtows her up ſo cloſe, that it's altogether impoſſible for any Perſon ſo much as to come to ſee whether there is any Leaks that may damnify the Goods or not.

Or otherwiſe, It's like that he gives no Body abſolute Charge of the Goods, to ſee and inſpect whether the Ship continues in a Capacity of ſecuring the Wares he has put on board, or to give Warning to the Carpenter, or Commander, to amend what he finds amiſs, ſo that the Caſe being properly conſider'd, I doubt not but the Damage will abſolutely fall upon the Merchant.

[illegible] It happens they meet an Enemy that comes up with them, and takes them, and it be proved that if the Men had ſtood by their Guns and Ammunition, they might have got clear, Shall the Men be damnified for not defending the Ship? If the Men had been ſhip'd upon that Condition to preſerve the ſaid Ship with their Lives and Fortune, it would have been diſobeying Command, and not having done according to what they Hired themſelves to do, if they had denied, but otherwiſe, I cannot perceive any Penalty can be placed upon them. For who can make the Men Satisfaction for their Lives and Limbs, the Widows for their Husbands, or the Children for their Fathers?

[illegible] But provided the Sails or Rigging are in fault by giving way, or otherwiſe the Ship had not run aſhoar, or had not been taken, Shall the Crew be damnified? No, except that they had refuſed to amend any Thing which they were order'd to do, and ſo have been guilty of the breach of Orders.

[illegible] It happens that a Ship being at an Anchor, is oblig'd to heave the Anchor on board, (term'd weighing an Anchor) and the Sailers refuſe to heave the Cap-ſtand, or Windleſs, upon which the Commander cuts the Cable, and the Anchor and part of the Cable is loſt, the Ship running into a Harbour is forced aſhoar

aſhoar and loſt, and it be proved, that if ſhe had had the Anchor that was cut away ſhe had been ſaved; Shall not the Men that refuſed, and diſobey'd Orders, be damag'd for it? Yes; it appears they ought to forfeit all their Wages for ſo refuſing. For they ought to have endeavour'd to do what lay in their power; and if one half ſhould prove obſtinate, the other half ought to have done as far as lay *in them*, *for it would have been an Excuſe for thoſe that did* their Duty, if the Damage had been done through the refuſal of the other

But in Caſe it ſhould happen, that all the Crew ſhould not be ſtrong enough to weigh the Anchor, and they finding themſelves obliged to loſe their Ship, or put her from her Anchor, and the Commander orders one of the Crew to cut the Cable, and he refuſe to do it, under the pretence that the Commander ought to ſtrike the firſt Stroke: Is not this Refuſal a Breach of Orders, and what the Perſon ſo refuſing may be lyable to be damnify'd for? It ſeems as if it was, for I cannot perceive but that it's really Lawful for any of the Ship's Crew (if the Commander order him) to cut the Cable, and part the Ship from her Anchor, as if the Commander had done it himſelf: But then it will be very proper for every one of the Ship's Crew to be by, and on Occaſion to be Evidence for the doing of the ſame by Order of the Commander, and then I am of Opinion, that the Perſon ſo order'd is ſafe in cutting, and not ſafe in refuſing

Sails blown away

In Caſe the Commander ſhould order the Topſails, or Courſes, to be handed, and the Men refuſe to hand them, by which means the Maſts are carried away, and the Ship taken or loſt; Shall not the Men be damag'd for not obeying Command? This is almoſt the ſame Caſe as the former.

Goods damnified, ſlipping of them

Provided the Goods are damnified in receiving on board, either by letting them fall into the Water, or in hoiſting on board the Tackles or Slings break, Shall the Crew be damag'd for theſe Faults? They ought, if they are proved to do it wilfully; but if they did their endeavour, there's no more can be expected of them, it muſt happen upon the Owner, for not providing ſuitable Strength, or Proviſion, to get the Merchants Goods, that he is paid Freight for, on board his Ship. But provided that the Goods are damnified before they be taken on board, Shall the Owner ſtand to the Damage? It ſeems unreaſonable they ſhould, notwithſtanding it would bear a Diſpute. And in ſuch Caſes it would be very proper for the Commander or Owner, to inſpect the Goodneſs of what Goods they take on board for their own Safety.

Men or Commander imbezelling the Goods.

In Caſe it happen that the Goods are waſted, or by either the Commander or ſome of the Crew, they are imbezel'd, Shall the Crew be damnified for ſuch Waſte, or will it fall on the Commander or Owner? It could be wiſh'd, that the Party ſo imbezelling might be diſcover'd, however if they cannot, I can't perceive how the Crew can be damag'd generally, for they took no manner of charge of the Security of the Goods, and therefore this Damage lyes principally at the Maſter or Commander's door, for he might have had proper and convenient Security for to debar any Perſons coming at them: Which Security if the Owner had refuſed they ought to have been at the Loſs themſelves.

Ship caſt away

But all things doing well, and the Ship coming near home is either taken, or run aſhoar and loſt, Shall the Men loſe, or have their Wages ſtop'd, becauſe the Ship is loſt?

If the Men were ſhip'd by the Voyage, that they were to be paid ſuch a Sum of Money when the Ship arriv'd at the ſame Place, or Harbour, where they firſt carried her from, I cannot perceive how they can expect their Wages if the Ship never come back to that Place, for it ſeems, that they in a manner inſured the Ship's coming ſafe home again with their Wages, ſo far that if the Ship never came home, they are never to have any Money for failing on board her

But if the Men are ſhip'd by the Month, I cannot perceive but that they may Lawfully demand their Money at every Month's end, and indeed it ſeems reaſonable that they ſhould demand it of him that ſhip'd them, if they expect to make it a due Debt: Or otherwiſe there may be ſomething ſaid for it, that the Crew did not expect their Wages till the Ship arrives at her unloading Port, or otherwiſe where they were ſhip'd on board

A Dealer a-shoar hires Servants, and his House burnt.

For it may be as well, or as reasonable, for a Man of great Dealings, that hires several Servants by the Day, Week, Month or Year, and it happen that his House is burnt down Shall the Servants lose their Wages? Yes, if they are Instrumental in doing of it, otherwise believe, they may recover their Wages, if the Master is any ways in a condition to pay them, and also in proportion to the Time they lived with the said Master, although the Time they were hired for is not actually expired

A Merchant hiring a Ship of an Owner

In Case a Merchant should hire a Ship to do such and such Services, and agrees to give the Owner so much Monthly or Yearly, the Owner is to find all Wear and Tear, sufficient and agreeable to secure a Ship of that Magnitude in every respect.

The Agreement is also, if the said Ship is lost by such and such Casualties, that the Merchant shall pay a certain Sum of Money for her, according to the Agreement

It happens that the Ship is drove upon a Lee-shoar; but seeing the Shoar first, she chops, or suddenly lets go her Anchors, and cuts away her Masts, by which means the Ship is saved Shall the Merchant pay the Damage the Ship sustains by cutting her Masts away? Here's a Query.

Says the Merchant, I promised to pay for the Ship if she was lost by Casualty, but not to be at the Loss of such Fancies, for who knows whether the Ship would have drove upon the Shoar if her Masts had not been cut away? Did the Ship drive before the Masts were cut away, after the Anchors were fast in the Ground?

No, says the Commander and Crew, we did not stay to Experience that; for we had but a small Drift, or a little distance between the Shoar and us, and in all probability, if the Anchors had once started, the cutting of the Masts away would not have done.

It would be really a great pity, that the Merchant should scruple the paying 500 *l* for saving 5000 *l*. However, it's no more than what is generally observed in divers Cases The Merchant believes, as not knowing by Experience, that the Commander imposes on him, and therefore is so far from paying the Damage, and commending the Commander for his Care, that he harbours an ill Opinion of him, and condemns him rather, believing it to be a rash Action.

Why then will the Damage rest upon the Owner? No, says the Owner, I will not pay for the Masts, and Damage sustain'd, since if the Ship had gone ashoar, I had been paid for the Ship. So that in all probability, the Loss must lye upon the Commander, or those that cut the Masts away, if they are any ways able to stand to the Loss, although in all probability, the Ship and all the Crew had been totally spoil'd if the thing had not been done

The same Parallel may be drawn in cutting a Boat from the Stern, or heaving away some other Incumberance, to lighten a Ship, and clear her from the Enemy. And in such Cases we may say with *Hudibras*

He that Kills himself,
Or knocks out his Brains,
I'll be hang'd
If he is blam'd.

THE

THE
Converting PART
IN
SHIP-TIMBER
Made Obvious.

HAVING in another Place, mention'd ſomething * in Relation to the Price and Value of Timber, from the Content and Faſhion of the Species; which is to ſay, The different Content that makes an equal Value in ſtraight Timber, compar'd with Compaſs, or regular crook'd Timber: I ſhall in this following Conſideration, ſhew a Reaſon for ſuch Unequality, in the different Magnitudes of Timber, equal in Goodneſs, and yet of equal Price.

The Number of Shipping in *England*, at this Time, is very great, and daily increaſes, both in the Publick, and alſo in the Merchants Service, and beſides the Building of New Shipping, it's found, That in the wear of moſt Shipping, they require continual, and very often large Reparations.

However, That is not what cauſes ſuch a Difference in the Price, between ſtraight and Compaſs Timber, but it may very reaſonable be allow'd, That it cauſes a general Riſe in the Price of all Timber, that's fitting for Ship Work; and therefore it muſt follow, That this Difference, between ſtraight and Compaſs Timber, is caus'd, by the Scarcity there will always happen between the Species; not only from the different Production, or Growth there is between one and another, but alſo through the different Number of Pieces there is in every Ship, far larger of Compaſs Timber, than what may reaſonably be call'd ſtraight Timber.

I ſhall therefore ſhew, What Parts in any Ship may be allow'd to be regular Compaſs Timber, and what crooked Timber may be allow'd as irregular Compaſs Timber, and not near ſo valuable as it's often judged to be. And alſo what ought to be accounted for as ſtraight; with the Advantage, or Diſadvantage, which ought to be with Indifferency conſider'd, in converting and dealing for ſuch Commodities.

The Keel of any Ship being generally ſtraight, and alſo made with Elm, *Keel.* which for its Plenty and Uſeleſneſs, is much cheaper than Oak, but better for the Service, however, its directly ſtraight, and ought to be accounted for ſo.

The Stern-poſt is alſo perform'd with a ſtraight Piece. *Stern-post.*

The Stem is crooked, and cannot be well perform'd otherwiſe, but muſt have *Stem.* principal Compaſs Timber; and alſo in a certain Number of Pieces, according to the Magnitude of the Ship: And therefore I ſhall now proceed to ſhew the Reaſon, Why there ought to be a Difference in ſtraight and Compaſs Timber, according to their ſeveral Bulks.

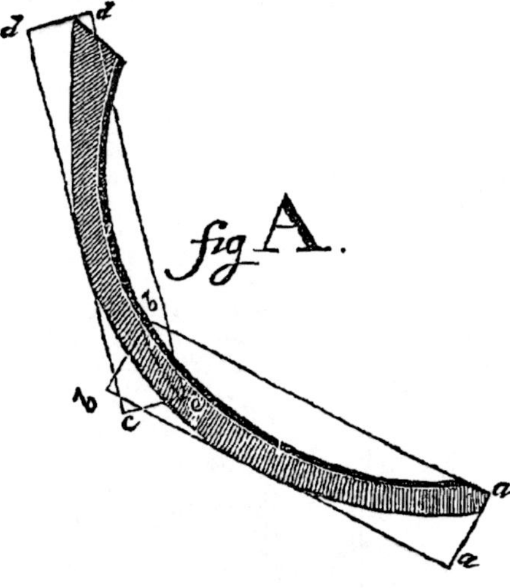

Figure *A*, repreſents the Stem of a Ship, which I allow to be of that ſize which is generally made in two Pieces, tho' it cannot be deny'd, but that it would be much ſtronger, if it was made out of one entire Piece. Let from *a*, *a*, to *b*, *b*, be the length of one Piece, and from *c*, *c*, to *d*, *d*, be the length of another Piece; and for a more clear Explanation of the matter, I ſhall imagine, That crooked or compaſs Timber could not be obtain'd; and really it need not be only imagin'd, for at divers Times it's really found ſo, and the Work often retarded for the want of ſuch a Part, ſince it ought not to be piec'd, eſpecially in the Wake of the Rabbits· Neither ought it be defective, by Reaſon of what is faſten'd to it; and the Difficulty that will undeniably happen, in ſhifting ſuch a Piece, as a Stem of a Ship

Therefore, If theſe Pieces were to be wrought out of ſtraight Timber, they would require two Pieces equal in bigneſs to the Squares; *a*, *a*, *b*, *b*, and *c*, *c*, *d*, *d*, according to the thickneſs requiſite in ſuch a Stem; which will be near equal to what you may obſerve by the Tinge.

That ſuch compaſs Pieces, which are capable of making ſuch a Stem in two Pieces, ought to be equal in Value to two ſtraight Pieces, whoſe bigneſs on the Superficies, ſhall be equal to the Parallelogram, *a*, *a*, *b*, *b*, and *c*, *c*, *d*, *d*, one way, and the otherways to be equally ſcantled, according to what is requiſite in ſuch a Stem, as the ſaid Figure *A* deſcribes in the Tinge; only minding that the Waſte (abating for the Converſion) ought to be deducted out of the Price of the ſtraight Pieces; provided it can be allow'd, That ſuch compaſs Pieces, converted out of large Straight, can be as ſerviceable, as thoſe compaſs Pieces that naturally grow ſo.

Now provided this Stem be, when nicely converted, and fitting for the Deſign, 36 Foot long, and 16 Inches ſquare, it will contain 64 Foot; but the ſtraight Pieces, that make ſuch a Stem, will contain 169 Feet; the Difference is 105 Foot; and the Extra charge of Sawing, will be four or five Shillings more, in converting the ſtraight Piece, than that which is circular: The Reaſon is thus, The ſtraight Piece will be large enough to divide into Halves the other way, ſince Timber grows very nearly ſquare.

However, Here will be near 100 Foot of Waſte cut off, to make ſuch ſtraight Pieces circular, which will be in ſix Pieces, and muſt be converted to ſome other uſes; but then the Value will be much diminiſh'd, of what it was in the large Piece: For ſet the Caſe, That the large Piece, of 169 Foot, be worth 3 *l* 9 *s*. *per* Load, or 17 *d per* Foot; and the Waſte being divided in ſix Pieces, containing each in the Medium 17 Foot and a half, be worth 1 *l* 12 *s per* Load, or 7 *d*. *per* Foot; firſt there will be 11 *l* 19 *s*. the Price of the Timber, and the Converſion will make 12 *l* 3 *s* only there will be 105 Foot to be taken out, at 7 *d per* Foot, which is 3 *l*. 1 *s* 3 *d* remains 7 *l* 17 *s*. 9 *d*. for 64 Foot, which will be 5 *l* 12 *s* 8 *d per* Load, or 2 *s* 5 *d*. halfpenny *per* Foot, which Obſervations will hold in ſuch principal Pieces as Stems. And now I proceed to the Tranſums, and faſhion Pieces.

The Tranſums and faſhion Pieces are not general; for in ſome Ships they are left out, and that is in Pink-ſtern'd Ships, generally call'd round-ſtern'd Ships· The Reaſonableneſs of ſuch Pieces, is only for creating large Accommodations, in the After-parts of the Ship, and that is, to make broad, or square-stern'd Ships, as they are term'd.

However, I shall refer it to be consider'd by the Master Builders, who have the Charge upon them, of the Conveniency, or Frugality there may be, either in continuing the said Fashion, or wholly leaving of it of; for undeniably, the After-part of any Ship may be built, and every way as well perform'd, without either Transum or fashion Pieces. And I shall now proceed to shew the Fashion of such Pieces, and the Value from thence.

The Figure *B*, is the shape of the upper or Wing-transum, which comes nearest to a Straight, of any other of the Transums.

Figure *C* is its opposite, the lower Transum, and also requires to be most circular, or in a manner Knee-timber.

Now if the upper Transum as Figure *B*, was to be made out of a straight Piece, it would require a Piece equal in bigness to the Parallelogram *a*, *b*, *c*, *d*, besides the Beveling caus'd by the rapering of such a Part of the Ship. However, This being a Part that is variously perform'd, some will work the Plank quite over this Transum, and others will by rabbiting the said Transum, work the Plank five or six Inches short of the upper Edge, according to the Magnitude of the Ship.

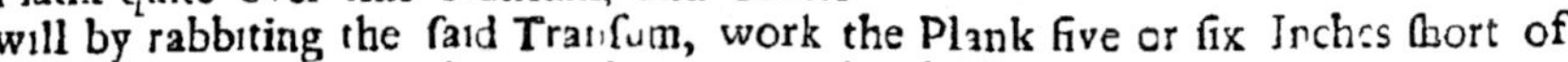

Now if the Plank is work'd quite over this Transum, I cannot see it at all unreasonable, for to joyn two Pieces together, as at the Line 1, 2, which will make the Transum something less in Value, but if the said Transum has a Rabbit work'd in it, and not entirely covered with Plank, then it ought to be made out of one Piece, otherwise it would not be firm Work, but would leak: However their will arise something of Charge in splicing, and scarphing of Pieces, which ought to be added into the Value of the Pieces that are intire, and deducted out of such Parts as are made in divers Pieces.

Figure *C*, and all the other Transums, may be consider'd after such a manner; but this Transum being the lowermost, and intirely cover'd with Plank without side, and therefore will allow of being pieced; for if it would not, it will require a Piece of Timber, equal to the Parallelogram made by 3, 3, o, o. However, since it may be made sufficiently strong with a Chock, as 8, 8, 9, 9, a Piece will suffice, that's equal to 5, 5, c, o, only observing that the Value of the Chock, 8, 8, 9, 9, with the Workmanship of joyning it, must be added in, which together, ought directly to shew the Price of such a Piece, that will make it intirely, as may be observ'd by the Tinge, and to be thick the other way, according to the Scantling of such a Part.

Then to the fashion Piece, as in Figure *D*, which shews one, for there are two fashion Pieces, equal and as exactly alike as they can be made, since they are for shaping the Stern, and making both Buttocks equal in Similitude, and these Pieces are always made in one Piece, notwithstanding there may be a small Piece joyn'd on, at the lower End. However, Considering the large bevelling that there is usually in these Parts (which sometimes is a great deal more than what is really needful to be [illegible] in such principal Pieces of Timber) it may very reasonably be allow'd, That such a Piece may

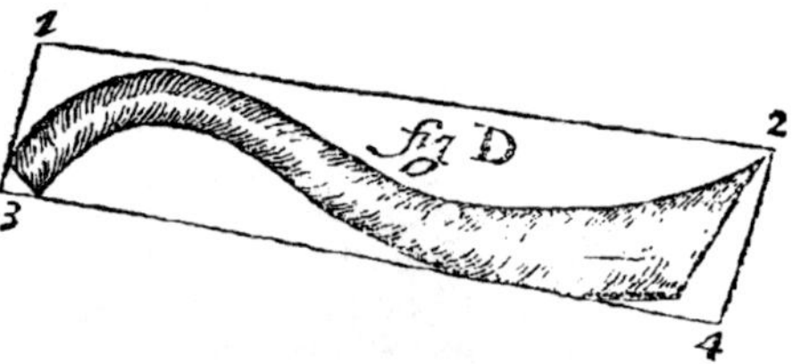

be equal in Value to a Parallelogram, made by the Lines 1, 2, 3, 4, and of the thickness, suitable to make such a fashion Piece, according to the Magnitude of the Ship · And now I proceed to the Floor-timber, since the Dead-wood may be perform'd with perfectly straight Timber; only the Knee which connex's the after Dead wood, which may be consider'd from that general Observation, I shall make on Knee-timber · As follows hereafter.

The Floor-timbers may, in some measure, be consider'd from what has been said of the Transums; nay, and something more may be said of piecing them, than of piecing the Transums.

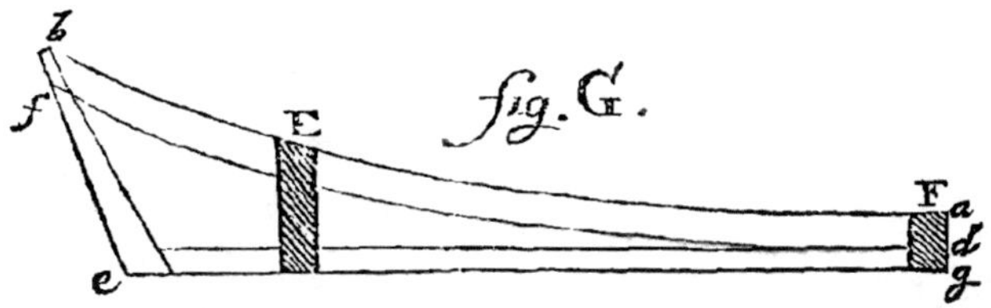

Supposing Figure G, to be the after or foremost Part of any Ship, *e*, *g*, being the upper Part of the Keel, *d*, *f*, the commencing of a Hollow, or rising straight Line, in the outer Part of the Timbers, and *a*, *b*, the cutting down Line, or upper Part of the Floor-timbers, or the Shape of the lower Part of the Hole. Let Figure *F*, be the Midship-timber, standing at *F*, in Figure *G*: It's manifest, That a straight Piece would make such Timbers, without any waste, more than to reduce the But to the bigness of the Top

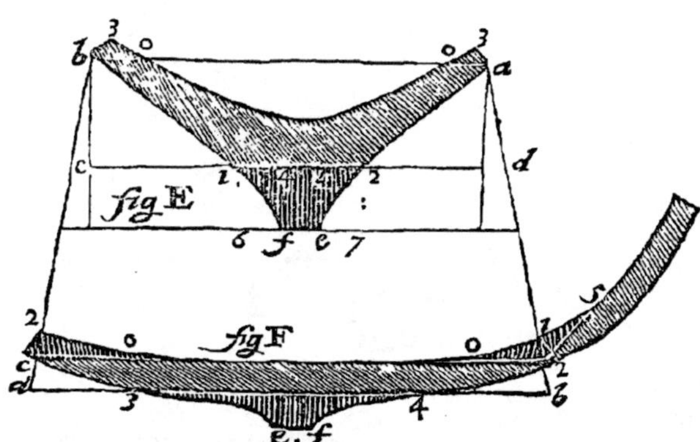

Figure *F*, the Part 3, 4, *e*, *f*, is a Chock put on, and so may o, 1, 2, and o, *c*, 2, nay, it would be much better for the Ship, if every Floor Timber-head, and second Foot-hook Heel, was served so throughout the whole Frame; as may be observ'd by 1, o, 5, 2, which is to scarf a Chock, that shall go Part upon the Head, and Part upon the Heel of every Timber, since it would unite the Parts, and strengthen the joining of the Timbers; which will farther appear, when the Plank is brought on, and treneld through Timber and Chock

Figure *E*, is placed at *E*, in Figure *G*, it being call'd a rising Timber, which is the Term that distinguishes such Floor Timbers, from those which are flat, and in the middle Part of the Ship, this being caused by the tapering of the Ship aft and forward; and such Timbers may in some measure be call'd Knee Timber, since they must be form'd out of Knees, notwithstanding the Chock 1, 2, *f*, *c*, will save considerably in such Timbers; and by piecing of them after that manner, it will mightily help the compassing, or extraordinary Bending; and will also cause them Parts to be more easily handled; since the Chock, 1, 4, *f*, may be fitted on (if the Timber stands on the Dead wood) after the principal Timber is placed to the Rising, and fastned; and so will the Chock, 4, 2, *e*.

The Chocks, *b*, 3, o, and o, 3, *a*, may be also placed accordingly, to the Rule afore mention'd, and therefore this Timber will be valuable, according

to

to a Superficies made by the Line, *a, b, c, d,* and the thickneſs the other way, ſutable to make ſuch a Floor Timber; but the Figure *F,* is only valuable, according to the length of ſuch a Piece, and the thickneſs ſuitable for ſuch a Floor Timber; only obſerving the Charge of piecing and ſcarphing, which will not be much in Conſideration of the Value *per* Foot, of ſound and ſerviceable Timber.

Next I come to the Foot-hooks, which are diſtinguiſh'd by a certain Number of Tires, according to the Magnitude of the Ship, term'd firſt or lower Tire, ſecond Tire, third Tire, fourth Tire, which is the greateſt Number there is in the biggeſt of our Shipping.

The Shape of the Foot-hooks are various, according to the Magnitude, and ſhape of the Ship.

As in Figure *I,* you may obſerve it to be the ſhape of a lower Foot-hook, in the Midſhips of the Ship, and Figure *H,* ſhews a lower Foot-hook, in the After-moſt, or foremoſt Part of the Ship; which difference in the Shape, is caus'd, by Reaſon of the Difference there is between the hanging or riſing Line, and the ſtraight Line, which makes the upper Edge of the Keel.

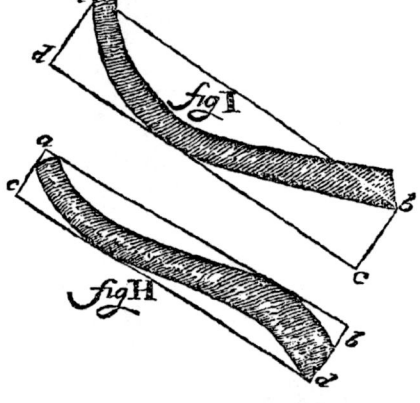

The Figure *I* is valuable, according to the Parallelogram *a, b, c, d;* and the thickneſs the other way, according to the Scantling approved on, for ſuch a Timber.

And Figure *H* is valuable, according to the Parallelogram *a, b, c, d,* and the thickneſs as aforeſaid.

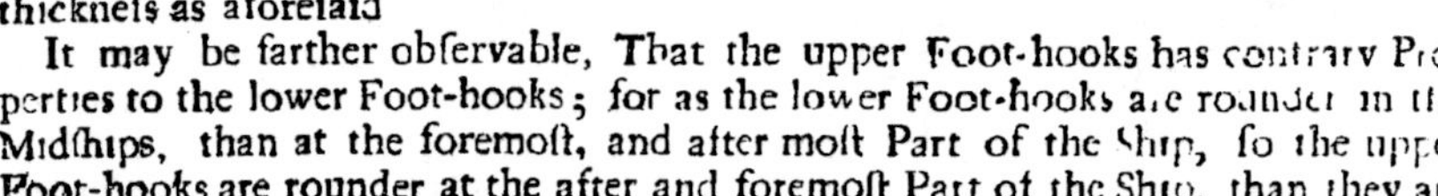

It may be farther obſervable, That the upper Foot-hooks has contrary Properties to the lower Foot-hooks; for as the lower Foot-hooks are rounder in the Midſhips, than at the foremoſt, and after moſt Part of the Ship, ſo the upper Foot-hooks are rounder at the after and foremoſt Part of the Ship, than they are in the Midſhips, according to the different tapering of the hanging Conoid, that forms the Ships Body; and each are valuable, according to their ſeveral and reſpective Parallelograms 1, 2, 3, 4, in Figure *L* and *M.*

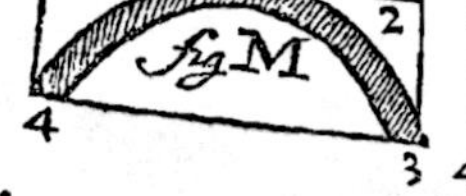

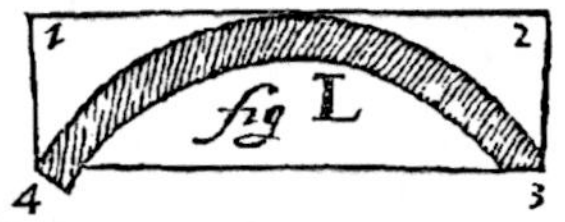

There is alſo double Foot-hooks, by ſome called long Timbers, both afore and abaft, which are alſo valuable, in direct Proportion, according to the Parallelograms, made by each Timbers reſpective length, and breadth, and depth.

There is one thing more, which may be plac'd amongſt the Foot-hooks; altho' they no other than imitate, and ſtand in the room of Floor Timbers, or half a Floor Timber; and are call'd half Timbers, as in the Figure *K,* where may at ſundry Times be obſerv'd, an unreaſonable Method in making ſuch Timbers, ſince they are plac'd againſt the Dead-wood, from *d,* to 6; which Dead-wood, ought to be join'd as firm, as if it had grew in one intire Piece, and alſo faſtned as well, and with as much Regard to Security, as it poſſibly can be made, and then

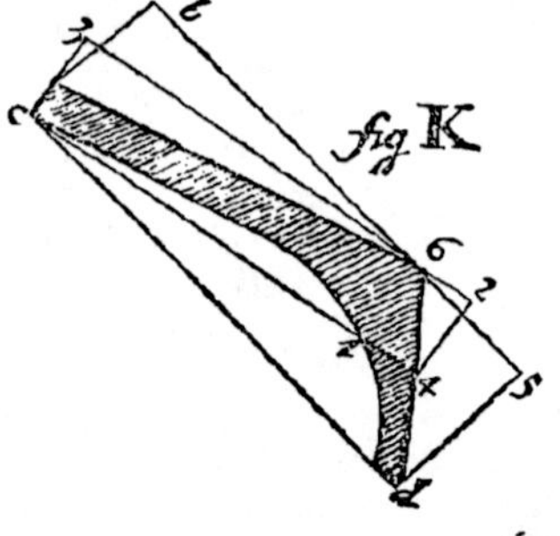

there

there will be no occaſion to be at ſuch an unreaſonable Expence, as to make ſuch extraordinary Compaſs half Timbers to ſecure the Dead-wood.

But farther, They are no ſtrength at all to the Dead-wood; ſince they are wrought ſo very thin, that they are rather deſtructive to the Work contiguous to them, as may be more fully illuſtrated, when Ships are old and pull'd to pieces; ſuch lower thin Foots are often broke and ſplit to pieces, with the boring of the Holes, and driving the Trenels; and of Conſequence, any Ship would be much better and ſtronger in thoſe Parts, if that chargeable, and inſignificant Faſhion, was wholly left off

For were ſuch Timbers work'd no lower than 4 and there well faſtned, and a Chock work'd below that, as 1, 4, *d*, it would be every whit as good Work, and the Charge but as 2 to 1, as may be ſeen by the Parallelograms *b*, *c*, 5, *d*, and 2, 4, 3, *c*

I now proceed to the Top-timbers, which are generally Timbers of a double Property, having the Curve reverted; which Faculty is chiefly uſed for beautifying that part of the Ship which is always in Sight · However, They ought to be thorowly conſider'd, for ſtrengthening the Ship upwards, and helping the Defects or Weakneſs, that's caus'd by cutting the Port-holes; for which Reaſon, as I ſhall ſhew in the Figures, they ought in ſome Places, to partake of a three-fold Faculty, as in ſome meaſure may be term'd ſide round, which is meant when the Sides are not ſtraight.

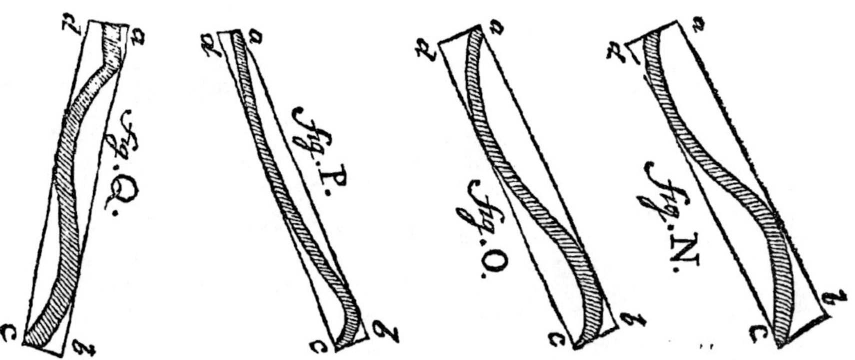

The Figures *N, O, P, Q*, ſhews a general ſhape of the Top-timbers; *N* being a Midſhip Timber, *P* an after Timber, *O* between them, and *Q* a foremoſt Timber, which different Shapes in Top-timbers aft, is caus'd by that Diſproportion there is between the narrowing of the main breadth, and the narrowing of the Top-timber breadth, to make greater Accommodation upwards for the Commander's Cabin; and the Difference between the Midſhips, and forward, is caus'd to make Proviſions to heave the Anchor from the Bow, and theſe Timbers will be in value, according to their ſeveral and reſpective Parallelograms, *a*, *b*, *c*, *d*, in Figure *N*, and *a*, *b*, *c*, *d*, in Figure *O*, and *a*, *b*, *c*, *d*, in Figure *P*; and *a*, *b*, *c*, *d* in Figure *Q*, and their ſeveral breadths the other way, according to the Scantling requiſite.

In the Figures *R*, *S*, *T*, you may observe what will, in divers Cases, be required to make the Port-holes, since the Timbers at first are equally spaced, beginning from the Midships forward, and from the Midships aft, so that by such exact Spacing, some Top-timbers would either direct themselves through, and stop a Port hole, or otherwise, be cut off to make room for the said Holes, which will be very detrimental And therefore such Timbers as are imitated by these Figures *R*, *S*, *T*, often prove very convenient to cast themselves (as its term'd) clear of such Port holes, and still retain their Strength and Substance, without being Grain cut; and therefore ought to be valued, this way, equal to a straight Piece of the bigness of the Parallelogram 1, 2, 3, 4, in the Figure *R*, and 1, 2, 3, 4, in the Figure *S*, and 1, 2, 3, 4, in the Figure *T*, besides the extra Value which ought to be set on them for their other Regular Crookeding, as is shew'd in the former Figures.

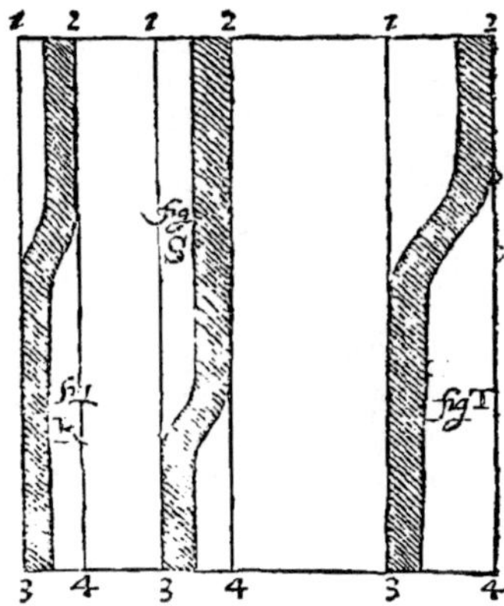

Such Cases, and what will farther appear as I proceed, would put every Person upon a Thought, that designs any Good to himself, or any that he is concern'd for, what will be materially requisite in Buying, Providing, and Receiving Timber, since the Difficulty doth appear so very obvious, that it is really a nice point to put a true and exact Value upon divers Pieces of Timber for Ship-work; and that no Person can be too well grounded in the Experimental Part, before he can be placed to have the least share in Bargaining, or Receiving such Materials.

Although I know it has been very often approved on by some, that any Country fellow, or a Clark, that never knew any thing of Ship-building, (or scarce knows Elm Timber from Oak) may be the properest Person for Measuring and Receiving such Goods, because he knows how to Measure, and set down the Contents, in order to make out a Bill

Which is a rare Qualification for a Man to be intrusted in such a weighty Concern, and to give Judgment in Receiving and Measuring some valuable Pieces of Timber · But to proceed, and shew the Defect a little farther, which is to the Plank without side

The Plank without board may be perfectly straight, or declining so little from such a Position, that a straight Plank may suffice to do the design'd Service, and therefore there will be no Occasion to make any consumption in Compass Timber, whose Scarcity cannot but be extreamly observed, and how very hard it is to obtain a convenient Quantity to carry on Ship-work, without very often being mightily retarded for want of such Goods.

Besides there ought to be a great deal of good Management in Receiving and Ordering Plank from four Inches downwards, that is to say, from four Inches thick to one Inch and half thick; for since a Ship is composed of divers Curves, some of which being almost Straight, and others altogether as Circular, there ought to be as much difference in the Value of Plank, as there is between Compass Timber, and that which is directly Straight

All our fore-most and after-most parts of Shipping in general is very Round, and will require the Plank to be very Round that covers such parts, however such Crookeding is generally forced with Fire and Water · For if such Stuff was to be made out of Timber, the Value ought to be allowed for such Pieces according to my preceeding Observations of Crooked Timber · Besides, there is a vast Difference in the Nature of Plank, some will bend much freer than others Nay, some sort of Plank will break before it will bend to any purpose, and others again being so very pliant, that you may bend it almost beyond credit.

The Faculties incident thereto will be very hard to demonstrate in every particular; however the principal are as follows:

First, To choose a Plank that has no Knots nor Defects.

Secondly, Let it be an outside Plank, and the ground-end, or butt, put to the greatest Bending

Thirdly, In Bending, if it be possible, lay the outside of the Plank next to the Fire, that the Water may be applied to that side which is next to the heart of the Tree.

Fourthly, Let the Plank be very even and smooth, and well tended with a quick Fire, and Water as hot as it can well be made.

And since the different Charge, and Facility in Bending of Planks, is so very much as has been observed, that at some times seven hundred Bavins has been burnt under one Plank to bend it for a medium Buttock, neither full nor thin. The Charge of the Bavins at 12 *s. per* Hundred is 4 *l.* 4 *s.* and the Value of the Plank not 40 *s.* Prime Cost, so that Planks of a more yielding nature ought to have a peculiar Value set on them, that will be bended much Rounder with half the Expence.

And therefore in receiving such Goods, it will be highly necessary to have a very able Shipwright continually at the Receipt, as has been formerly customary, and for the Reason of sorting such Goods, and order the stowing of them separate, and not lay them up after such a manner, that will oblige twenty Shipwrights to rumage a whole Day to find one for their purpose, amongst a number of mix'd Planks.

And also to lay Planks equal in Length and Thickness by themselves, and also of equal Breadth by themselves. Observing the different Strength there will be in Shipping, by working Planks throughout the whole Ship, if it be possible, directly equal, both in Length and Breadth.

I now proceed to the Wales, which in the Midships may be straight, and perform'd with such Timber, but the following Pieces and Harpings are crooked, and ought to be valued accordingly Not but that after one Wale is fastened, and the Strake between the other, let it be upper or lower Wale, may on occasion be bent by Fire, and forced to the Shape of the Ship. And as to the different Charge in performing it, I shall mention as follows, to shew how the Value of Crooked Stuff may be farther adjusted

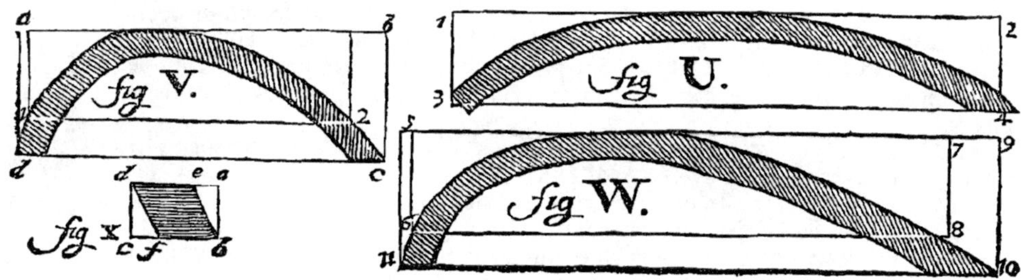

Figure *V*, shews the Shape of a Harping the foremost Piece of either Lower Wales, or Channel Wales.

I shall imagine this Piece in its natural Rounding to be from *a*, *b*, to 1, 2, but the Shape of the Bow requires it to Round from *a*, *b*, to *c*, *d*, and unless such a Piece can be forced, it will not do for that Service · However, it's Experimentally found that it will with this Proviso, that proper means are used, and that the Ship is in such a Condition, as will bear the Force which is requisite to bend it, without disordering the Frame of the Ship.

I shall again imagine, that such a Piece which is shew'd in Figure *V*, being clear and free from Knots, and other visible Defects, and withal so pliant, that eight Hours burning or heating with Fire and hot Water, and tended with five Men,

Men, burning fifty Bavins an Hour, will make ſuch a Piece in a condition to work, it will increaſe the Value of ſuch a Piece that naturally grows to the Work, by the Charge of four hundred Bavins, and the five Men for eight Hours, beſides that extra Proviſion which will be requiſite to ſet the ſaid Piece to its Work, over and above the Proviſion that may ſuffice to ſet any Piece that naturally grows to that Shape which will be required.

But inſtead of ſuch a good natur'd Piece, there ſhould happen to be a Piece of hard knotty Timber, that would require ſixteen Hours lying upon as good a Fire, and as well tended as the other, and perhaps broke at laſt.

This I ſay ought to be another material Conſideration, what Judgment is requiſite in Purveying and Receiving of Timber.

And this Charge of Bending by Fire, and the Hazard you run, will in all probability make ſuch a Piece that grows to the natural Rounding, ſince by the Parallelogram *a, b, c, d,* be valuable in direct Proportion, (or rather more) as the Parallelogram *a, b, c, d,* is to the Parallelogram *a, b,* 1, 2.

Figure *V* is term'd a following Piece, the next piece to the Harping, that is uſed on the Round of the Bow, which Piece may be conſidered from the preceeding Conſiderations of the Harpings.

Figure *W* may alſo imitate the after piece of Wales, and indeed there is a material Conſideration in working ſuch pieces, that require two Edges to be directly Horizontal, and the other Edges upon ſome certain Angle between the Horizon, and a perpendicular from the Horizon, as may be ſeen in the Figure *x*; that *a, b, c, d,* are the Horizontal parts, and *e, b, d, f,* ſhew the Angle the Ship's body makes with the Horizon.

Let us imagine, that *c, a,* is the proper Thickneſs ſuch a Piece ought to be, and if it was placed in any part of the Ship that was perpendicular to the Horizon, ſuch a Thickneſs would ſuffice; but ſince it's placed at ſome certain Angle between, ſuch a Piece ought to be of that ſubſtance, which may be ſeen by the Parallelogram *a, b, c, d,* and in Value as the Parallelogram 5, 11, 9, 10, although the natural Curve made by ſuch a part may be bounded by the Parallelogram 5, 7, 6, 8, as may be ſeen in the Figure *W*.

And what has been ſaid of the Lower Wale, may be referable to the Channel Wales, alſo the Plank below to the Plank aloft. And now I proceed to the Work within-ſide, or in-board Work, where firſt I ſhall begin with the Kelſon.

The Kelſon ought to be intire for Breadth and Depth, and to ſcarph or overlaunch the Keel, if it be poſſible, that the Scarphs of the Kelſon ſhall be fitted over the middle part of the Keel's Scarphs, which will be moſt certainly a ſtrengthening to the lower part of the Ship, but may be perform'd with ſtraight Pieces.

The Foot-waleing follows of courſe to the Kelſon, which Foot-waleing is wrought of divers Scantlings (term'd Thick Stuff) according to the weakneſs of the Ship, or the extra ſtrength which is requir'd where it's wrought.

The Thick Stuff is cut out of principal Timber, it ought to be thoroughly conſider'd in converting of it, ſince every ſuperficial Foot of Foot waleing that's wrought on board the largeſt Ship is valued at 2 *s.*

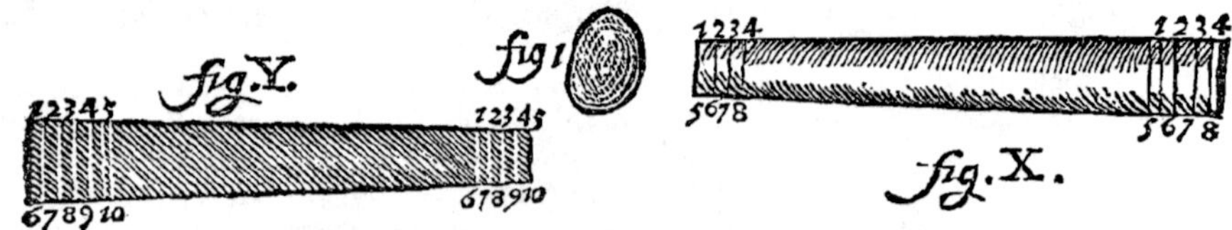

As in Caſe there was a certain ſtraight Tree to be converted, as in Figure *X* and *Y*, and that the ſaid Tree did not grow directly Round but Oblong, as in Figure 1, ſo that there could be cut out one way 4 ſix Inch pieces, and the other way but 3 ſeven Inch pieces, it would be more advantagious to cut out 4

ſix

ſix Inch pieces, ſince the extra breadth in the middle would do but little Service, it being an uncontroulable Maxim, that all Plank, or Thick Stuff, that's wrought on any Ship's bottom in the middle part, ought to be directly Straight, and of parallel Breadth, both to add Strength, and alſo for good Husbandry: Nay, if the Piece was Round, and to be cut after ſuch a manner, the Management would appear in the ſix Inch pieces.

For ſet the Caſe, there was a Piece of 20 Foot long, and 2 Foot broad, then there would be wrought of the ſix Inch Stuff 80 Foot of Timber, and of the ſeven Inch Stuff but 70 Foot, or 10 Foot difference. But in Caſe there was 3 eight Inch pieces cut the other way, as there might be, provided the Length was ſuitable to the Thickneſs, then the Converſion would be better in the eight Inch Stuff than in the ſix Inch Stuff, by Reaſon of what would be expended more in the ſix Inch Stuff than in the eight Inch Stuff, by reaſon of often Converſion.

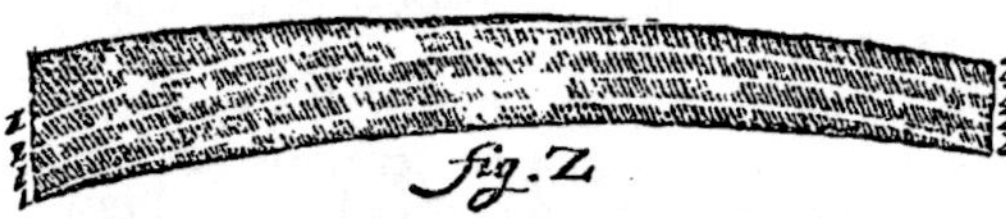

In the Figure Z, may be ſeen what Conſiderations ought to be in Compaſs Pieces, ſince it's much more valuable than ſtraight Pieces.

You ought to cut ſuch Pieces by the Lines 1, 2. and not according to the ſhape of the Tree, although it would be ſomething Grain-cut However ſuch a ſmall matter would not prejudice the Converſion, in proportion to the Help and Advantage there might be attributed to the Strength of the Ship, by ſuch a Regular and Circular Converſion.

It may alſo be farther obſerved, That in ſome particular Pieces, that are to be placed in a winding or twiſted Poſition, and not upon a direct Plan, it would be much better, in converting ſuch Pieces, to cut one Cut in the middle of the Piece, or near the middle, that might help their Obliquity, otherwiſe you run more Hazard in forcing a Twiſt in any piece of Timber, than if you was to force a Regular Rounding upon a direct Plan, in a much greater proportion of Bending.

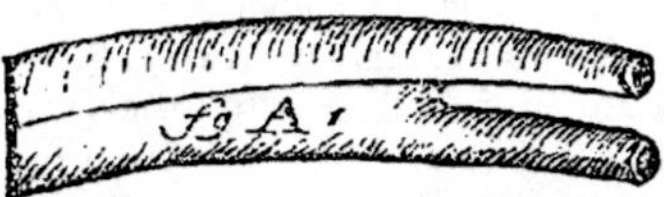

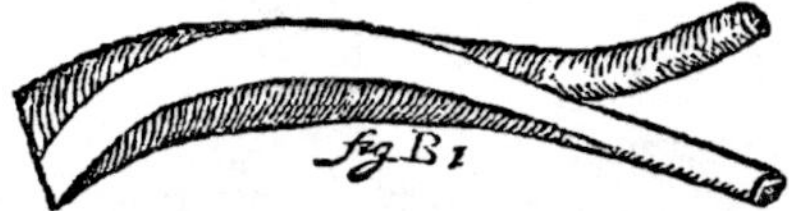

In Figure *A* 1, may be ſeen what meaſures ought to be taken in cutting ſuch Pieces, that have two Forks, or Top ends, grow from one Butt; for if the Butt is not over-big, it would be better to help the Length and Compaſs of two pieces, than to cut off the two Top ends, and wholly depend on converting the Butt.

In Figure *B* 1, it may be obſerved, of ſuch a Piece that hath two Tops, and one grows irregular, notwithſtanding, if the Butt be not over-big it would be better to make a Compaſs-piece of the greateſt Extent as may be, by Help of the Butt and one Top.

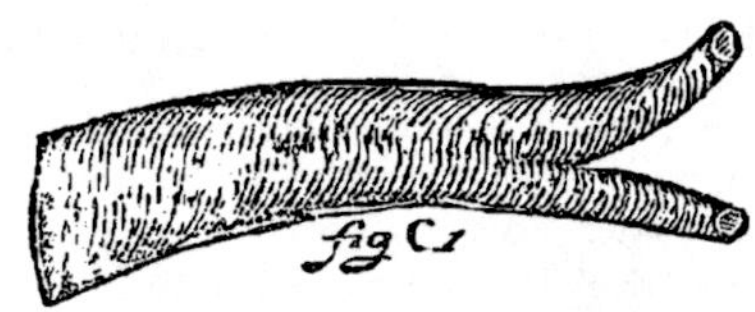

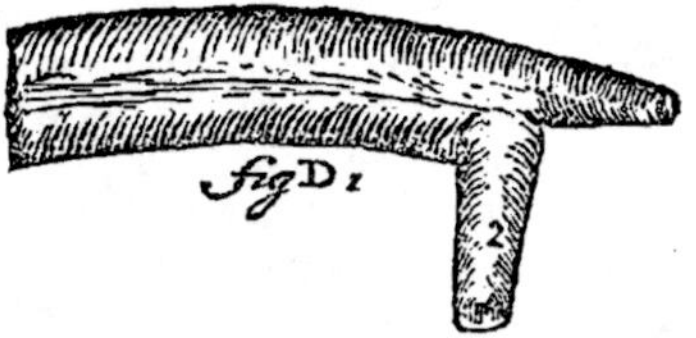

But in Figure C 1, where the Butt is very large, in ſuch Caſes it would be much better to cut off the Tops, and ſave the Butt

Alſo

Alſo in Figure *D* 1, it will be very material where ſuch Ends grow out, as 2, which will make a Knee. To ſave ſuch a Knee, and convert the other Part to ſmaller Uſes, according to what it will bear; all which may be more fully conſider'd, from what has been already ſaid, and hereafter ſhall be ſaid: And I proceed to the Floor Riders.

The Floor Riders may, in ſome meaſure, be properly call'd ſo, from their ſtriding the Kelſon. They are principal Supports to the firſt Floor of the Ship, in laying on the Ground, and alſo in the uneaſineſs which is caus'd by the Sea.

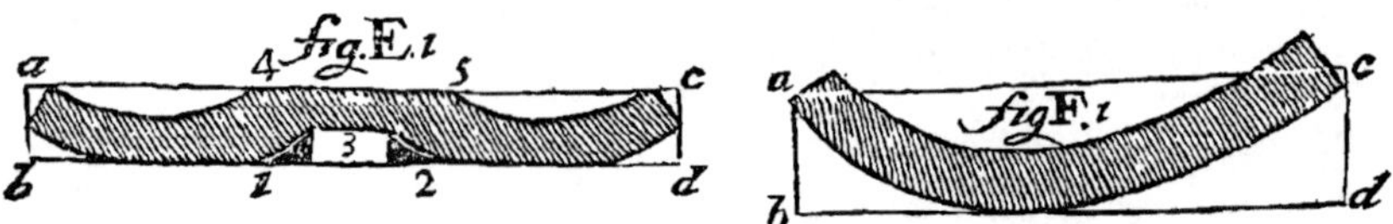

Figure *E* 1, ſhews the ſhape of a Floor-rider; and that ſuch a Piece is valuable, as the Parallelograms *c*, *d*, *a*, *b*, ſince it cannot be perform'd with a leſs Piece, for in Caſe a Piece grew directly according to the Shadow, or Tinge, it ought to be valu'd equal to a Piece, that's as ſquare as the ſaid Parallelograms; for it muſt be ſcor'd for the Kelſon 3; and ought to have ſubſtance upwards, to help that defect; only the breadth the other way, ought to be charg'd according to preceding Obſervations.

Figure *F* 1, ſhews the ſhape of a Foothook-rider, which will be valuable, according to the Parallelograms, *a*, *b*, *c*, *d*; and the thickneſs the other way, according to the Scantling requiſite

Obſerving, That it will not be at all convenient to piece ſuch Parts in the middle of them, but at the Ends they may, as was aforeſaid of Timbers And now to the Beams.

The Beams are Parts that chiefly unites the two ſides of the Ship together, and may be variouſly conſider'd, according to their lengths, and extream rounding in the ſame, more in one Deck than in another Alſo it's general, for the longeſt and largeſt of ſuch Parts, to be made in two Pieces, term'd ſcarphing of Beams, by over-launching the Parts, and coaking and bolting the ſame together.

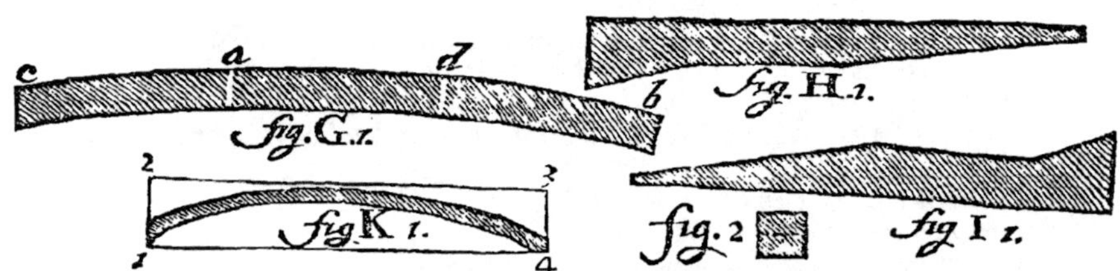

In Figure *G* 1, may be ſeen the ſhape of the largeſt Beam in a Ship, near 500 Tuns, which is 14 Inches one way, and 12 inches the other way, and 31 Foot long, containing near 36 Foot and a half of converted Timber

Now in making ſuch Beams out of rough Timber, it has been obſerv'd, That two Pieces has been expended of rough Timber (according to the Cuſtom of ſquaring in the River) which being converted with all the Frugality imaginable, has been before converted near 70 Foot, notwithſtanding, I'll reckon the two together at 130 Foot; ſo that the Product has not been as 1 to 3, but as 7 to 25, the Charge of ſcarphing them will be 40 *s* that's 31 *s*. Iron, and 9 *s* Workman's Wages, ſo that there may be 40 Foot of Timber added more to 130, which is 170, at 12 *d per* Foot, is, 8 *l*. 10 *s*. the Proportion will then bear as 3 is to 14, that the Charge will be near as 5 to 8, that if the whole Beam coſts

5 *l* the converted Beam will cost 8 *l*. Which Observation, nicely consider'd and adjusted, will be very material for such Gentlemen, that have long large Timber at a great distance from the Water; since here is fairly given for Beams of this bigness, near 4 *s* 7 *d per* Foot, and more than 11 *l* 5 *s per* Load, which will quit Cost for to bring Timber by Land a considerable way. And this Observation will also be of Use toward several other valuable Pieces in a Ship.

Figure *H* 1 and *I* 1, shews the shape of such rough Pieces, which in Figure *G* 1, reaches from *a* to *b*, and from *c* to *d*.

K 1, shews the shape of other Beams, smaller, and much rounder than the large Beams, and ought to be valu'd as such, according to the Parallelograms, 1, 2, 3, 4, but then Elm or Fir, which is cheaper and lighter than Oak, may do; and be as proper for such Beams, as Elm Strings is to fix them in. Besides, As the Custom is to cause an Extra-rounding in such Beams, purely to beget heights between Deck and Deck, so it's also customary to cut them bigger fore and aft, than they are up and down, for the same Faculty, as may be seen in Figure 2; and therefore it will be very proper, in such Cases, to consult in the squaring of the Timber, that there may be no Waste made, but that the Proportion of such small Beams, may be as 1 to 2, as may be seen in the Figure.

The large Beams cannot be reckon'd compass Timber, since Timber perfectly straight, may do for such Parts, for the substance of the Butt, compared with the Top, in Timber truly squar'd, will suffice to compass those Pieces, as in Figure *G* 1. I now proceed to the Knees.

And, First, To the Knee of the Head, since it's most material, and ought to be principally consider'd, by Reason that a defect in such a Part, may not only endanger the loosing of the Head, and Parts contiguous, but also the Ship it self; since it principally secures the Equiping belonging to such Machines.

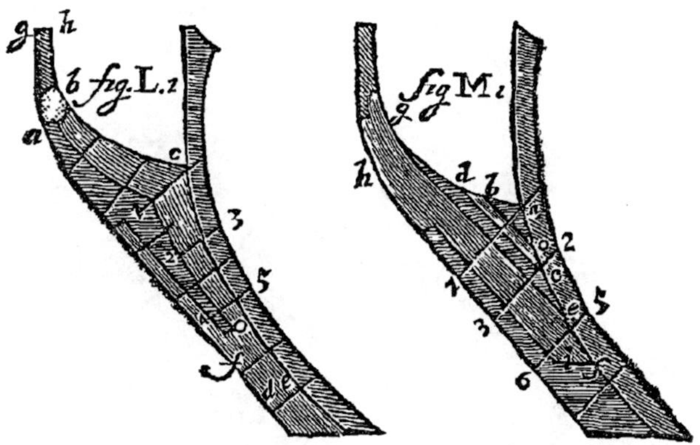

Such Knees are variously perform'd, as may be seen in Figure *L* 1, and *M* 1: Some Men will endeavour, if it's possible, to have the principal Piece fit entirely to the Stem, without putting Chocks between, as may be seen in Figure *L* 1. That *a*, *b*, *c*, *d*, *e*, is the principal Piece which fits intirely to the Stem, without any other Piece from *c* to *e*; and such a Piece is properly call'd a Knee, since it bears the Similitude of one. The Part *a*, *b*, *g*, *h*, is joyn'd on with a flat Scarph, and can be made as firm as can be requir'd

Also the Parts, *a*, *g*, *o*, may be brought on so artificially, that it will be good Work; and so will *f*, *d*, *e*, which is the upper end of the Gripe, and will be much stronger than the other Fashion, which appears in Figure *M* 1.

It may be seen in the Figure *M* 1, that not one Piece in it has the least Similitude of a Knee, altho' it's call'd so, from which it must be allow'd, That it's only a made Knee, since the Parts are every one of them perfectly straight Pie-

ces.

ces, the first grand Piece is, *f, g, h, i, e,* and no more of that Part fits on the Stem, than from *e* to *f*, all the other Parts are brought on in smaller Parts, as *g, e, d, c, b, o,* and is really a very dangerous fashion in making Heads so, as will appear by comparing the Figures: For First, The Bolts in *L* 1, is but from 1, *c*, and 2, 3, and 4, 5, but in Figure *M* 1, they are from *a*, 1, and 3, 2, and 6, 5, which are much longer, and consequently much weaker with equal bigness, and if the bigness is augmented to make them of equal strength, then they will be dearer and heavier, besides, the Hole will weaken the Knee more than the smaller Bolts will.

The Violence of the Sea, will also have more Power of the principal Piece in *M* 1, than in *L* 1, and the Chocks, tho' ever so well joyn'd, will shrink, and become loose; which in extreme agitating of the Ship, caus'd as well from forcing the Motion, as the Turbulency of the Sea, may endanger the spliting of the Stem of the Ship, and of Consequence be a Means to cast the Ship away.

And notwithstanding the principal Piece in *L* 1, is compass Timber, and the other straight, yet according to our preceding Observations, the Value will increase, according to the Parallelograms made by each Knee, which if they are every ways equal in bigness, their Price will be also equal as to the Timber, but the Workmanship will be something more in *M* 1, than in *L* 1, and consequently *M* 1, will be dearer to purchase than *L* 1, in every respect.

Figure *N* 1, shews the fashion of a large and substantial Knee, that stands and secures the Stern-post, and the Keel together. It is part of the Dead-wood, and since it may be reasonable to have a Piece (term'd a Britch) put on, as 1, 2, 3, it will only be valuable, according to the Parallelograms *a, b, c, d*; and the bigness the other way, according to the scantling requisite.

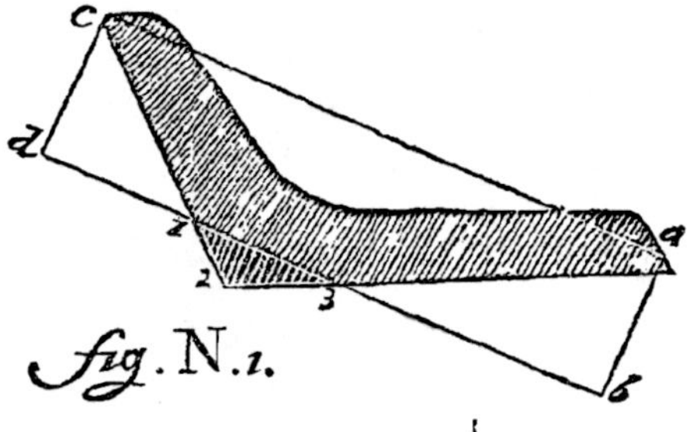

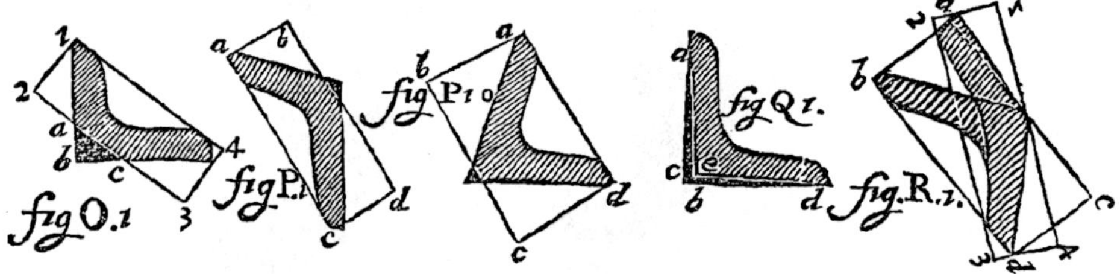

Figure *O* 1, is a lodging Knee's Shape: A Knee that lies on the Clamps that bear the Beams, and may be piec'd, as *a, b, c*: and will be valuable, according to the Parallelograms 1, 2, 3, 4

P 1, is the Figure of a hanging Knee, which ought not to be piec'd to extreme; and therefore all such Knees, and Standers, as may be seen by the other Figure *P* 1, o, will be valuable, according to the Parallelograms, *a, b, c, d*, in each.

Since the strain of any Ship thwartships, caus'd by rowling, is at some Times very violent; and since the Standers and hanging Knees support that strain, or the extraordinary labouring sideways, they ought to be very strong, and as well fastned, which cannot so well be in divers Pieces

Figure *Q* 1, shews how ill Management may be in using such Limbs, for in Case there was any Part of the Ship that required a Knee, that made such an Angle,

Angle, as *e, a, d*, if inſtead of taking ſuch a Knee, there ſhould be one taken that would make the Tinge or Shadow, it would be a great Waſte, and a piece of Miſmanagement, as it will farther appear in Figure *R* 1. That ſome Knees require no more compaſs, than is contain'd in the Parallelograms 1, 2, 3, 4, and then it would be very unreaſonable to uſe a Knee, that would compaſs as much as is contain'd in the Parallelograms *a, b, c, d,* which will appear to be almoſt of a double Value, or as the Parallelograms 1, 2, 3, 4, is to the Parallelograms *a, b, c, d.*

b *a* *fig. S1* *c* *d*

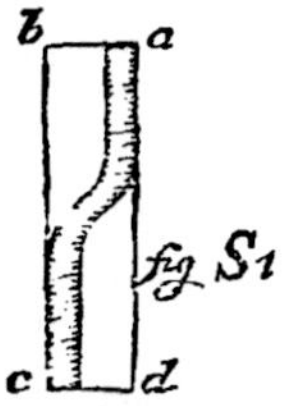

There is one thing more that may be conſider'd in the Value of Knee timber, which will appear in Figure *S* 1, which is what is term'd Dagger knees, or Knees with Caſts, which are only us'd, when the Beams of the Decks, either through Negligence, or Ignorance, is plac'd in the Wake of the Port-holes, or in other Caſes, to be fix'd againſt a Timber, that the Bolts which faſten the Knees, may be drove through a principal Timber: All which may be prevented, with taking Care to place the Timbers before the Plank is brought on.

However, If ſuch Knees are requir'd, and the Service cannot be perform'd without having ſuch ſhap'd Limbs, they ought to increaſe the Value of each according to the Parallelograms *a, b, c, d*; beſides the Value caus'd by the compaſſing of thoſe Parts the other way, as is demonſtrated in the other Figures

From all which general Obſervations, it will appear, That there is very few Pieces in a Ship, that are requir'd ſo irregular, but that they may be nicely adjuſted, and a true Value put upon them, without gueſſing at the Price, or leaving the matter ſo very intricate, that one Man may have room to over-reach another Nay, indeed, Was it not for the Cat-head, which for the Conveniency of making room on the Forecaſtle, there's not one Piece of any Ship, that would abſolutely give an Advantage to provide an irregular Piece of Timber, for to compoſe her with

And it may be heartily wiſh'd, That there was not that ill-conveniency in a Ship, ſince it gives way for ſeveral hundred Pounds worth of irregular and uſeleſs Timber to be provided, eſpecially where the Damage, or Loſs, lights not on the Shoulders of them that provides and receives it: That is, In allowing abundance of Timber to be compaſs, according to the length extreme, and bigneſs of each reſpective Piece, when in reality it's not near ſo valuable, as that which is perfectly ſtraight, but muſt be cut off, at every irregular bending, before it can be brought to Uſe

Not but that there may be ſome Pieces, which is ſide round Pieces, or Pieces truly circular each ways, that may be very uſeful in Ship-work: All which will require the beſt of Judges to adjuſt ſuch intricate Caſes, and allow of no Perſon to have the leaſt Imployment in providing, inſpecting and receiving Timber, but ſuch as are true bred, and very accurate Shipwrights.

A LIST of the Royal Navy, *with the Number of Men, and Guns, carried in War.*

First Rates

Ships Names	Men	Guns
ROyal Sovereign	815	100
Royal George	815	100
Royal William	780	100
Britannia	815	100
London	780	100
Queen	780	100
Royal Ann	780	100
	5565	700

Second Rates

Ships Names	Men	Guns
ST George	660	90
Prince George	660	90
Prince	660	90
Princess	660	90
Union	660	90
Marlborough	660	90
Barfleur	660	90
Blenheim	660	90
Namure	660	90
Ramellies	660	90
Neptune	660	90
Sandwich	660	90
Vanguard	660	90
Katherine	660	90
	9240	1260

Third Rates

Ships Names	Men	Guns
NAssau	460	70
Orford	460	70
Russel	460	70
Devonshire	520	80
Boyne	520	80
Grafton	460	70
Bedford	460	70
Berwick	460	70
Bredah	460	70
Buckingham	460	70
Burford	460	70
Cambridge	520	80
Captain	460	70
Chichester	520	80
Cornwall	460	70
Cumberland	520	80
Defiance	400	66
Dorsetshire	520	80
Dreadnought	400	66
Dunkirk	400	66
Elizabeth	460	70
Essex	460	70
Prince Frederick	460	70
Hampton Court	460	70
Humber	520	80
Ipswich	460	70
Kent	460	70
Lancaster	520	80
Lenox	460	70
Monk	400	66
Monmouth	400	66
Newark	520	80
Norfolk	520	80
Northumberland	460	70
Ranelaugh	460	70
Revenge	460	70
Royal Oak	460	70
Rupert	400	66
Shrewsbury	520	80
Somerset	520	80
Sterling-Castle	460	70
Suffolk	460	70
Torbay	520	80
Warspight	400	66
Yarmouth	460	70
	21060	3252

Fourth Rates

Ships Names	Men	Guns
ADvice	280	50
Anglesea	280	50
Antelope	280	50
Assistance	280	50
August	365	60
Argyle	280	50
Bristol	280	50
Burlington	280	50
Canterbury	365	60
Centurion	280	50
Chatham	280	50
Chester	280	50
Colchester	280	50
Crown	280	50
Dartmouth	280	50
Deptford	280	50
Dragon	280	50
Exeter	365	60
Falkland	280	50
Falmouth	280	50
Greenwich	280	50
Guernsey	280	50
Hampshire	280	50
Jersey	280	50
Kingston	365	60
Leopard	280	50
Litchfield	280	50
Lyon	365	60
Mary	365	60
Medway	365	60
Montague	365	60
Moor	365	60
Newcastle	280	50
Nonsuch	280	50
Norwich	280	50
Nottingham	365	60
Panther	280	50
Pembroke	365	60
Plymouth	365	60
Portland	280	50
Preston	280	50
Rippon	365	60
Rochester	280	50
Romney	280	50
Ruby	280	50
Salisbury	280	50
St Albans	280	50
Severn	280	50
Southampton	280	50
Strafford	280	50
Sunderland	365	60
Superbe	365	60
Sutherland	280	50
Swallow	280	50
Tilbury	280	50
Tyger	280	50
Warwick	280	50
Weymouth	280	50
Winchester	280	50
Windsor	365	60
Woolwich	280	50
Worcester	280	50
York	365	60
	19093	3370

Fifth Rates

Ships Names	Men	Guns
ADventure	190	42
Bedford-Gally	135	32
Bridgewater	155	36
Charles-Gally	190	42
Diamond	190	42
Dolphin	155	36
Dover	190	42
Enterprize	190	42
Experiment	135	32
Feversham	190	42
Folkstone	190	42
Fowey	190	42
Gosport	190	42
Garland	155	36
Hastings	190	42
Hector	190	42
Kinsale	155	36
Lark	190	42
Launceston	190	42
Looe	190	42
Lowestoft	135	32
Ludlow-Castle	190	42
Lime	135	32
Mary-Gally	190	42
Mermaid	155	36
Milford	155	36

Ships Names.	*Men*	*Guns*
Pearl	190	42
Pool	135	32
Portsmouth	190	42
Roebuck	190	42
Royal Ann Gally	190	42
Rye	135	32
Saphire	190	42
Scarborough	135	32
Sheerness	135	32
Shoreham	135	32
Soilings	190	42
Southsea-Castle	190	42
Sweepstakes	190	42
Winchelsea	155	36
	6860	1548

Sixth Rates.

Alborough	110	24
Biddiford	100	20
Blanford	100	20
Deal-Castle	110	24
Flamborough	115	24
Fox	115	24
Gibraltar	100	20
Glascow	110	20
Greyhound	110	20
Hind	110	20
Lively	110	20
Nightingal	115	24
Carolina	60	12
Phœnix	115	24
Port-Mahone	110	20
Queenborough	115	24
Rose	110	20
Seaford	115	24
Sea-horse	110	20
Solbay	115	24
Speedwell	110	20
Squirrel	115	24
Success	110	20
Valeur	115	24
	2605	516

Fireships

Ships Names	*Men*	*Guns*
Griffin	45	8
Owners Love	45	8
Ann & Christopher	45	8
Castle	45	8
Cressant	45	8
Eagle	45	8
Firebrand	45	8
Flame	45	8
Fortune	45	8
Hawk	45	8
Holmes	45	8
Hunter	45	8
Joseph	45	8
Lightning	45	8
Peace	24	6
Providence	24	6
Phœnix	45	8
Roebuck	45	8
Sampson	40	6
Sarah	20	4
Strombolo	45	8
Spanish-Merchant	36	6
Spy	45	8
Terrible	45	8
Vesuvius	45	8
Vulcan	45	8
Vulture	45	8
Unister	45	8
Wivenhall	25	6
	1204	

Boombs

Mortar	65	18
Serpent	65	18
Firedrake	65	18
Salamander	30	4
Basilisk	30	4
Blast	30	4
Furnace	30	4
Granada	30	4
Kitchin	30	6
	375	

Yachts.

Ships Names	*Men*	*Guns*
William *and* Mary	40	12
Mary	30	8
Bolton	14	6
Charlotte	30	8
Cleaveland	30	8
Dublin	40	12
Fubbs	40	12
Henrietta	30	8
Jemmy	4	4
Isabella	30	8
Katharine	30	8
Isle of Wight	6	4
Queenborough	4	4
Littleton	6	4
Navy	14	6
	348	

Advice-Boats, Sloops, and Brigantines

Drake	85	14
Ferret	80	14
Discovery	35	8
Dispatch	35	8
Fly	35	8
Hazard	80	14
Jamaica	80	14
Shark	80	14
Swift	80	14
Tryal	80	14
	670	

The whole Number of Ships, Men and Guns.

Ships	*Num*	*Men*	*Guns*
First Rates	7	5565	700
Second	14	9240	1260
Third	45	21060	3252
Fourth	63	19093	3370
Fifth	40	6860	1548
Sixth	24	2605	516
Fireships	29	1204	
Boombs	9	375	
Yachts	15	348	
Advice-Boats	10	670	
		67020	10646

Number of Men to Man all His Majesty's Royal Navy, is Sixty Seven Thousand and Twenty

Number of Guns for all the Men of War, is Ten Thousand Six Hundred Forty Six

But some of the Fireships, and small Frigats, are Sold since the War

A

A TABLE TO THE First PART.

AN Account of the Lines made use of, in designing the Figure of a Ship, according to the Solid of least Resistance, Pag 1

Observations on placing the Midship-timber and also the Mast's-place, 2

An Index to the Parts of a first siz'd Ship, 3 4

The Figure and Demonstration of a three Deck Ship, by a Scale of Feet and Inches, 4. 5

Calculations for finding the Contents, and placing the Masts, 6

A Consideration of the Weight of Water, resisted by a Ship, and of the Masts, and Security for them, as Stays and Shrouds, 7. 8. 9 10

The Figure of a Yatcht, ibid

The Proportion that the Rigging has to the Masts, and the Area of Canvas suitable for Sails, 11

The Shape and Proportion of Ships Sails, 12 13

Proportion of the Guns and Anchors for any Ship, 14

Calculations to size the Anchors and Cables, 15

For proportioning the Men, agreeable to each Ship, 16

Calculations for the Masts and Yards, and the Figure of a Hoy, 17, 18

Several Schemes and Tables to fashion, and also for the Magnitude of the Masts and Yards, 19. 20 21

Tables for the Parts of the Anchors, and an Index to the Parts, 22

Figures of Anchors, and of setting the Arms, Pag. 23

An Observation of the size of Anchors, and the Cables; and the Figure of the second siz'd Ship, 24

An Index of the Parts of the second, and third siz'd Ship, with the Figure of the third siz'd Ship: All drawn by the first siz'd Ship's Scale, 25. 26

The Proportion and Index for the third and fourth size, 27. 28

The Figure of the fourth siz'd Ship 29

The Index for the fifth size, 30

The Figure of the fifth siz'd Ship, 31

The Proportion of the fifth siz'd Ship's Parts, and an Index for the sixth size, 32

The Figure of the sixth siz'd Ship, 33

The Proportion of the sixth siz'd Ship's Parts; and the Figure of my Proportional Compasses, 34

Parallels for finding the Scantling, by the Cube, and Square Root, 35

The Scantling, or General Proportion for every Part of six sizes in Ships; and how to gain the Scantling of any other Ship from them, 36 37 38 39 40. 41 42 43. 44 45

Tables for the Dimensions of Masts and Yards, Caps, and Cross, and Trusletrees for Ships, from fourty six Foot broad, to twenty Foot broad, with an Account of the Variety of Authors, 46 47 48 49

The Dimensions and Value of making six Sets of Masts, from a Ship of fourty

nine

nine Foot broad, to one of twenty four Foot broad; with every Material belonging thereto moſt conciſe, Pag 50. 51 52 53. 54 55
The Dimenſions and Proportions of Ketches, and Hoy's-maſts, 56
Of Boat's-maſts, with Shoulder mutton-ſails, Bermudas, and Smack-ſails, 57
A Table of the Porportions for tranſporting rough Maſts, for the Uſe of Shipping in General, 58
An Explanation of the Table, and of Cheeking-maſts, 59 60
Of Scarphing-yards, ibid
Rules to perform the making of made Maſts, or putting divers Pieces together, to make one intire large Maſt, 61 62
How to bevel a Crutch of a Hoy's-Maſt, with a Half-ſprit; and how to ſet off the Quarters of Maſts, and Yards, by Gunter's *Line,* ibid
Some Rules to adjuſt the Uſe and Faſhion of the Main-capſtern, 63 64
The Proportions, ibid
The Jeer capſtern accordingly, 65
How to improve the Shape, and Make, of the Capſterns, 66
How to ſet off the Squares, and reducing the Barrel, and of the Uſe of ſmall Capſterns or Crabs, 67
Of the Windleſs, or Horizontal Capſterns; with Obſervations on the Uſe, and forcing Power in ſuch Machines, 68 69
The Scale of Feet and Inches, 69
Some Reaſons ſet forth by Mr. John Cocks, *about the Shipwrights Charter,* 70. 71. 72. 73. 74
References in the Margin of each Page, Pag. 74
The Nature of Contracting for Building any New Ship, with proper References in the Margin of each Page, from 75. to 96
Material Reaſons for drawing full Contracts, and what Uſe and Advantage it may be of to both Parties, 96. 97
Material Caſes that may happen in Building, rebuilding and ſailing of Ships, which being minded, may very probably be a Means to hinder litigious Diſputes; with proper References in the Margins, from 98 to 116
Rules to convert Timber for Shipping to its various uſes, alſo how to ſet a true and proper Value on Compaſs timber, compar'd with ſuch as is ſtraight, from 117. to 130
Interrogations to adjuſt the Value of Compaſs timber; with proper Signatures of the Stem in a Ship, 117. 118
Faſhion pieces and Tranſums, 119
Floor-timbers and Foot hooks, 120, 121
Half-timbers, ibid
Top-timbers, 122, 123
Side-round-timbers, ibid
Harpins and following Pieces, 124
Converting Thick ſtuff, and Knees, 125. 126
Riders and Beams, 127
Knees of the Head, 128
Other Knee-timber, 129
Side-round-knees, &c. *With ſome Reaſons to prove none fitting to convert, adapt or receive Timber, but a very able and experienc'd Shipwright,* 130

The End of the Firſt Part.

CPSIA information can be obtained
at www.ICGtesting.com
Printed in the USA
LVOW09s0753060717
540204LV00066B/1092/P